NURSING KEY TOPICS REVIEW

Fluids and Electrolytes

NURSING KEY TOPICS REVIEW

Fluids and Electrolytes

ELSEVIER

Senior Content Strategist: Jamie Blum
Senior Content Development Specialist: Heather Bays
Publishing Services Manager: Deepthi Unni
Project Manager: Haritha Dharmarajan
Design Direction: Margaret Reid

Printed in the United States of America

Last digit is the print number: 9   8   7   6   5   4   3   2   1

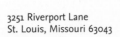

3251 Riverport Lane
St. Louis, Missouri 63043

Working together
to grow libraries in
developing countries

www.elsevier.com • www.bookaid.org

Reviewers

Angie Atwood, PhD, RN
Assistant Professor of Nursing
School of Nursing
Campbellsville University
Campbellsville, Kentucky

Michelle Bonnheim
Nursing Student
California State University, Fresno
Fresno, California

Joanna Cain, BSN, BA, RN
Auctorial Pursuits, Inc.
President and Founder
Boulder, Colorado

Kim Clevenger, EdD, MSN, RN, BC
Baccalaureate Program Coordinator
Associate Professor of Nursing
Morehead State University
Morehead, Kentucky

Beth Cofini, MANE, RN
School of Nursing
Jersey College
Teterboro, New Jersey

Sally Fitzgerald, MSN, RN
Professor of Nursing
Community College of Beaver County
Monaca, Pennsylvania

Crystal Gallardo
CNA Nursing Assistant
Cypress College
Cypress, California

Tiffany Jakubowski, BSN, RN, CMSRN, ONC
Instructor
Health Professions
Front Range Community College
Westminster, Colorado

Christina D. Keller MSN, RN, CHSE
Instructor
School of Nursing
Radford University Clinical Simulation Center
Radford, Virginia

Katelynn Landers
Nursing Student
Brockton Hospital School of Nursing
Brockton, Massachusetts

Angela Lanzoni
Nursing Student
Brockton Hospital School of Nursing
Brockton, Massachusetts

Reagan Lizardi
Nursing Student
Polk State College
Winter Haven, Florida

Michelle Luckett
Nursing Student
Polk State College
Winter Haven, Florida

Lisa McDavid, MSN, RN
Associate Professor of Nursing
Associate Degree Nursing Program
Center for Health, Education, and Research
Morehead State University
Morehead, Kentucky

Nancy Noble, MSN
Associate Professor
College of Professions, Department of Nursing
Marian University
Fond du Lac, Wisconsin

Karla Psaros
Nursing Student
Brockton Hospital School of Nursing
Brockton, Massachusetts

Gina Rena
Nursing Student
Polk State College
Winter Haven, Florida

Elizabeth Rudshteyn, MSN, RN
RN Program Chair
School of Nursing
Jersey College
Teterboro, New Jersey

Cianna Simpson
Nursing Student
Brockton Hospital School of Nursing
Brockton, Massachusetts

Briana Sundlie
Nursing Student
Cypress College
Cypress, California

Dokagari Woods, PhD, RN
Assistant Professor & Director of Undergraduate
    Program
Tarleton State University
Stephenville, Texas

The *Nursing Key Topics Review* book series was developed and designed with you, **the nursing student**, in mind. We know how difficult nursing school can be! How do you focus your study? How can you learn in the most time-efficient way possible? Where do you go when you need help?

We asked YOU, and this is what we learned:

- You think textbooks are useful, but they can be overwhelming (also . . . heavy).
- You want quick and easy access to manageable levels of nursing information.
- You like questions and rationales to challenge you and to make sure you know what you need to know.

Nursing Key Topics Review is your solution, whether you are looking for a textbook supplement or an NCLEX® examination study aid. Review questions interspersed throughout the text make it easy to test your knowledge. The bulleted outline format allows for quick comprehension. A mobile app with key points lets you take your review with you anywhere you go!

In short, *Nursing Key Topics Review* helps you narrow down what is important and tells you what to focus on. Be sure to look for all the titles in the series to make your studies more effective . . . and your journey a little bit lighter!

Table of Contents

NURSING KEY TOPICS REVIEW

Fluids and Electrolytes

Concepts of Body Fluids 1

BODY FLUIDS OVERVIEW

Water
- Makes up 60% to 65% of the total body water (TBW)
  - 65% of TBW is intracellular fluid (ICF)
  - 35% of TBW is extracellular fluid (ECF)
- Moves freely among body compartments
- Distributed by osmotic and hydrostatic forces
- Under normal conditions, water loss equals water gain, and the body's water volume remains constant.

Body Fluids
- Maintaining fluid and electrolyte balance is an essential part of life.
  - Needed for all body systems to function
  - Largest single constituent of the body
- The volume, concentration, and composition of body fluids must be maintained.
- Homeostasis
  - Compensatory mechanisms maintain a steady state in the body.
  - Regulation of water and minerals in the body occurs through osmoregulation.
  - Composition and volume of body fluids need to be kept within a narrow range.
  - Consistency is maintained through osmosis, diffusion, filtration, and active transport.
- A loss of 20% of the body's fluid content may be fatal and can lead to irreversible health problems or death.

Electrolytes
- Electrolytes are substances found in the ICF and the ECF.
  - Molecules split into ions when placed in water.
- Without electrolytes, the body cannot maintain homeostasis.
- Major electrolytes found in the body
  - Potassium
    - Abbreviation: K
    - Reference range: between 3.5 and 5.0 mEq/L
      - Hyperkalemia: Potassium concentration is higher than the normal range.
      - Hypokalemia: Potassium concentration is lower than the normal range.
  - Sodium
    - Abbreviation: Na^+
    - Reference range: between 135 and 145 mEq/L
      - Hypernatremia: Sodium concentration is higher than the normal range.
      - Hyponatremia: Sodium concentration is lower than the normal range.
  - Calcium
    - Abbreviation: Ca

- Reference range: between 8.5 and 10.5 mg/dL
  - Hypercalcemia: Calcium concentration is higher than the normal range.
  - Hypocalcemia: Calcium concentration is lower than the normal range.
- Chloride
  - Abbreviation: Cl^-
  - Reference range: between 95 and 105 mEq/L
    - Hyperchloremia: Chloride concentration is higher than the normal range.
    - Hypochloremia: Chloride concentration is lower than the normal range.
- Phosphorus
  - Abbreviation: P
  - Reference range: between 2.8 and 4.5 mg/dL
    - Hyperphosphatemia: Phosphorus concentration is higher than the normal range.
    - Hypophosphatemia: Phosphorus concentration is lower than the normal range.
- Magnesium
  - Abbreviation: Mg
  - Reference range: between 1.5 and 2.5 mEq/L
    - Hypermagnesemia: Magnesium concentration is higher than the normal range.
    - Hypomagnesemia: Magnesium concentration is lower than the normal range.
- Electrolytes are distinguished by their electrical charge.
  - Positive
    - Cations
      - Potassium
      - Sodium
      - Magnesium
      - Calcium
  - Negative
    - Anions
      - Chloride
      - Phosphate
      - Bicarbonate (HCO_3^-): Reference range: between 24 and 30 mEq/L
  - Sources of electrolytes: fruits; vegetables; grains; red meat; poultry; fish; fluids; supplements
  - Mechanisms that maintain electrolyte balance in the body: diffusion; active transport; osmosis
  - Functions of electrolytes: maintain homeostasis; regulate fluid; maintain acid-base balance.

APPLICATION AND REVIEW

1. Of the total percentage of TBW, how much is found in the intracellular spaces?
   1. 35%
   2. 55%
   3. 65%
   4. 85%
2. The consistency of body fluids needed to preserve homeostasis is maintained through which processes? *(Select all that apply.)*
   1. Osmosis
   2. Diffusion
   3. Filtration
   4. Active transport
   5. Passive transport

3. Which conclusion concerning prognosis should the nurse determine when told that it has been estimated that a client has lost 22% of his or her total body fluids?
   1. The client needs immediate intravenous fluid therapy.
   2. Such a loss is associated with irreversible health problems.
   3. The transfer of ECF into the intracellular spaces has begun.
   4. Although a significant amount of fluids has been lost, the client is not yet in danger.
4. Which substances are considered major electrolytes required for human body homeostasis? *(Select all that apply.)*
   1. Potassium
   2. Sodium
   3. Calcium
   4. Chromium
   5. Iron
5. Which serum sodium level supports the existence of hypernatremia in a teenaged client?
   1. 5.4 mEq/L
   2. 8.8 mg/dl
   3. 104 mEq/L
   4. 147 mEq/L
6. Which is the accepted abbreviation for the electrolyte potassium?
   1. Cl^-
   2. K
   3. Na^+
   4. P
7. Which serum magnesium level would suggest the client is experiencing hypomagnesemia?
   1. 1.3 mEq/L
   2. 1.7 mEq/L
   3. 2.4 mEq/L
   4. 2.8 mEq/L
8. Which electrolytes are referred to as cations? *(Select all that apply.)*
   1. Barcarbonate
   2. Calcium
   3. Chloride
   4. Magnesium
   5. Potassium
9. The nurse demonstrates an understanding of an anion when making which statement?
   1. "Sodium is classified as an anion."
   2. "An anion binds with only other anions."
   3. "Anions produce a negative electrical charge."
   4. "The majority of all major electrolytes are anions."

See Answers on pages 16–18.

Fluid and Electrolyte Balance

- Kidneys
  - Responsible for maintaining balance of fluids and electrolytes and the control of output
  - Remove waste materials and excessive substances from ECF
  - Excrete water and reabsorb or release sodium, potassium, HCO_3^-, and hydrogen ions, which regulates intracellular and extracellular concentrations
  - Antidiuretic and aldosterone hormones help the kidneys regulate urine output.
    - Antidiuretic hormone (ADH)
      - Affects ECF
      - Secreted by the posterior pituitary gland
      - Considered the water conservation hormone
        - Increased production of ADH
          - Increase in urine saving
          - Increase in amounts of water reabsorbed by the kidney through osmosis
    - Aldosterone hormone
      - Regulates extracellular volume by affecting renal control of sodium and potassium

- Secreted by the adrenal cortex
- Acts on the distal portion of the renal tubules to increase reabsorption (saving) of sodium, chloride, and water and the secretion of potassium and hydrogen
  - Sodium retention leads to retention of extracellular volume.
- Renin
  - Kidney enzyme
  - Produces angiotensin I, which causes some vasoconstriction
  - Angiotensin II
    - Angiotensin I is converted into angiotensin II.
    - Creates selective vasoconstriction, which will redirect blood flow to the kidneys and improve renal perfusion
    - Stimulates the release of aldosterone when the serum sodium concentration is low
- Functions
  - Transports nutrients, electrolytes, and oxygen to cells
  - Carries water products away from cells
  - Regulates body temperature
  - Lubricates joints and membranes
  - Acts as a medium for food digestion
- Throughout the body, the cell membranes and capillary walls are selectively permeable.
  - Water and some solutes freely pass through barriers.
  - Other solutes require an active transport system.

Fluid Distribution

- Infants
  - Increased body water
    - Approximately 75% to 80% of body weight
      - ICF 40%
      - ECF 35%
        - Approximately 15% greater than the average adult
      - Decreased fat
  - More susceptible to changes in body water, attributable to high metabolic rate and greater body surface area in proportion to body size
- Children
  - At approximately 2 years of age, the proportion of body weight that is fluid decreases.
- Adults
  - Fluid is approximately 60% of body weight.
- Obese adults
  - Very little water is contained in adipose (fat) cells.
  - Individuals with increased body fat will have less TBW.
  - Obese adults will be more susceptible to fluid imbalances.
- Older adults
  - Fluid may be reduced 45% to 50% of body weight in adults older than 65 years of age.
  - Body fluid changes in older adults.
    - Ability to regulate sodium and water balance is reduced in older adults.
    - Older adults typically have increased tissue loss.
    - Fever and dehydration may lead to significant fluid balance problems in this client population.
      - Dehydration can be caused by sodium or water loss.

Fluid Loss

- Whenever the loss of water from the body exceeds intake, water is extracted from the extracellular compartment.
- Water volume decrease
  - Concentration of sodium and other electrolytes increase in plasma.
    - This concentration increases osmotic pressure in the extracellular compartment.
- Older adults and young children
  - These populations may not have the ability to compensate and adjust to fluid changes.
- Two types of fluid loss
  - Sensible: can be measured
    - Examples
      - Urine
        - Approximately 1400 to 1800 mL (60%) of daily water is lost through urine in the healthy adult.
        - Normal urine output (mL/24 hr)
          - Newborn: 50 to 350
          - Infant: 350 to 500
          - Child: 500 to 1000
          - Adolescent: 700 to 1400
          - Adult man: 800 to 1800
          - Adult woman: 600 to 1600
      - Feces
        - Approximately 100 mL (2%) of daily water is lost through feces in the healthy adult.
  - Insensible: cannot be measured
    - Oxidation accounts for approximately 300 to 500 mL (10%) of body water loss each day in the healthy adult.
    - Examples
      - Fluid loss through the skin
        - Perspiration through exercise and fever
      - Fluid loss through the respiratory tract
        - Increased respiratory rate increases the amount of fluid loss.
- Signs of severe water deficit: weakness; confusion; hypotension (decreased blood pressure); tachycardia (increased heart rate); delirium
- Types of fluid volume deficits
  - Dehydration
    - Significant decrease in fluid intake and/or loss of body fluid without replacement
    - Three types of dehydration
      - Isotonic dehydration
        - Isotonic dehydration is the most common type of dehydration.
        - Loss of fluid and electrolytes is approximately balanced in proportion.
        - Loss is sustained by the extracellular compartment.
        - Physical signs: gray skin color; cold temperature; poor turgor; dry feel; dry mucous membranes; absent tearing and salivation; sunken eyeballs; sunken fontanel; subnormal or elevated body temperature; rapid pulse; rapid respirations; irritable or lethargic behavior
      - Hypotonic dehydration
        - Electrolyte deficit is greater than the fluid deficit.
        - ECF is hypotonic; it moves into the intracellular space.

- ECF volume decreases.
- Symptoms of this deficit are more severe.
- Physical signs: gray skin color; cold temperature; very poor turgor; clammy feel; slightly moist mucous membranes; absent tearing and salivation; sunken eyeballs; sunken fontanel; subnormal or elevated body temperature; very rapid pulse; rapid thicken respirations; lethargic or comatose behavior and/or convulsions
- Hypertonic dehydration
  - Deficit of fluids is greater than the deficit of electrolytes.
  - Fluid shifts out of the intracellular space and into extracellular space.
  - Symptoms are not as apparent.
  - Neurological disturbances become evident.
  - Physical signs: gray skin color; cold or hot temperature; fair turgor; doughy feel; parched mucous membranes; absent tearing and salivation; sunken and/or soft eyeballs; sunken fontanel; subnormal or elevated body temperature; moderately rapid pulse; rapid respirations; significant lethargy with extreme hyperirritability on stimulation
- Causes
  - Insensible water loss
    - Perspiration
    - High fever
    - Heatstroke (increased body temperature to 40.6º C or 105º F)
    - Symptoms: cerebral edema; seizures; delirium; coma; increased pulse; increased respiratory rate; hypotension; anxiety; confusion; impaired sweating; listlessness
    - Treatment
      - Oxygen therapy
      - Intravenous (IV) normal saline (NS)
      - Do NOT use lactated Ringer (LR) solution; the liver cannot metabolize it, which can worsen lactic acidosis.
      - Continuous core temperature monitoring
      - Monitor for seizures, and administer benzodiazepine drugs as needed.
    - Sodium and potassium depletion
  - Gastrointestinal (GI) loss: vomiting; diarrhea; suction; fistula drainage
  - Diabetes insipidus: causes large volumes of urine output
  - Osmotic diuretic agents: inhibit reabsorption of water and sodium
  - Hemorrhage (heavy discharge of blood)
  - Overuse of diuretic agents
  - Inadequate fluid intake
  - Third-spacing fluids: burns; intestinal obstruction
- Moderate symptoms
  - Flushed, dry skin
  - Decreased urine output
    - Urine characteristics
      - Increased specific gravity
      - Urine color between dark-yellow and amber
  - Dry mucous membranes
  - Skin turgor: tenting
  - Thirst
  - Weight loss

- Restlessness
- Lethargy
- Severe symptoms
  - Dry, cracked tongue
  - Soft, sunken eyeballs
  - Thready pulse
  - Tachycardia: heart rate >100 beats per minute (bpm)
  - Decreased central venous pressure (CVP)
  - Postural hypotension
  - Rapid respiratory rate
  - Lethargy; may progress to coma
  - Absence of tearing or sweating
  - Oliguria or very concentrated urine
  - Hemoconcentration
    - Increased hematocrit (Hct)
    - Blood urea nitrogen (BUN)
    - Electrolyte imbalances
- Diagnostic findings
  - Urine-specific gravity >1.020
  - Elevated hemoglobin (Hgb) and Hct levels
  - Elevated potassium levels
- Treatment includes restoring fluid loss.
  - IV fluid replacement
    - Isotonic solutions (0.9% NS)
    - Balanced solutions for initial treatment (LR solution)

APPLICATION AND REVIEW

10. The nurse notes in the medical record that a client is unable to produce sufficient qualities of angiotensin II to support renal perfusion. The nurse suspects the problem results from a deficiency in what renal enzyme?
    1. ADH
    2. Angiotensin I
    3. Aldosterone
    4. Renin
11. Which client is at greatest risk for fluid imbalances?
    1. 9-year-old child who is developmentally challenged
    2. 20-year-old young adult with a fractured left femur
    3. 45-year-old adult with a history of tobacco use
    4. 67-year-old older adult who is diagnosed as obese
12. Which older adult is at greatest risk for developing dehydration?
    1. 90-year-old client who has recently undergone cataract surgery
    2. 85-year-old client who is cognitively impaired
    3. 79-year-old client with a history of osteoporosis
    4. 69-year-old client with symptoms of viral gastroenteritis
13. Which client is at greatest risk for a fluid imbalance because of an insensible fluid loss?
    1. A toddler recovering from influenza
    2. An older adult who is experiencing polyuria
    3. A teenager with severe seasonal nasal allergies
    4. A middle-aged adult diagnosed with chronic diarrhea

14. What interventions would the nurse implement to monitor a client for possible severe water deficit?
    1. Listening to the client's apical heart rate
    2. Taking the client's blood pressure every 4 hours
    3. Asking the client to confirm his or her name each time care is given
    4. Offering the client his or her favorite beverage with meals and snacks
    5. Monitoring the client for indications of a red, itchy rash initially noted on the face
15. Which signs and symptoms would suggest a client is experiencing a heatstroke? *(Select all that apply.)*
    1. Observable seizure
    2. Profuse sweating
    3. Above normal pulse rate
    4. Disoriented to time and place
    5. Abnormally low blood pressure
16. Which intervention, prescribed for a client who experienced a sunstroke, should the nurse question?
    1. Supplemental oxygen therapy
    2. Continual monitoring of the core temperature
    3. IV infusion of LR solution
    4. Arranging for serum sodium and potassium diagnostic tests

See Answers on pages 16–18.

Fluid Volume Excess

- Too much fluid goes into the body with the failure to eliminate.
- When excess fluid is retained, it causes a dilution of the ECF and water moves into the ICF.
- Edema may exist; however, edema and fluid volume excess are not the same.
- Fluid volume causes
  - Compulsive water drinking
    - Fluid intoxication: rapid infusion of IV fluids
    - Excessive isotonic or hypotonic IV fluids
    - Retention of fluids
    - Renal failure
    - Cushing syndrome (also called hypercortisolism)
      - Adrenal gland disease
      - Condition resulting from exposure to high-cortisol levels for a long period
        - Long-term use of corticosteroids
        - Syndrome of inappropriate antidiuretic hormone (SIADH) secretion
        - Primary polydipsia
          - Excessive fluid intake in the absence of physiological stimuli to drink
        - Interstitial-to-plasma fluid shift
  - Symptoms: edema; peripheral pitting; positive jugular vein distension (JVD); respiratory difficulties (shortness of breath [SOB]; moist breath sounds; coughing); weight gain; altered mental status (AMS); lethargy; muscle cramps; nausea; cerebral edema
  - Diagnostic findings: hyponatremia; decreased specific gravity; low Hct and Hgb levels; decreased serum osmolarity
  - Treatment goal: decrease the amount of fluid in the cells
    - Hypertonic IV fluids
    - Diuretic agents: to increase renal excretion of water and sodium; to reverse osmotic gradient, and to pull water out of the cells

Fluid Balance

- The required amount of water is present in the body and is distributed among the various body fluid (e.g., ICF, ECF) compartments.
- Fluid balance
  - When water intake equals water loss
- Fluid imbalance
  - Inseparable from electrolyte balance
  - Necessary part of homeostasis
  - Regulation of fluid balance: thirst mechanism; hypothalamus; pituitary glands; adrenal glands; kidneys; GI system
- Fluids are taken into the body through three sources.
  - Oral (ingested) liquids
    - Largest quantity of water taken into the body
    - Thirst is the primary factor that determines fluid intake.
      - Conscious desire for water
      - Thirst stimulation
        - Osmoreceptors in the hypothalamus
          - These cells are stimulated by an increased in the osmotic pressure of body fluids, which initiates thirst.
      - Decrease in the ECF volume
        - The body initiates thirst as a way to regain balance.
      - Decrease in salivation
        - Dryness in the mouth will result in decreased salivary secretion and increased thirst.
          - Water in foods
          - Oxidation of foods
- Daily maintenance fluid requirements
  - Body weight of 1 to 10 kg: 100 mL/kg
  - Body weight of 11 to 20 kg: 1000 mL + 50 mL/kg for each kg over 10
  - Body weight of >20 kg: 1500 mL + 20 mL/kg for each kg over 20
- Certain individuals are likely to need additional fluid intake.
  - Infants
  - Clients with a cerebral injury, a confused status, an elevated temperature, or burns, as well as clients who have undergone a tracheostomy
  - Older adults
- Intake versus output
  - Generally, the amount of liquids ingested in a 24-hour period is approximately equal to the amount of fluids excreted in the same 24-hour period.
  - Average fluid intake over a 24-hour period for an adult: 2200 to 2700 mL
  - Average daily fluid intake and output
    - Gains
      - Ingested liquids: 1100 to 1400 mL
      - Water in foods: 800 to 1000 mL
      - Water from oxidation: 300 mL
    - Loss and location
      - Kidneys (sensible fluid loss): 1200 to 1500 mL
      - Skin (insensible fluid loss): 500 to 600 mL
      - Lungs (insensible fluid loss): 400 mL
      - GI (sensible fluid loss): 100 to 200 mL

APPLICATION AND REVIEW

17. Which event is a common trigger of Cushing syndrome?
    1. Too rapid infusion of IV fluids
    2. Development of type 2 diabetes mellitus
    3. Long-term use of corticosteroidal agents
    4. Chronic renal failure
18. Which assessment findings support a possible diagnosis of excessive fluid volume? (*Select all that apply.*)
    1. Pitting edema in the legs and feet
    2. Positive JVD
    3. SOB
    4. Flaccid muscles
    5. Weight loss
19. Which organs have a role to play in the regulation of fluid balance in the human body? (*Select all that apply.*)
    1. Hypothalamus
    2. Pituitary glands
    3. Adrenal glands
    4. Kidneys
    5. Heart

See Answers on pages 16–18.

Extracellular Fluid

- Approximately one-third of the body water is ECF.
  - In an adult, approximately 15% of the total body weight is ECF.
    - Interstitial fluid
      - Makes up three-quarters of the ECF.
      - Makes up 11% of the total body weight.
    - Intravascular fluid
      - Makes up one-quarter of the ECF.
      - Makes up 4% of the total body weight
- Components
  - Sodium is the major electrolyte in ECF.
- ECF has three primary compartments.
  - Interstitial fluid
    - Also known as the "third space"
    - Fluid in the space between the cells and the lymph glands
  - Intravascular fluid
    - Fluid found in blood plasma
    - Within the blood vessel
  - Transcellular fluid
    - Part of ECF
    - Small amounts of fluid are contained in the cerebrospinal fluid, GI tract, and in the pleural, synovial, and peritoneal fluids.
      - Synovial joint fluid
      - Fluid in the pericardial sac around the heart
      - Fluid in the eye (intraocular)
    - No impact on fluid and electrolyte balances
- Functions: carries nutrients and oxygen to the cells; carries waste materials from the cells; keeps cells moist; bathes the cells

Intracellular Fluid

- ICF contains water and dissolved solutes and proteins.
  - Solutes are electrolytes needed for proper body functioning.
- Approximately two-thirds of the TBW is ICF.
- In an adult, approximately 40% of body weight is ICF.
- ICF is found inside the cell.
- Movement of water in and out primarily occurs by osmosis.
- Components
  - Potassium
    - Is the primary electrolyte in ICF
    - Works to maintain balance
  - Magnesium
  - Phosphate
- Compartment: ICF compartment usually does not experience rapid changes in osmolarity.
- Functions: transports food within the cells; brings waste products from the cells so they may be excreted from system; maintains integrity (shape and size) of the cell

Constituents of Body Fluids

- Atoms
  - Basic units of matter and defining structure of elements
  - Made up of three particles
    - Protons: positively charged particles
      - The number of protons in an atom defines what element it is.
        - Carbon atoms have six protons.
        - Hydrogen atoms have one proton.
        - Oxygen atoms have eight protons.
      - Heavier than electrons and weigh more than 1800 electrons
      - Reside in the nucleus at the center of the atom
    - Neutrons: uncharged particles found in all atomic nuclei
      - Number of neutrons in a nucleus determines the isotope of that element; for example, hydrogen has three isotopes.
      - Heavier than electrons
      - Reside in the nucleus at the center of the atom
    - Electrons: negatively charged and electrically attracted to positive-charged protons
      - Tiny, compared with protons and neutrons
        - 1800 times smaller than either
        - Extremely lightweight
        - Exist in a cloud that orbits the nucleus
        - Electron cloud has a radius 10,000 greater than the nucleus.
  - Atoms always have an equal number of protons and electrons.
- Ions
  - Atoms or molecules that have gained or lost one or more valence electrons, giving the ion a net-positive or net-negative charge
  - Two types
    - Anion
      - Negative charge
      - If there are more electrons than protons

- Cation
  - Positive charge
  - If the chemical species has more protons than electrons
- Predicting anions and cations
  - Predictions can be made based on its position on the periodic table.
  - Cations
    - Alkali metals
    - Alkaline earths
    - Typically, most metals: iron; gold; mercury
  - Anions
    - Halogens
    - Typically, most other nonmetals: oxygen; nitrogen; sulfur
- Writing chemical formulas
  - Cation is listed before anion. For example: NaCl
  - The sodium atom acts as the cation, whereas the chlorine atom acts as the anion.
- Anion gap
  - A difference exists between the primary measured cations and the primary measured anions in serum.
  - Reference range of the anion gap: 3 to 11 mEq/L
  - Normal value for serum anion gap: 8 to 16 mEq/L
    - Can be defined as low, normal, or high
    - Decreased (low) anion gap may suggest
      - Hypoalbuminemia (decreased albumin)
      - Plasma cell dyscrasia
      - Monoclonal protein
      - Bromide intoxication
      - Normal variant
    - Normal anion gap may suggest
      - Loss of HCO_3^- (through diarrhea)
      - Recovery from diabetic ketoacidosis
      - Ileostomy fluid loss
      - Carbonic anhydrase inhibitors: acetazolamide; dorzolamide; topiramate
      - Renal tubular acidosis
      - Arginine and lysine in parenteral nutrition
      - Normal variant
    - Elevated (high) anion gap may suggest
      - Methanol
      - Uremia
      - Diabetic ketoacidosis
      - Propylene glycol
      - Isoniazid intoxication
      - Lactic acidosis
      - Ethanol ethylene glycol
      - Rhabdomyolysis
      - Salicylates
- Flow of currency
  - Anode
    - Positively charged electrode

- Attracts electrons or anions
- Source of positive charge or an electron acceptor
- Cathode
  - Negatively charged electrode
  - Attracts cations or positive charge
  - Source of electrons or an electron donor; may accept positive charge
- Helpful hint
  - Cathode attracts cations
  - Anode attracts negative charge

Movement of Fluids

- Fluids and solutes move constantly throughout the body.
- Movement of fluids maintains homeostasis and balance in the body.
- Solutes
  - Substances that are dissolved
  - Particles, usually salt
- Solvent
  - Solution in which the solute is dissolved
  - Liquids, usually water
- Solution
  - Solute and solvent mixed together
- Diffusion
  - Process by which a solute may spread throughout a solution
  - Process by which a solute spreads from an area of higher concentration to an area of lower concentration
- Facilitated diffusion
  - When a carrier substance is needed to transport another substance across a membrane
- Osmosis (Figure 1.1)
  - Solvent molecules move across a selectively permeable membrane.
  - Solvent molecules are moved to an area where a decreased concentration of solvent is present.
  - The result of osmosis is two solutions, separated by a membrane, that are more nearly equal in concentration of solutes.

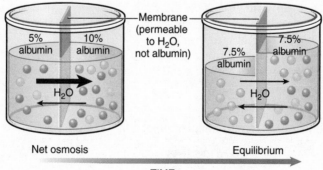

FIGURE 1.1 Osmosis through a semipermeable membrane. (From Lewis, S. L., Bucher, L., Heitkemper, M. M., & Harding, M. [2017]. *Medical-surgical nursing: Assessment and management of clinical problems,* [10th ed.]. St. Louis: Elsevier.)

- Filtration
  - Filtration is a process during which both solutes and solution move together in response to fluid pressure to create equilibrium.
  - Tissue perfusion is an example.
    - Water, nutrients, and waste products are exchanged at the capillary bed.
    - Difference in hydrostatic pressure is between the capillaries and the tissue space.
- Active transportation
  - When molecules move "uphill" against concentration and osmosis
  - When energy from adenosine triphosphate (ATP) and a carrier molecule, adenosinetriphosphatase (ATPase), are needed

Types of Solutions (Table 1.1)

- Isotonic solutions
  - Have the same osmolarity as normal body fluids
    - Concentration of solute particles: between 250 and 375 milliosmoles per liter (mOsm/L)
  - Isotonic solutions help by expanding the fluid in the ECF space.
  - Fluid has equal tonicity, and no exchange of fluid occurs at the cell membrane.
    - Establishes equilibrium
  - Examples: 0.9% NS; LR solution; 5% dextrose in water (D_5W)
  - Common uses: to replace fluid loss; to maintain fluid
  - Conditions to monitor
    - Fluid volume overload
    - Decreased Hgb and Hct levels
      - Dilution by overexpansion of intravascular compartments
    - D_5W allows free water to be distributed, which may lead to increased ICF and to cerebral edema.
  - Isotonic fluid loss
    - Can cause dehydration and fluid volume deficit
    - Examples of isotonic fluid loss: perspiration (sweating); blood loss; wound drainage
    - Will not cause swelling or shrinking of cells.
  - Excessive isotonic solutions can result in hypervolemia (fluid overload).
- Hypotonic solutions
  - When one fluid contains less solutes when compared with other another fluid
  - Pushes fluid from the vascular space into cells
    - Helps hydrate the cells
    - Decreases the amount of fluid in the circulatory system
    - Less concentrated than ECF
    - Causes cells to swell
  - Examples of hypotonic solutions are 0.45% (½) NS and distilled water, which does not have solutes in it.

TABLE 1.1   Concepts of Hypertonic, Isotonic, and Hypotonic Solutions

Hypertonic	Isotonic	Hypotonic
Osmolarity > body fluid	Osmolarity = body fluid	Osmolarity < body fluid
Shifts fluid into blood plasma; moves fluid from tissues.	Keeps fluid in intravascular volume.	Shifts fluid from intravascular area to tone tissue cells.

- Common uses: to lower serum sodium levels; to expand and hydrate cells
- Conditions to monitor: wet breath sounds; increased blood pressure; fluctuation of serum sodium levels
- Contraindicated in certain client populations
  - Clients with intracranial pressure (ICP)
    - Solution will increase the fluid shift into the brain cells and result in greater cerebral swelling.
  - Clients with burns
    - Abnormal fluid shifts from the extracellular space into the intracellular space.
- Hypertonic solutions
  - Contain more solutes as compared with other fluids
  - Pull fluids from the inside of the cell into the vascular space
    - Causes extracellular space to expand
    - Assists in restoring circulation volume
  - Cause cells to shrink
  - Examples: 10% dextrose in water ($D_{10}W$); 3% NS; 0.45% dextrose in NS (D_5 ½ NS); 5% dextrose in NS (D_5NS);
  - Common uses: to treat hypovolemia and hyponatremia
  - Conditions to monitor: wet breath sounds; increased blood pressure; fluctuation of serum sodium levels

Intravenous Solution Tonicity

- D_5W: Isotonic solution
- $D_{10}W$: Hypertonic solution
- ½ NS: Hypotonic solution
- NS: Isotonic solution
- 3% NS: Hypertonic solution
- D_5 ¼ NS: Isotonic solution
- D_5 ½ NS: Hypertonic solution
- D_5NS: Hypertonic solution

APPLICATION AND REVIEW

20. If the goal is to shift fluid from the intravascular spaces into the cells, which IV fluid should be prescribed?
    1. 3% NS
    2. ½ NS
    3. D_5 ¼ NS
    4. D_5W

See Answer on pages 16–18.

Measurement of Osmotic Pressure

- Osmolality
  - Concentration of a solution is expressed as the total number of solute particles per kilogram.
- Osmolarity
  - Concentration of a solution is expressed as the total number of solute particles per liter.

- Specific gravity (relative density)
  - Ratio of the density of a substance to that of a reference substance
  - Example:
    - Will tell whether the object will sink or float in water
      - Water acts as the reference substance.
- Hydrostatic pressure (turgor pressure)
  - Is defined as the pressure that is exerted by a fluid at equilibrium at a given point within the fluid, attributable to the force of gravity
  - Increases in proportion to the depth measured from the surface, attributable to the increasing weight of fluid exerting downward force from above
- Osmotic pressure
  - Is defined as the amount of pressure that, when applied to a hypertonic fluid, will stop osmosis from occurring across a semipermeable membrane
- Pressure gradient
  - Is defined as the quantity that describes which direction and at what rate the pressure most rapidly increases
  - Higher pressure to lower pressure

ANSWER KEY: REVIEW QUESTIONS

1. **3 Water makes up 60% to 65% of the body's TBW with 65% of that amount being stored in the intracellular spaces.**
   1 35% of the body's TBW is found in the extracellular spaces. **2** 55% of the body's TBW is stored in the intracellular spaces. **4** 85% of the body's TBW is stored in the intracellular spaces.
   Client Need: Physiological Integrity; **Cognitive Level:** Knowledge; **Integrated Process:** Teaching and Learning

2. **Answers: 1, 2, 3, 4**
   The consistency of body fluids that are necessary to maintain the required steady state (homeostasis) is achieved through a combination of osmosis, diffusion, filtration, and active transport.
   5 Passive transport is not a method for maintaining body fluids in the process of homeostasis.
   Client Need: Health Promotion and Maintenance; **Cognitive Level:** Understanding; **Integrated Process:** Teaching and Learning

3. **2 A loss of 20% of the body's fluid content may be fatal since it can lead to irreversible health problems.**
   1 Although a loss of 20% of the body's fluid content requires fluid replacement, the response does not address prognosis; a loss of 20% of the body's fluid content may be fatal since it can lead to irreversible health problems. **3** The conclusion should be related to prognosis; a loss of 20% of the body's fluid content may be fatal since it can lead to irreversible health problems. **4** The client is in danger; loss of 20% of the body's fluid content may be fatal since it can lead to irreversible health problems.
   Client Need: Physiological Integrity; **Cognitive Level:** Analysis; **Nursing Process:** Evaluation

4. **Answers: 1, 2, 3**
   Potassium, sodium, and calcium are among the major electrolytes found in the human body.
   4 Chromium is a trace mineral needed by the body but only in small quantities (less than 20 mg/day). **5** Iron is a trace mineral needed by the body but only in small quantities (less than 20 mg/day).
   Client Need: Physiological Integrity; **Cognitive Level:** Knowledge; **Integrated Process:** Teaching and Learning

5. **4 The normal range for serum sodium concentration is 135 to 145 mEq/L; 147 mEq/L would be above normal, indicating hypernatremia.**
   1 The normal range for serum potassium concentration is 3.5 to 5 mEq/L; 5.4 mEq/L would be above normal, indicating hyperkalemia. **2** The normal range for serum calcium concentration is

8.5 to 10.5 mg/dl; 8.8 mg/dL would be within normal limits. **3** The normal range for serum chloride concentration is 95 to 105 mEq/L; 104 mEq/L would be at the high normal limit.

Client Need: Physiological Integrity; **Cognitive Level:** Comprehension; **Integrated Process:** Teaching and Learning

6. **2 K is the accepted abbreviation for the electrolyte, potassium.**

   1 Cl^- is the abbreviation for the electrolyte, chloride. **3** Na^+ is the abbreviation for the electrolyte, sodium. **4** P is the abbreviation for the electrolyte, phosphorus.

   Client Need: Physiological Integrity; **Cognitive Level:** Knowledge; **Integrated Process:** Teaching and Learning

7. **1 Normal serum magnesium level is 1.5 to 2.5 mEq/L; 1.3 mEq/L would indicate a lower-than-normal level (hypomagnesemia).**

   2 Normal serum magnesium level is 1.5 to 2.5 mEq/L; 1.7 mEq/L would indicate a normal level of magnesium. **3** Normal serum magnesium level is 1.5 to 2.5 mEq/L; 2.4 mEq/L would indicate a normal level of magnesium. **4** Normal serum magnesium level is 1.5 to 2.5 mEq/L; 2.8 mEq/L would indicate a higher-than-normal level (hypermagnesemia).

   Client Need: Physiological Integrity; **Cognitive Level:** Comprehension; **Integrated Process:** Teaching and Learning

8. **Answers: 2, 4, 5**

   Calcium, magnesium, and potassium are identified as being cations.

   1 HCO_3^- is referred to as an anion. **3** Chloride is referred to as an anion.

   Client Need: Physiological Integrity; **Cognitive Level:** Comprehension; **Integrated Process:** Teaching and Learning

9. **3 Distinguished by their electrical charge, electrolytes that produce negative charges are called anions.**

   1 Sodium is a cation; capable of producing a positive electrical charge. **2** The term anion does not refer to binding property; rather, it refers to the ability to produce a negative electrical charge. **4** The majority of major electrolytes are not anions.

   Client Need: Physiological Integrity; **Cognitive Level:** Evaluation; **Integrated Process:** Teaching and Learning

10. **4 Renin is a kidney enzyme that produces angiotensin I, which, in turn, is converted into angiotensin II.**

    1, 2, 3 ADH, angiotensin and aldosterone are hormones, not enzymes.

    Client Need: Physiological Integrity; **Cognitive Level:** Application; **Integrated Process:** Teaching and Learning

11. **4 Adults who are obese have very little fluid contained in their adipose (fat) cells, resulting in a below normal level of TBW, which contributes to the risk of fluid imbalance. The effect of the client's older age (an increase in tissue loss) also increases the risk for dehydration.**

    1 The 9-year old child is not at an abnormally high risk for fluid imbalance, and developmental challenges do not increase the risk. **2** Neither age nor physical condition places this 20-year-old young adult at risk for fluid imbalances. **3** Although smoking is a general health risk, it does not significantly increase this 45-year-old adult's risk for fluid imbalance.

    Client Need: Physiological Integrity; **Cognitive Level:** Analysis; **Nursing Process:** Evaluation

12. **4 An older adult who is experiencing the symptoms of viral gastroenteritis, especially a fever, is at an increased risk for dehydration.**

    1, 2, 3 Although age is a factor, cataract surgery, cognitive impairment, and osteoporosis do not increase this client's risk for dehydration.

    Client Need: Physiological Integrity; **Cognitive Level:** Analysis; **Nursing Process:** Evaluation

13. **3 Insensible fluid loss cannot be measured; fluid loss through respirations are an example of such a loss. Nasal allergies and their effect on respirations, especially mouth breathing, would increase the risk of dehydration.**

    1 Influenza, and the resulting vomiting and possible diarrhea, is a risk for sensible (measurable) fluid loss. **2** Polyuria (excessive urination) is a risk for sensible (measurable) fluid loss. **4** Chronic diarrhea is a risk for sensible (measurable) fluid loss.

    Client Need: Physiological Integrity; **Cognitive Level:** Analysis; **Nursing Process:** Evaluation

14. **Answers: 1, 2, 3**

    Signs of severe water deficit include confusion, hypotension (decreased blood pressure), and tachycardia (increased heart rate).

4 Administering fluids would not be considered a monitoring intervention. 5 A red, itchy rash is not associated with a water deficit.

Client Need: Physiological Integrity; **Cognitive Level:** Analysis; **Nursing Process:** Evaluation

15. **Answers: 1, 3, 4, 5**

    The signs of a heatstroke include seizures, increased pulse rate, confusion, and hypotension.

    2 Impaired sweating is a sign of heatstroke.

    Client Need: Physiological Integrity; **Cognitive Level:** Analysis; **Nursing Process:** Evaluation

16. **3 IV LR solution should not be administered; it worsens lactic acidosis.**

    1, 2, 4 Treatment for sunstroke includes oxygen therapy, continuous core temperature monitoring, and establishing baselines for serum sodium and potassium.

    Client Need: Physiological Integrity; **Cognitive Level:** Appling; **Nursing Process:** Evaluation

17. **3 Cushing syndrome, also called hypercortisolism, is triggered by long-term exposure to cortisol and/or corticosteroids.**

    1 Although too rapid an infusion of IV fluids can trigger fluid intoxication, it will not cause Cushing syndrome. 2, 4 Type 2 diabetes mellitus and chronic renal failure are not triggers for Cushing syndrome.

    Client Need: Physiological Integrity; **Cognitive Level:** Applying; **Nursing Process:** Evaluation

18. **Answers: 1, 2, 3**

    Signs and symptoms of excessive fluid volume include peripheral pitting edema, positive JVD, and SOB (dyspnea).

    4 Muscle tetanus (cramps), not flaccidness, is associated with excessive fluid volume. 5 Weight gain, not weight loss, is associated with excessive fluid volume.

    Client Need: Physiological Integrity; **Cognitive Level:** Comprehension; **Nursing Process:** Assessment

19. **Answers: 1, 2, 3, 4**

    The balance of fluids in the body is regulated by the hypothalamus, pituitary and adrenal glands, and kidneys.

    5 Although the heart is responsible for circulating blood, it is not directly associated with regulating fluid balance.

    Client Need: Physiological Integrity; **Cognitive Level:** Comprehension; **Integrated Process:** Teaching and Learning.

20. **2 A hypotonic solution, such as ½ NS, is needed to shift fluids from the intravascular spaces into the cells.**

    1 A hypertonic solution, such as 3% NS, is needed to shift fluids into blood plasma and out of the cells. 3, 4 An isotonic solution, such as either D_5 ¼ NS or D_5W, is needed to keep fluids in the intravascular spaces.

    Client Need: Physiological Integrity; **Cognitive Level:** Comprehension; **Integrated Process:** Teaching and Learning

Fluid and Electrolyte Balance and Imbalance $\quad$ 2

FLUID AND ELECTROLYTE BALANCE AND IMBALANCE OVERVIEW

Electrolytes

- Definition
  - An electrolyte is an element of compound that, when melted or dissolved in a solution (water), separates into ions and carries an electrical current.
    - Electrically charged particles (ions)
      - Anion: negative ion
      - Cation: positive ion
    - Positive changes attract negative charges; similar charges repel one another.
  - Electrolytes are substances that dissociate (separate).
  - Intracellular, interstitial, and intravascular compartments contain electrolytes.
  - Whenever an electrolyte moves out of a cell, another moves in and replaces it.
- Function
  - Electrolytes are responsible for maintaining health and function in all body systems.
  - Physiological processes, for which electrolytes are essential, include neuromuscular function, body fluid osmolality, acid-base balance, and distribution of body fluids and electrolytes.
  - Electrolytes play a major role in maintaining cellular excitability and impulse transportation.
  - For normal cell function, a specific kind and amount of certain electrolytes must be available.
    - In both extracellular fluid (ECF) and intracellular fluid (ICF), even a small alteration has the potential to cause major health problems.
- Measuring electrolytes
  - Nurses are not concerned with how much the electrolytes weigh; rather, they want to know how many ions are available or what the chemical interaction is.
    - Nurses want to know the chemical activity of the electrolytes in a solution.
    - Chemical combining power of an electrolyte reveals how many ions are available.
  - Chemical combining power
    - Number of ions available
  - Milliequivalent (mEq) is a unit of measure that expresses the combining activity of an electrolyte.
    - One mEq of any cation will always chemically react with one mEq of any anion.
- Sources of electrolytes
  - Electrolytes can be found in fruits, vegetables, and grains; red meat, poultry, and fish; fluids; and supplements.
  - Sources of sodium: table salt; seasonings; spices; saltine crackers; pretzels; potato chips; canned soda beverages; pickles; pickled foods; sardines and herring; potatoes and other white vegetables
    - Processed foods: hot dogs; cold cuts; beef jerky; canned soup
  - Sources of potassium: bananas; dark greens; leafy vegetables; raisins; salt substitutes; all-bran cereals; potatoes; dried beef (beef jerky); dried fruit

- Sources of calcium
  - Dairy products: milk; cheese; yogurt; sour cream; cottage cheese; ice cream
  - Canned seafood: salmon; sardines; oysters
  - Fruit juices that are labeled "fortified"
  - Dark green, leafy vegetables: spinach; kale; rhubarb; collard greens; broccoli
- Sources of phosphorus: milk; cheese; eggs; meat; fish; fowl; nuts; dried fruit
- Sources of magnesium: whole grains; nuts; seeds; bananas; oranges; peanut butter; chocolate
  - Green vegetables are the best source of magnesium and include broccoli, spinach, squash, avocados, and potatoes.
  - Magnesium is commonly found in tap water and is a mineral.
- Common electrolytes
  - Sodium
    - Sodium is the major cation in ECF.
    - Its primary role is to maintain fluid volume in the body.
    - Its normal laboratory value is between 135 and 145 mEq/L.
    - Sodium changes the osmotic pressure by changing the concentration levels.
    - Water follows sodium.
    - Adrenal cortex regulates sodium and releases aldosterone to increase sodium reabsorption by maintaining ECF volume and by excreting potassium.
    - Functions
      - Regulates osmolality
      - Aids in maintaining blood pressure (BP)
      - Balances the volume of water in the body
      - Works with other electrolytes to promote nerve impulses to muscles and tissues
      - Aids with acid-base balance
  - Potassium
    - Potassium is the primary cation in the ICF.
    - Kidneys are the primary regulators.
    - Functions
      - Maintains fluid balance in cells
      - Contracts skeletal, cardiac, and smooth muscles
      - Breaks down carbohydrates and fats
      - Maintains cellular growth
      - Maintains acid-base balance
  - Calcium
    - Cation
    - Found in bones and teeth
    - Most abundant mineral found in the body
    - Controlled by the parathyroid hormone (PTH) (Figure 2.1)
      - Excreted by the parathyroid gland
      - Vitamin D
      - Calcitonin
    - Vitamin D is necessary for calcium absorption.
    - Functions
      - Maintains muscle tone
      - Secretes hormones

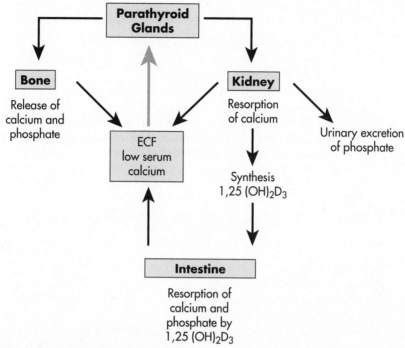

FIGURE 2.1   Mechanism of parathyroid hormone. (From Price, S. A., Wilson, L. M. [2012]. *Pathophysiology: Clinical concepts of disease processes,* [6th ed.]. St. Louis: Mosby.)

- Transmits nerve impulses
- Contracts the skeletal and heart muscles
- Is necessary for strong bone and teeth development
- Aids in BP regulation
- Is an enzyme co-factor in clotting cascade
  - Assists in the formation of blood clots
  - Releases of thromboplastin from platelets
- Phosphorus
  - Anion
  - Normal laboratory value: between 2.5 and 4.5 mg/dL
  - Most abundant anion in the ICF
  - Balance requires adequate renal functioning.
    - Kidneys are the primary route for excretion.
  - Functions
    - Intermediary in metabolism of protein, carbohydrates, and fats
    - Muscle contraction
    - Transport of fatty acids
    - Acidification of urine
    - Acids-base buffering
      - Binds with hydrogen (in urine)
      - Primary urinary buffer
  - Maintains the function of the red blood cells (RBCs)

- Magnesium
  - Cation
  - A clear understanding of what organs control which levels in the body is not available. The kidneys assist in controlling high levels of magnesium by excreting through feces and conserving by storing in bone.
  - Only 1% of magnesium is found in the ECF.
  - Functions
    - Co-enzyme in metabolizing carbohydrates and proteins
    - Muscular irritability and contractions, directly acting on the myoneural junction
    - Maintenance of strong and healthy bones

APPLICATION AND REVIEW

1. Exposure to what physical factor is required to cause an electrolyte to separate into ions?
   1. Cold
   2. Heat
   3. Water
   4. Electrical current
2. Which critical body processes rely heavily on the function of electrolytes? *(Select all that apply.)*
   1. Distribution of body fluids
   2. Cognitive mood stability
   3. Neuromuscular function
   4. Body fluid osmolality
   5. Acid-base balance
3. What foods and beverages are good sources of electrolytes? *(Select all that apply.)*
   1. Roasted chicken breast
   2. Bowl of vegetable soup
   3. Glass of iced water
   4. Slice of raisin toast
   5. Fish taco
4. A client is encouraged to include more potassium in his daily diet. Which food choice shows that the client is demonstrating an understanding of the appropriate food choices?
   1. Banana and all-bran cereal for breakfast
   2. Cup of vanilla yogurt for a bedtime snack
   3. Sardines and crackers for an afternoon snack
   4. Egg salad sandwich and a glass of milk for lunch
5. Which electrolyte is the most common extracellular cation?
   1. Sodium
   2. Potassium
   3. Magnesium
   4. Aldosterone
6. A nurse reviewing a client's diagnostic laboratory reports would be unconcerned about which sodium result?
   1. 118 mEq/L
   2. 126 mEq/L
   3. 138 mEq/L
   4. 148 mEq/L
7. An imbalance related to potassium is likely to result in what disorder?
   1. Ineffective cardiac contractions
   2. Pathological bone fractures
   3. Impaired fat metabolism
   4. Poor denture formation

See Answers on pages 37–39.

Fluid and Electrolyte Balance

- Homeostasis
  - Homeostasis is defined as a steady state of the body, which allows the internal systems of the body to maintain an equilibrium or balance, despite external conditions. It is maintained by adaptive responses.

- An equal number of cations and anions is necessary to maintain homeostasis.
- To function at an optimal level, body cells must contain electrolytes and fluids.
- Examples of the processes include:
  - Temperature regulation
    - Body regulates temperatures to maintain an internal temperature of approximately 98.6º F (37º C).
    - Compensatory mechanisms
      - Sweating cools the body on a hot day.
      - Shivering produces heat on a cold day.
  - Osmoregulation: regulation of the amounts of water and minerals in the body by the kidneys
  - Excretion of metabolic waste: excretory organs (kidneys)
  - Regulation of pH levels: exchange of oxygen and carbon dioxide
  - Regulation of blood glucose levels: liver and insulin secreted by the pancreas
- Stress
  - Disturbs homeostasis and causes the body to attempt to adapt to the stressor
  - Stimulates the hypothalamic, pituitary, and adrenal (HPA) glands
  - Physical stress: hypoglycemia; trauma; exposure to extreme temperatures; infections; heavy exercise
  - Psychological stress: acute anxiety; chronic anxiety; anticipation of stressful situations
- Significance of fluid balance
  - Required amount of water is present and distributed among various body fluid compartments (ICF and ECF).
  - Fluid balance is inseparable from electrolyte balance.
  - Fluid balance is a necessary component in maintaining homeostasis.
  - Sources of fluids
    - Ingested liquids: water; other fluids
    - Intravenous fluids (IVFs)
    - Foods: fruits; vegetables
  - Functions of body water
    - Transportation: nutrients; electrolytes; oxygen to cells
    - Waste: water products carried away from the cells
    - Body temperature regulation
    - Lubricant: joints; membranes
    - Medium food digestion
- Control of electrolytes
  - Regulated in the body by their degree of concentration
  - Mechanisms that maintain electrolyte balance in the body
    - Diffusion: moves molecules from an area of higher concentration to an area of lower concentration; no energy is required
    - Active transport
      - Moves molecules across the concentration gradient
      - Requires adenosine triphosphate (ATP)
      - Sodium-potassium pump: sodium moves out of the cell as potassium moves into the cell to maintain steady balance
    - Osmosis: water moves from an area that contains more water (diluted area) to an area that has less water.
- Osmoreceptors: located in the hypothalamus; initiate a stimulus that senses the need for fluid intake (thirst)

- Thirst
  - Fluid balance is regulated in the body by the thirst mechanism, as well as the hypothalamus, pituitary and adrenal glands, kidneys, and gastrointestinal (GI) system.
  - Thirst is initiated when the body's fluid level decreases.
  - Osmoreceptors initiate this stimulus.
- Fluid volume
  - ICF
    - Makes up approximately two-thirds of the body's water
    - Located within the body's cells
    - Accounts for approximately 40% of body weight
    - Examples: lymph system fluid; pleural fluids; synovial fluids; cerebrospinal fluid; GI system and peritoneal fluids; blood and plasma
  - ECF
    - Makes up approximately one-third of the body's water
    - Interstitial fluid is found between the cells
    - Has two primary compartments:
      - Interstitial fluid: found in space between the cells and lymph glands
      - Intravascular fluid: found in blood plasma
- Blood volume
  - Amount of blood circulating inside the circulatory system and stored in certain organs
  - A typical adult has blood volume of approximately 5 liters.
  - Females generally have less blood volume than males.
  - Regulated by the kidneys
- Intravascular volume
  - Volume of blood in an individual's circulatory system
  - Includes ICF and ECF
- Edema
  - Excess fluid in the interstitial spaces
  - Under normal circumstances, the interstitial fluid volume is regulated. When balance is not possible (attributable to an underlying health issue), the interstitial spaces can become filled with excess fluid.
- Aldosterone
  - Secreted by the adrenal cortex that affects ECF volume
  - Regulates the ECF volume by affecting the renal control of sodium and potassium
  - Released by the adrenal cortex
    - Overactive adrenal glands
      - Should the adrenal glands become overactive and secrete more aldosterone, a serious imbalance may occur.
        - Cushing syndrome: disorder in which the adrenal glands are overactive; symptoms are the result of the excretion of potassium and the retention of sodium, chloride, and water.
    - Underactive adrenal glands
      - Should the adrenal glands be extremely underactive, the excretion of potassium will decrease and the levels of sodium, chloride, and water will decrease as a result of these ions being lost in urine.
        - More potassium will be retained in the body.
        - Large amounts of urine will be excreted.

- ▪ Clients with hypoactive adrenal glands
  - ○ Acquired immunodeficiency syndrome (AIDS)
  - ○ Metastatic cancer
  - ○ Adrenalectomy
- Aldosterone acts on the distal portion of the renal tubules to increase the reabsorption of sodium, chloride, and water and the secretion of potassium and hydrogen.
  - ▪ With sodium retention comes water retention, which promotes the regulation of ECF volume.
- With an increased production of aldosterone, the kidneys retain more sodium, chloride, and water.
- An increased production of aldosterone also causes a loss of potassium.
- Production of aldosterone is not completely understood. In a healthy individual, increased production occurs when there is low fluid volume, low blood sodium, and/or high blood potassium.
- Antidiuretic hormone (ADH)
  - Names explains the action: *anti* means against; *diuretic* means increased secretion of urine.
  - ADH is a water conservation hormone; an increase in the production of ADH will result in an increase of urine saving.
  - The hypothalamus makes ADH, and the posterior pituitary gland stores and secretes ADH.
  - ADH production is regulated by changes in osmotic pressure, which stimulates a retention of fluid to correct an increase in osmotic pressure.
  - ADH regulates fluid volume in the body.
  - When released, the kidneys reabsorb water, increasing urine concentration and inhibiting ADH. Kidneys inhibit the reabsorption of water, thus diluting the urine.
  - ADH regulates osmotic pressure of ECF by regulating the amount of water reabsorbed from the body by the renal tubules, which makes the tubules more permeable to water.
    - ▪ Increased water permeability allows the water to return to the circulating system and leads to dilution of blood and an increase in osmolarity.
- Atrial natriuretic peptide (ANP)
  - Peptide hormone that assists in reducing an expanded ECF volume
  - Causes increased renal sodium excretion
  - Primarily synthesized in the cardiac muscle cells in the walls of the atria of the heart
  - Secreted in response to atrial distention
  - Circulated in the plasma
  - Elicits natriuretic, diuretic, vasorelaxant, and antimitogenic effects, which results in a reduction of body fluid and BP regulation
- Renin (angiotensinogenase)
  - Enzyme that is secreted and stored in the kidneys and stimulates the formation of angiotensin in the blood and tissues, which then stimulates the release of aldosterone from the adrenal cortex
  - Release of renin is stimulated by sympathetic nerve activation and renal artery hypotension and is due to sympathetic hypotension or renal artery stenosis.
    - ▪ Decreased sodium delivered to the distal tubules of the kidney
  - Initiative enzyme for the renin-angiotensin system and responsible for the production of angiotensin I

- Responsive to a decrease in renal perfusion as a result of a decreased extracellular volume
- Angiotensin I
  - Angiotensinogen is first created by the liver and then broken up by renin, resulting in the production of angiotensin I.
  - Stimulates the release aldosterone from the adrenal cortex
  - Acts to cause vasoconstriction, causing blood vessels to become narrower and increasing BP
  - Converted into angiotensin II
- Angiotensin II
  - As angiotensin I passes through the bloodstream, it turns to angiotensin II by the action of angiotensin-converting enzyme (ACE).
  - Binds to many receptors in the body and affects several systems
    - Can increase BP by constricting blood vessels
    - Can trigger thirst or the desire for salt
    - Responsible for the release of the pituitary gland's ADH
  - Functions
    - Constricts resistance vessels, which increases systemic vascular resistance and arterial pressure
    - Acts on the adrenal cortex, which promotes the release of aldosterone and, in turn, acts on the kidneys to increase sodium and fluid retention
    - Stimulates sodium reabsorption at the renal tubular sites
    - Increases sodium and water retention by the body
    - Stimulates thirst in the brain
    - Stimulates the release of vasopressin (ADH) from the posterior pituitary gland, which increases fluid retention by the kidneys
    - Stimulates cardiac and vascular hypertrophy
    - Aids in the release of norepinephrine from sympathetic nerve endings and inhibits norepinephrine reuptake; enhances sympathetic adrenergic function
- Problems with angiotensin
  - High angiotensin
    - Can cause the body to retain too much fluid
    - Elevated blood pressure
    - Not due to other problems
    - May cause the heart to grow, which will lead to heart failure
    - Angiotensin blockers may assist by blocking the receptor sites that take up angiotensin. Side effect of this problem can be too much potassium retention.
  - Low angiotensin
    - May prevent the regulation of blood volume and pressure
    - Increases retention of potassium
    - May lead to a loss of sodium and an increase in urine output, which can lead to low BP (hypotension)
  - Nursing interventions
    - Knowing potential problems associated with angiotensin levels
    - How to balance angiotensin levels
    - Risk factors of angiotensin blockers
    - Therapeutic angiotensin levels

APPLICATION AND REVIEW

8. Which body system has the greatest role in maintaining homeostasis?
   1. Musculoskeletal
   2. GI
   3. Cardiac
   4. Renal
9. Which physiological processes stimulate a response by the HPA glands and brings about an effect on homeostasis? *(Select all that apply.)*
   1. Infection
   2. Exposure to extreme heat
   3. Decrease in serum glucose
   4. Anticipation of a stressful situation
   5. Trauma in the form of organ damage
10. What information concerning the process of active transport is true when considering its role in maintaining electrolyte balance? *(Select all that are true.)*
    1. Is responsible for moving water internally.
    2. Requires ATP to function.
    3. Requires no source of supplemental energy.
    4. Is responsible for the function of the sodium-potassium pump.
    5. Moves molecules from higher to lower areas of concentration.
11. What must be triggered to affect the sensation of thirst?
    1. Osmosis
    2. Osmoreceptors
    3. Sodium-potassium pump
    4. Increase in sodium consumption

See Answers on pages 37–39.

ELECTROLYTE IMBALANCE

- Sodium
  - Plays a primary role in the body's fluid balance and also on the functioning of the body muscles and the central nervous system (CNS)
  - Normal range: between 135 and 145 mEq/L
    - Hypernatremia: sodium level higher than 145 mEq/L
      - Possible causes (Box 2.1)
        - Diabetes insipidus
        - Dehydration: fever; vomiting; diarrhea; Cushing syndrome; extensive and/or excessive exercise; prolonged exposure to environmental heat; diaphoresis
      - Signs and symptoms (Box 2.2): agitation; restlessness; thirst; edema; dry mucous membranes; confusion; seizure and coma (severe cases)
      - Goals of treatment: correction and management of the underlying causes and dietary sodium restrictions
      - Treatment: oral rehydration therapy; IVF replacement
      - Complications: rapid reduction may lead to rapid flow of water, which can result in cerebral edema, permanent brain damage (central pontine myolysis), and possible death.
      - Nursing interventions
        - Restrict sodium intake
        - Know the foods that are high in salt: butter; bacon; canned food; cheese; hot dogs; processed foods; lunch meat; table salt
        - Maintain client safety; individuals may be confused and/or agitated

| **BOX 2.1** | Causes of Hypernatremia (Hyperosmolality Imbalance) |

Insufficient Water Intake

Unable to perceive or respond to thirst (e.g., comatose, confused)

Nothing by mouth without sufficient intravenous (IV) maintenance

Unable to swallow (e.g., cerebrovascular accident)

Excessive Water Loss

Nonrenal

- Fever or diaphoresis or both
- Burns
- Hyperventilation
- Prolonged use of mechanical ventilator
- Watery diarrhea

Renal

- Diabetes insipidus (central, nephrogenic)
- Head trauma (particularly basal skull fracture)
- Neurosurgery
- Infection (encephalitis, meningitis)
- Brain neoplasm
- Osmotic diuresis

- Glycosuria in uncontrolled diabetes
- Urea diuresis in high-protein tube feedings
- Mannitol

Sodium Gain

Seawater drowning

Excessive use of IV sodium salts

- Hypertonic saline (3% or 5%)
- Excessive IV sodium bicarbonate used to treat cardiac arrest
- Isotonic saline

Accidental replacement of sugar with salt in infant formula

Therapeutic abortion with accidental entry of hypertonic saline into circulation

Types of Hypernatremia

Associated with normal extracellular fluid (ECF) volume

Associated with ECF volume depletion

Associated with ECF volume excess

From Price, S. A., & Wilson, L. M. (2012). *Pathophysiology: Clinical concepts of disease Processes,* (6th ed.). St. Louis: Mosby.

| **BOX 2.2** | Hypernatremia: Clinical Features |

Signs and Symptoms

Neurologic

- Early: lethargy, weakness, irritability
- Severe: agitation, mania, delirium, seizures, coma
- Increased deep tendon reflexes
- Nuchal rigidity

Thirst

Elevated body temperature

Flushed skin

Dry, sticky mucous membranes

Tongue rough, red, and dry

Laboratory Findings

Serum sodium >145 mEq/L

Serum osmolality >295 mOsm/kg

Urine osmolality usually >800 mOsm/kg (specific gravity >1.030)

From Price, S. A., & Wilson, L. M. (2012). *Pathophysiology: Clinical concepts of disease Processes,* (6th ed.). St. Louis: Mosby.

- ○ Give hypotonic fluids slowly
  - ○ Risk to brain tissue is increased, attributable to shifting fluids back into the cell.
  - ○ Cells are dehydrated with hypernatremia.
  - ▪ Prevention: low sodium diet
- ▪ Hyponatremia: sodium level lower than 135 mEq/L
  - ▪ Possible causes: syndrome of inappropriate antidiuretic hormone (SIADH); medications: diuretics; antidepressants; water intoxication; result of disease; thyroid gland disorder; cirrhosis; heart failure; pneumonia; renal failure; cerebral disorders; cancer; severe diarrhea and/or vomiting; diabetes insipidus; Addison disease; hypothyroidism; primary polydipsia

- Signs and symptoms: confusion; nausea and/or vomiting; muscle weakness; seizures; headaches; low energy level and/or fatigue; restlessness; irritability
- Goal of treatment: to correct and manage the underlying causes
- Treatment: diuretic medications; fluid restrictions; IV sodium; Addison disease (hormone replacement may be necessary)
- Complication: If sodium levels drop too rapidly, the individual is at risk of cerebral edema.
- Nursing interventions: monitor cardiac, respiratory, neuromuscular, renal, and GI status
- Prevention: treatment of conditions, which may contribute to hyponatremia (adrenal gland insufficiency)
- Potassium
  - Abundant intracellular electrolyte
  - Promotes and facilitates electrical impulses responsible for normal functioning of the brain and also muscular contractions
  - Normal range: between 3.7 and 5.2 mEq/L
    - Hyperkalemia: potassium level higher than 5.2 mEq/L
      - Possible causes: renal disease; some medications
      - Signs and symptoms: nausea; muscular weakness; fatigue; paralysis; life-threatening cardiac dysrhythmias
      - Goal of treatment: correction and management of the underlying causes
      - Treatment:
        - Dietary restrictions of potassium-containing foods;
        - Potassium-lowering medication (kayexalate to promote GI sodium absorption, which causes potassium secretion)
        - Renal dialysis
      - Complications: can be life threatening
      - Nursing interventions
        - Monitor cardiac, respiratory, neuromuscular, renal, and GI status.
        - Hold or stop any IV or oral potassium supplements.
        - Initiate a potassium-restricted diet, including foods high in potassium: potatoes; pork; tomatoes; avocados; strawberries; spinach; fish; mushrooms; cantaloupe; carrots; raisins; bananas
      - Prevention
        - Adjust diet to decrease potassium dietary load.
        - Manage medications that exacerbate hyperkalemia.
    - Hypokalemia: potassium level lower than 3.7 mEq/L
      - Possible causes (Box 2.3)
        - Commonly the result of bodily fluid loss: diarrhea; vomiting; diaphoresis
        - Medications: diuretics; laxatives
        - Diabetic ketoacidosis (DKA)
      - Signs and symptoms
        - Mild symptoms or asymptomatic
        - Moderate or severe symptoms: muscular weakness; tingling and/or numbness; muscle spasms; fatigue; dizziness and/or light-headedness; palpitations; constipation; bradycardia; cardiac arrest (severe cases)
      - Goals of treatment: to correct and manage the underlying causes
      - Treatment: supplemental potassium
      - Complication: cardiac arrest (severe cases)

| BOX 2.3 | Causes of Hypokalemia |

Decreased Dietary Intake of Potassium

Seriously ill client with nothing by mouth for several days without a potassium supplement added to an intravenous (IV) infusion

Starvation, tea and toast diet

Alcoholism

Gastrointestinal Loss

Protracted vomiting, nasogastric suction

Diarrhea, chronic laxative abuse

Ileostomy, fistulas

Villous adenoma of the colon

Renal Loss

- Diuretic drugs (thiazides, furosemide)
- Some renal diseases
  - Diuretic recovery phase of acute renal failure
  - Renal tubular acidosis

Diabetic acidosis leading to osmotic diuresis

Healing stage of severe burns

Excessive mineralocorticoid effect

- Primary or secondary hyperaldosteronism
- Extracellular fluid (ECF) volume deficit (by far, the most common cause)
- Cushing syndrome; corticosteroid therapy
- Licorice ingestion (aldosterone-like activity)
- Swallowing chewing tobacco (contains large amounts of licorice)

Antibiotics (carbenicillin, aminoglycosides)

Magnesium depletion

Increased Loss in Sweat During Heat Stress

Heavily perspiring individual not acclimated to heat

Shift of Potassium Into Cells

Metabolic alkalosis

Treatment of diabetic ketoacidosis (DKA) with insulin and glucose

From Price, S. A., & Wilson, L. M. (2012). *Pathophysiology: Clinical concepts of disease Processes,* (6th ed.). St. Louis: Mosby.

- ■ Nursing interventions: monitoring cardiac, respiratory, neuromuscular, renal, and GI status; checking serial potassium levels
- ■ Prevention: eating a diet rich in potassium
- Calcium
  - Essential for bone health and other functions
  - Normal range: between 8.5 and 10.6 mg/dL
    - ■ Hypercalcemia: calcium level higher than 10.6 mg/dL.
      - ■ Possible causes
        - ○ Hyperparathyroidism (endocrine disorder)
        - ○ Medications: thiazidine diuretics; lithium
        - ○ Certain forms of cancer of the lungs
        - ○ Paget disease
        - ○ Multiple myeloma
        - ○ Non–weight-bearing activity
        - ○ Elevated levels of calcitriol; can occur with sarcoidosis and tuberculosis
      - ■ Signs and symptoms: thirst; anorexia; renal stones; parenthesis; urinary frequency; bone pain; confusion; abdominal pain; muscular weakness; depression; fatigue; constipation; nausea and/or vomiting; lethargy
      - ■ Goal of treatment: to correct and manage the underlying causes
      - ■ Treatment
        - ○ IV fluid hydration
        - ○ Medications: prednisone; diuretics; bisphosphonates
        - ○ Severe cases may require dialysis.
      - ■ Complications
        - ○ Increased pain level; analgesia administration may be helpful.
        - ○ Pathogenic bone fractures can occur, secondary to the bone decalcification.

- Nursing interventions
  - Magnesium levels are highly associated with calcium levels.
    - It is necessary to correct and treat magnesium levels before calcium levels can be corrected.
  - Keep client hydrated, which will help decrease the chances of renal stone formation.
  - Assess for flank or abdominal pain and strain to look for stone formation.
  - Monitor cardiac, neuromuscular, renal, and GI status.
- Prevention
  - Decrease calcium-rich foods.
  - Assess the client's intake of calcium-preserving drugs: thiazides; supplements; vitamin D.
- Hypocalcemia: calcium level lower than 8.5 mg/dL
  - Possible causes
    - Renal disease
    - Inadequate dietary calcium
    - Vitamin D deficiency (vitamin D is essential for the absorption of calcium)
    - Low magnesium level
    - Hypoparathyroidism
    - Eating disorders
    - Pancreatitis
    - Medications: anticonvulsants; alendronate; ibandronate bisphosphonates; rifampin; phenytoin; phenobarbital; corticosteroids; plicamycin
  - Signs and symptoms: muscular aches and/or pains; tingling sensation in feet, fingers, tongue, and lips; bronchospasm (leads to respiratory problems); seizures; tetany; cardiac arrhythmias
  - Goal of treatment: to correct and manage the underlying causes
  - Treatment: calcium supplements, coupled with vitamin D
  - Complications: life-threatening cardiac arrhythmias
  - Nursing interventions
    - Monitoring cardiac and respiratory status
    - Providing client safety (at increased risk for bone fractures)
    - Providing seizure precautions
    - Administering calcium with vitamin D supplements after meals or at bedtime with a full glass of water
  - Prevention
    - Encourage intake of foods high in calcium: yogurt; sardines; cheese; spinach; collard greens; tofu; milk; rhubarb
- Magnesium
  - Plays an essential role in the body's enzyme activities, brain neuron activities, contraction of skeletal muscles, relaxation of respiratory smooth muscles, and in the metabolism of calcium, potassium, and sodium
  - Normal range: between 1.7 and 2.2 mg/dL
    - Hypermagnesemia: magnesium level higher than 2.2 mg/dL
      - Possible causes: renal failure; diabetic acidosis; dehydration; hyperparathyroidism; Addison disease; excessive and/or prolonged use of magnesium-containing laxatives or antacids
      - Signs and symptoms: nausea and/or vomiting; weakness; cardiac arrhythmias; respiratory disturbances (possible respiratory paralysis); CNS depression; hypotension
      - Goal of treatment: to correct and manage the underlying causes

- Treatment
  - Cessation of causative agents
    - Magnesium-containing laxatives
    - Renal dialysis
  - Administration of calcium gluconate, calcium chloride, and IV dextrose and insulin
- Complications: abnormal heart rhythms
- Nursing interventions
  - Monitor cardiac, respiratory, neuromuscular, renal, and GI status.
    - Watch for electrocardiographic (ECG) changes.
  - Provide client safety; client may be lethargic or drowsy.
- Prevention: avoiding magnesium antacids and laxatives in clients with renal failure and avoiding foods high in magnesium
- Hypomagnesemia: magnesium level lower than 1.7 mg/dL
  - Possible causes
    - Uncontrolled diabetes
    - Prolonged use of diuretics
    - Hypoparathyroidism
    - Diarrhea
    - GI disorders (Crohn disease)
    - Severe burns
    - Malnutrition
    - Alcoholism
    - Medications: cisplatin; cyclosporine; amphotericin; proton pump inhibitors (PPI); aminoglycoside antimicrobial drugs
  - Signs and symptoms: muscular weakness; tingling and/or numbness; seizures; muscle spasms; cramps; fatigue; nystagmus (involuntary eye movement may cause the eye to move rapidly)
  - Goals of treatment: to correct and manage the underlying causes
  - Treatment: pain management; administration of IV fluids and magnesium
  - Complications: pain and discomfort
  - Nursing interventions
    - Monitor cardiac, respiratory, neuromuscular, renal, and GI status.
    - Assess potassium levels.
      - If potassium level is low, magnesium levels will be hard to raise.
    - Closely monitor magnesium levels; the client can become magnesium toxic.
      - Depression
      - Loss of deep tendon reflexes
    - Maintain seizure precautions.
  - Prevention: encouraging foods rich in magnesium: avocados; green leafy vegetables; peanut butter; pork; potatoes; oatmeal; nuts; oranges; milk
- Phosphate
  - Necessary for the formation of bone and teeth
  - Plays an important role in the body to make protein for growth, maintenance, and repair of cells and tissues
  - Normal range: between 0.81 and 1.45 molecules per liter (mol/L)
    - Hyperphosphatemia: phosphate level higher than 1.45 mol/L
      - Possible causes: severe and/or advanced renal disease; hypothyroidism; DKA; rhabdomyolysis (destruction of muscular tissue); systemic infections

- Signs and symptoms
  - Weakness
  - Muscle spasms and/or cramping
  - Tetany
  - Crystal accumulations in the circulatory system and in the body's tissues may lead to severe itching and palpable calcifications in the subcutaneous tissue.
- Goal of treatment: to correct and manage the underlying causes
- Treatment
  - Restrict dietary foods containing phosphates: milk; egg yolks.
  - Administer phosphate binder medications to make it hard for the body to absorb phosphates (e.g., lanthanum, sevelamer).
- Complications: impaired circulation; cerebrovascular accident; myocardial infarction (MI); atherosclerosis
- Nursing intervention: phosphate binders administered with or immediately after meals
- Prevention: avoiding use of phosphate medications (laxatives, enema) restricting foods high in phosphate
  - Hypophosphatemia: phosphate level lower than 0.81 mol/L.
  - Possible causes: severe burns; diarrhea; severe malnutrition; hyperparathyroidism; pronounced alcoholism; lymphoma; leukemia; hepatic failure; genetic predisposition; osteomalacia; prolonged use of certain diuretics; prolonged use of aluminum antacids; long-term use of theophylline
  - Signs and symptoms: respiratory alterations (respiratory alkalosis); irritability; cardiac dysrhythmias; confusion; coma; death
  - Goal of treatment: to correct and manage the underlying causes
  - Treatment: oral and IV potassium phosphate; increased intake of high phosphorous foods (milk, eggs)
  - Complications
    - Assess renal status (blood urea nitrogen [BUN], creatinine) before administering phosphorous.
      - If kidneys are not functioning properly, the client will not be able to clear the phosphate.
  - Nursing interventions
    - Monitor cardiac, respiratory, neuromuscular, renal, and GI status.
    - Administer oral phosphorus with vitamin D supplement.
      - Vitamin D aids in the absorption of phosphate.
    - Provide client safety.
      - Individual is at risk of bone fractures.
  - Prevention: encouraging foods high in phosphate and low in calcium: fish; organ meats; nuts; chicken; pork; beef; whole grains
- Chloride
  - Is an essential part of the digestive juices, which are needed to maintain proper balance of body fluids
  - Normal range: between 97 and 107 mEq/L
    - Hyperchloremia: chloride level higher than 107 mEq/L
      - Possible causes: dehydration; renal disease; diabetes; certain medications (supplemental hormones, some diuretics); vomiting; diarrhea; hyponatremia; hyperparathyroidism

- Signs and symptoms: pitting edema; extreme thirst; vomiting; diarrhea; dehydration; dyspnea; Kussmaul respirations (deep, labored breathing pattern); tachypnea; hypertension; decreased cognition; coma
- Goal of treatment: to correct and manage the underlying causes
- Treatment: cautious fluid administration; elimination of problematic medications; correction of any renal disease and hyperglycemia
- Complications: can adversely affect the oxygen transportation in the body
- Nursing interventions
  - Fluids must be administered with caution. Too rapid of rehydration may lead to cerebral edema and other complications.
- Prevention
  - Intake of magnesium and potassium rich foods
  - Avoid foods high in chloride.
  - Adequate hydration
  - Avoid caffeinated products.
  - Reduce or avoid alcohol.
  - Start treatment immediately in diabetes, liver disorder, and kidney disorder.
- Hypochloremia: chloride level lower than 97 mEq/L
  - Possible causes: vomiting; hypoventilation; metabolic alkalosis; respiratory acidosis; cystic fibrosis; hyponatremia; respiratory acidosis; high bicarbonate levels
  - Signs and symptoms: dehydration; muscular spasticity; nausea and/or vomiting; hyponatremia; tetany; muscular weakness and/or twitching; respiratory depression; diaphoresis; elevated temperature
  - Goal of treatment: to correct and manage the underlying causes
  - Treatment: administration of chloride replacements; possible administration of hydrochloride acid and a carbonic anhydrase inhibitor, such as acetazolamide
  - Complications: respiratory arrest; seizures; coma
  - Nursing interventions
    - Monitor cardiac, respiratory, neuromuscular, renal, and GI status.
    - Provide client safety (individual may have increased agitation or irritability)
  - Prevention
    - Offering foods high in chloride, such as table salt or sea salt; seaweed; rye; celery; olives; lettuce tomatoes
    - Administering dietary supplements.

APPLICATION AND REVIEW

12. What assessment data support the diagnosis of moderate hypokalemia? *(Select all that apply.)*
    1. Fatigue
    2. Constipation
    3. Tachycardia
    4. Muscle spasms
    5. Muscle weakness
13. In what activity should a client be engaged to minimize his or her risk for developing hypercalcemia?
    1. Eat a banana each day.
    2. Get a pneumonia vaccination.
    3. Have regular thyroid screening.
    4. Avoid all forms of tobacco smoking.

14. The risk for hypercalcemia is increased for which client?
    1. A 24-year-old young adult who abuses laxatives.
    2. A 40-year-old woman diagnosed with Addison disease
    3. A 56-year-old man diagnosed with multiple myeloma
    4. A 72-year-old older adult diagnosed with chronic renal disease

15. A client has a serum calcium level of 8.3 mg/dL. Which assessment questions should the nurse ask to help identify the possible cause of this result? *(Select all that apply.)*
    1. "Are you taking any form of anticonvulsant medication therapy?"
    2. "Have you ever been diagnosed with an eating disorder?"
    3. "Do you take a diuretic medication regularly?"
    4. "How much dairy products do you consume weekly?"
    5. "Do you experience chronic diarrhea?"

16. A client with a serum magnesium level of 1.5 mg/dL demonstrates appropriate dietary selections when ordering what soup for dinner? *(Select all that apply.)*
    1. Baked potato
    2. Kale and bean
    3. Broccoli cheese
    4. Chicken noodle
    5. Fish chowder

17. The nurse recognizes that a client with a phosphate level of 0.79 mol/L should be encouraged to select which sandwich for lunch?
    1. Grilled chicken
    2. Grilled cheese
    3. Vegetable
    4. Hot dog

18. A client's serum chloride level of 95 mEg/L increases the risk of which disorders? *(Select all that apply.)*
    1. Metabolic alkalosis
    2. Respiratory acidosis
    3. Respiratory alkalosis
    4. Lymphoma
    5. Leukemia

See Answers on pages 37–39.

Fluids and Fluid Imbalances

- Hypervolemia
  - Fluid overload
  - Abnormal increase in the volume of fluid in the body
  - Possible causes: hypernatremia (increased sodium in the body); excess fluid supplementation that the body is unable to manage effectively; hepatic failure; renal failure; heart failure
  - Signs and symptoms: hypertension; shortness of breath; dyspnea; adventitious breath sounds (crackles, rales); abdomen ascites; distended, pulsating jugular veins; peripheral edema (in the hands, feet, ankles); tachycardia; strong, bounding pulses
  - Goal of treatment: to correct and manage the underlying causes
  - Treatment
    - Restrict fluid and sodium intake.
    - Decrease the amount of fluid in the cells.
    - May need to administer hypertonic IV solutions.
    - Administer diuretic medications.
    - Increase renal excretion of water and sodium, which reverses the osmotic gradient and pulls water out of the cell.
  - Complications
    - Congestive heart failure

- Hyponatremia
- Pulmonary edema
- Nursing interventions
  - Monitor mentation changes; change in mentation is an early sign of cerebral edema.
  - Accurately record the client's daily weight.
  - Monitor the client's intake and output (I&O) of fluids.
  - Limit the intake of water and sodium.
  - Elevate the head of the bed.
  - Encourage ambulation.
  - Monitor electrolytes, especially sodium and potassium.
  - Assess for underlying conditions that may promote fluid retention.
    - Heart failure
    - Renal failure
    - Cushing syndrome
  - Administer corticosteroids for a prolonged period.
    - SIADH
    - High salt intake
  - Teach the individual how to limit oral fluid intake.
  - Educate the individual on the symptoms associated with water retention.
    - Rapid weight gain is the best indication of fluid retention and overload (1 L of fluid = 2.2 kg [1 pound]).
- Prevention
  - Track fluid intake.
  - Follow fluid intake guidelines.
  - Manage thirst with sugar-free candies, ice chips, frozen grapes
  - Limit sodium intake.
- Hypovolemia
  - Deficit of bodily fluids
  - Possible causes: severe dehydration; bleeding and/or hemorrhage; vomiting; diarrhea
  - Signs and symptoms
    - Tachycardia, hypotension, oliguria, tachypnea, confusion, fainting
  - Goal of treatment: to correct and manage the underlying causes
  - Treatment
    - Administer IV rehydration with fluids.
    - Place the client in the Trendelenburg position.
      - Body is laid supine (flat on the back) with the feet higher than the head by 15 to 30 degrees.
    - Administer plasma expander, blood, and blood products.
  - Complications: decreased cardiac output; metabolic acidosis; hypovolemia shock; multi-system failure; coma; death
- Nursing interventions
  - Identify individuals at risk.
  - Monitor vital signs, including assessment for postural hypotension.
  - Measure and document the I&O of fluids, evaluating urinary output and specific gravity.
  - Accurately record the client's daily weight.
  - Monitor serum laboratory values for concentrations of hematocrit (Hct), BUN, and sodium.
  - Monitor hemoglobin (Hgb) and Hct (H&H) levels.

  - Monitor the client's level of consciousness (LOC).
  - Evaluate the individual's response to fluid replacement.
- Prevention: encouraging increased oral intake of fluids, at least 64 ounces of water daily

APPLICATION AND REVIEW

19. A nurse should assess a client experiencing hypernatremia for what underlying condition?
   1. Hyperparathyroidism
   2. Cushing syndrome
   3. Seizures
   4. Diarrhea
20. Which nursing interventions should be implemented for a client who is diagnosed with severe dehydration? *(Select all that apply.)*
   1. Assess for postural hypotension.
   2. Assess and document weight daily.
   3. Monitor Hgb and Hct levels.
   4. Assess for adventitious breath sounds.
   5. Measure and document I&O of fluids.

See Answers on pages 37–39.

ANSWER KEY: REVIEW QUESTIONS

1. **3 An electrolyte, when melted or dissolved in a solution (water), separates into ions.**
   1 Exposure to water, not cold, will result in an electrolyte separating into ions. **2** Exposure to water, not heat, will result in an electrolyte separating into ions. **4** Exposure to water, not an electrical current, will result in an electrolyte separating into ions.
   Client Need: Physiological Integrity; **Cognitive Level:** Understanding; **Integrated Process:** Teaching and Learning

2. **Answers: 1, 3, 4, 5**
   Physiological processes, for which electrolytes are essential, includes neuromuscular function, body fluid osmolality, acid-base balance, and distribution of body fluids and electrolytes.
   2 Cognitive mood stability is not heavily reliant on electrolytes but rather relies on hormones.
   Client Need: Physiological Integrity; **Cognitive Level:** Understanding; **Integrated Process:** Teaching and Learning

3. **Answers: 1, 2, 4, 5**
   Electrolytes can be found in fruits, vegetables, poultry, fish, breads, and red meat.
   3 Water contains no electrolytes unless they are added.
   Client Need: Physiological Integrity; **Cognitive Level:** Understanding; **Integrated Process:** Teaching and Learning

4. **1 Bananas and all-bran cereal are good sources of potassium.**
   2 Yogurt is a good source of calcium. **3** Sardines and most crackers are high in sodium. **4** Eggs are a good source of phosphorus, whereas milk is a good source of calcium.
   Client Need: Physiological Integrity; **Cognitive Level:** Evaluation; **Nursing Process:** Evaluation

5. **1 Sodium is the major cation in ECF.**
   2 Potassium is an abundant intracellular electrolyte. **3** Only 1% of magnesium is found in ECF. **4** Aldosterone is a hormone secreted by the adrenal cortex that affects ECF volume.
   Client: Teaching and Learning

6. **3 Serum sodium levels between 135 and 145 mEq/L are normal.**
   1 Since serum sodium levels between 135 and 145 mEq/L are normal, 118 mEq/L is dangerously low. **2** Since serum sodium levels between 135 and 145 mEq/L are normal, 126 mEq/L is dangerously low. **4** Since serum sodium levels between 135 and 145 mEq/L are normal, 148 mEq/L is high.
   Client Need: Physiological Integrity; **Cognitive Level:** Applying; **Nursing Process:** Analysis

7. **1 One of the primary functions of potassium is associated with cardiac muscle contraction.**

     2 Calcium is associated with bone and teeth formation and maintenance. **3** Phosphorus is associated with the metabolism of protein, carbohydrates, and fats. **4** Calcium is associated with bone and teeth formation and maintenance.

     Client Need: Physiological Integrity; **Cognitive Level:** Apply; **Nursing Process:** Analysis

8. **4 The renal system is involved in several functions related to homeostasis, including osmoregulation, excretion, and pH regulation.**

     1 Although all systems are affected by homeostasis, the musculoskeletal system is not significantly associated with maintaining homeostasis. **2** Although all systems are affected by homeostasis, the GI system is not significantly associated with maintaining homeostasis. **3** Although all systems are affected by homeostasis, the cardiac system is not significantly associated with maintaining homeostasis.

     Client Need: Physiological Integrity; **Cognitive Level:** Understanding; **Integrated Process:** Teaching and Learning

9. **Answers: 1, 2, 3, 5**

     Physiological events, including infection, temperature exposure, hypoglycemia, and physical trauma, stimulate a response by the HPA glands, which, in turn, affects homeostasis.

     4 Anticipation of stress is a psychological trigger that stimulates the HPA glands.

     Client Need: Physiological Integrity; **Cognitive Level:** Applying; **Integrated Process:** Teaching and Learning

10. **Answers: 2, 4**

     2 Active transport requires the presence of ATP to function. **4** Active transport is responsible for the function of the sodium-potassium pump.

     1 Water is moved via osmosis. **3** Diffusion requires no energy source. **5** Diffusion moves molecules from higher to lower areas of concentration.

     Client Need: Physiological Integrity; **Cognitive Level:** Understanding; **Integrated Process:** Teaching and Learning

11. **2 Thirst is initiated when the body's fluid level decrease and, in turn, the osmoreceptors are stimulated.**

     1 Osmosis is the mechanism that moves water, but it is not directly involved in the stimulation of thirst. **3** The sodium-potassium pump moves sodium out of the cell, allowing for potassium to move in. **4** Although sodium consumption can alter fluid distribution, it is the stimulation of osmoreceptors that triggers thirst.

     Client Need: Physiological Integrity; **Cognitive Level:** Understanding; **Integrated Process:** Teaching and Learning

12. **Answers: 1, 2, 4, 5**

     Signs and symptoms of hypokalemia include fatigue, constipation, muscle spasms, and muscle weakness.

     3 Bradycardia, not tachycardia, is a symptom of hypokalemia.

     Client Need: Physiological Integrity; **Cognitive Level:** Understanding; **Nursing Process:** Assessment

13. **4 Hypercalcemia is associated with certain forms of lung cancers; avoiding tobacco smoking minimizes the risk for developing lung cancer.**

     1 Hypokalemia is treated with the increase of potassium-rich foods such as bananas. **2, 3** Hyponatremia is associated with both hypothyroidism and pneumonia.

     Client Need: Health Promotion and Maintenance; **Cognitive Level:** Applying; **Integrated Process:** Teaching and Learning

14. **3 Hypercalcemia is associated with multiple myeloma.**

     1 Hypokalemia is associated with the overuse of laxatives. **2** Hyponatremia is associated with Addison disease. **4** Hyperkalemia is associated with renal disease.

     Client Need: Physiological Integrity; **Cognitive Level:** Analysis; **Integrated Process: Nursing Process:** Assessment

15. **Answers: 1, 2, 4**

     A calcium level of 8.3 mg/dL is indicative of hypocalcemia; possible causes include inadequate dietary calcium, anticonvulsant medication therapy, and an eating disorder.

     3 Diuretic medication therapy can result in a depletion of potassium, not calcium. **5** Diarrhea can result in a depletion of potassium, not calcium.

     Client Need: Physiological Integrity; **Cognitive Level:** Analysis; **Nursing Process:** Assessment

16. **Answers: 1, 2, 3**

    A client with a serum magnesium level of 1.5 mg/dL is experiencing hypomagnesemia and should eat foods high in magnesium, such as potatoes, and leafy greens, such as kale and broccoli.

    4 Chicken is not a good source of magnesium. **5** Fish is not a good source of magnesium.
    Client Need: Physiological Integrity; **Cognitive Level:** Evaluation; **Nursing Process:** Evaluation

17. **1 A client with a phosphate level of 0.70 mol/L is experiencing hypophosphatemia. Foods high in phosphate include chicken.**

    2 Cheese is not a food source high in phosphate. **3** Eggs are not a food source high in phosphate. **4** Although hot dogs may contain some beef or pork, they are not a food source high in phosphate.
    Client Need: Physiological Integrity; **Cognitive Level:** Applying; **Nursing Process:** Implementation

18. **Answers: 1, 2**

    A client with a chloride level of 95 mEq/L is experiencing hypochloremia and should be monitored for possible metabolic alkalosis and respiratory acidosis.

    3 Respiratory alkalosis is associated with hypophosphatemia. **4** Lymphoma is associated with hypophosphatemia. **5** Leukemia is associated with hypophosphatemia.
    Client Need: Physiological Integrity; **Cognitive Level:** Analysis; **Nursing Process:** Analysis

19. **2 Cushing syndrome could be an underlying condition that would promote hypernatremia and the resulting fluid retention.**

    1 Hyperparathyroidism is a possible cause of hyperchloremia. **3** Seizures are a complication of hypochloremia. **4** Diarrhea is a possible cause of hypophosphatemia.
    Client Need: Physiological Integrity; **Cognitive Level:** Application; **Nursing Process:** Assessment

20. **Answers: 1, 2, 3, 5**

    Severe dehydration is a possible cause of hypovolemia (deficit of bodily fluids). Nursing interventions include assessing for postural hypotension, monitoring weight daily, monitoring Hgb and Hct levels, and monitoring I&O of fluids.

    4 Hypervolemia could result in fluid accumulation in the lungs, causing adventitious breath sounds.
    Client Need: Physiological Integrity; **Cognitive Level:** Applying; **Nursing Process:** Planning

3 Concepts of Fluid Volume Deficit and Excess

FLUID VOLUME DEFICIT AND EXCESS OVERVIEW

Intake versus Output (Figure 3.1)

- Oral intake
  - Ingestion of fluid
    - Approximately 60% of water comes into the body through drinking, totaling 1400 to 1800 mL in the average adult.
    - The infant body is approximately 70% water.
  - Ingestion of solid food contains water.
    - Approximately 30% of the body water comes from solid food.
    - Between 700 and 1000 mL of water per day enters the body in the form of solid food.
- Fluid output
  - Two types
    - Insensible (cannot be measured)
      - Approximately 10% of body water, or between 300 and 500 mL, is lost through oxidation each day.
      - Fluid loss through skin via perspiration
        - Exercise and fever increase fluid loss through the skin.
        - Sodium is the primary solute lost through sweating.
        - Sweat losses can range from 0 to 1000 mL/hr, depending on the environment and the condition of the client.
        - Approximately 500 mL per day of body water is lost through normal evaporation.
      - Fluid loss through the respiratory tract via respirations
        - 300 mL/day of fluid is normally lost through the lungs.
        - Increased respirations increase the amount of fluid loss via the respiratory system.
    - Sensible (can be measured)
      - Urine
        - 60% of daily water, or approximately 1400 to 1800 mL, is lost through urine in a healthy adult.
        - Output should be approximately 1 mL of urine for each kilogram of body weight per hour.
      - Feces
        - Approximately 100 mL to 200 mL of water is normally excreted in feces each day and accounts for 2% of the total body water.
        - Approximately 8 L of fluid circulates daily through the gastrointestinal system.
        - Diarrhea can dramatically increase the amount of fluid loss through the gastrointestinal system, increasing the risk of developing a fluid volume deficit.
      - Drains
      - Emesis
  - Measuring fluid volume status
    - Blood pressure (BP)
      - Used to assess fluid volume

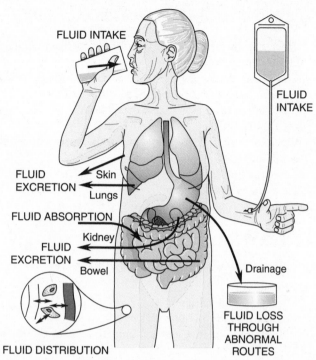

FIGURE 3.1 Fluid homeostasis. (From Banasik, J. L., & Copstead, L. C. [2019]. *Pathophysiology*, [6th ed.]. St. Louis: Elsevier.)

- Can be taken using a sphygmomanometer and stethoscope
- Can be assessed with an electronic BP machine
- May be assessed with direct lines using arterial catheters
- Arterial lines
  - Inserted in an artery
  - Connected to a transducer that translates fluid wave pressures into electronic numbers for monitoring
  - Provide continuous BP monitoring
  - May be used to obtain blood samples.
- Pulmonary artery catheters
  - Inserted in the subclavian or intrajugular vein
  - Tip of catheter located in pulmonary artery
  - Provides measurements for pulmonary artery wedge pressure (PAWP), pulmonary artery pressure, central venous pressure, and cardiac output, all of which provide a broad picture of the client's fluid volume status.
- Central venous catheter
  - Measures the pressure of the blood inside the superior vena cava—central venous pressure (CVP)
  - Inserted and positioned above the right atrium in the superior vena cava
  - Normal range: between 2 and 8 mm Hg
  - Increased CVP is indicative of fluid volume overload.

1. Which assessment data are directed at the documentation of a postsurgical client's insensible fluid output?
   1. Bed linen is changed two times because of the client's diaphoresis.
   2. Client has passed two formed stools in 12 hours.
   3. 600 mL of urine was voided over 8 hours.
   4. Client vomited 60 mL of clear emesis.
2. Which method of venous fluid status measurement can also be used to secure diagnostic blood samples?
   1. Arterial line
   2. Central venous catheter
   3. Pulmonary artery catheter
   4. Electronic sphygmomanometer

See Answers on pages 62–64.

FLUID VOLUME DEFICIT

Pathophysiological Factors of Fluid Volume Deficit

- Dehydration
  - Deficient fluid volume
  - Loss of water from the body's cells
  - Older adults, infants, and children are more at risk to develop dehydration.
    - Clients who cannot obtain fluids without help and have a self-care deficit in obtaining fluids are at risk of dehydration.
  - Dehydration is classified on the basis of the ratio of fluid-to-electrolyte loss.
    - Types
      - Isotonic dehydration
        - Occurs when loss of water and solutes from the extracellular fluid (ECF) compartment are equal
        - No shift of fluid from the intracellular space to the extracellular space
        - Usually caused by vomiting and diarrhea
      - Hypotonic dehydration
        - Develops when the loss of sodium exceeds the loss of water
        - Osmotic shift of water from the extracellular fluid (ECF) space to the intracellular fluid (ICF) space
        - Usually caused by gastrointestinal fluid loss
      - Hypertonic dehydration
        - Occurs when water loss exceeds the amount of sodium lost from the extracellular space
        - Osmotic shift of water from the ICF space to the ECF space
        - May be caused by excessive sweating or diuresis
        - A lack of water in the extracellular space causes fluid to shift out of the cells into the extracellular space.
        - Cells shrink and cannot maintain their shape, obtain nutrients, or remove waste products.
- Hypovolemia
  - Loss of fluids and solutes from the extracellular space
    - Also known as fluid volume deficit
    - Deficient fluid in the vascular compartment

BOX 3.1 Signs and Symptoms of Clinical Dehydration

Absence of sweat and tears
Coma
Confusion and lethargy
Decrease in postural blood pressure with concurrent increased heart rate
Decreased skin turgor
Dryness of oral mucous membranes
Flat neck veins when supine or neck veins that collapse during inspiration (older children and adults)
Hard stools
Hypovolemic shock
Increased serum sodium concentration

Lightheadedness, dizziness, or syncope upon standing
Longitudinal furrows in the tongue
Oliguria
Prolonged capillary refill time
Prolonged small-vein filling time
Rapid, thready pulse
Soft, sunken eyeballs
Sudden weight loss
Sunken fontanel (infants)
Thirst

From Banasik, J. L., & Copstead, L. C. (2019). *Pathophysiology*, (6th ed.). St. Louis: Elsevier.

- Water loss accompanied by the loss of electrolytes
  - The ratio of water and electrolytes remains the same.
- May be acute or chronic
- Can rapidly develop, depending on the cause
- Clinical symptom development can be rapid with increased severity if the body does not have time to compensate for fluid and electrolyte loss.
- Caused by excessive loss of fluids: vomiting; diarrhea; fever; hemorrhage; drainage from nasogastric (NG) tubes; excessive sweating; excessive urination; diabetic ketoacidosis; renal failure; medications such as diuretics
- Can occur when the output of fluid exceeds the intake of fluid
- More serious for the newborn and older adult populations
- Results from the loss of body fluids and/or decreased fluid intake
- Decreased circulating fluid volume can also develop from third-space fluid shifts.
- With increased volume loss, CVP and PAWP decrease.

Signs and Symptoms of Fluid Volume Deficit

- Dehydration (Box 3.1)
  - Signs and symptoms: dizziness; thirst; fever; dry skin; dry mucous membranes; poor skin turgor; concentrated urine; increased heart rate; decreased BP
- Hypovolemia
  - Signs and symptoms: tachycardia; hypotension and/or orthostatic hypotension; pale, cool skin; delayed capillary refill; confusion, restlessness, anxiety, loss of consciousness; seizure; coma; dry mucous membranes; decreased elasticity of skin; thirst (older adult clients may not experience thirst); decreased urine output

APPLICATION AND REVIEW

3. Which statement is accurate when considering the process of dehydration?
   1. Fluid and solvents are lost from the body's extracellular space.
   2. Dehydration occurs when the output of fluid exceeds the intake of fluid.
   3. Dehydration is related to the third-spacing process.
   4. Dehydration results when the body's cells lose water.

4. What intervention focused on managing a direct cause should the nurse consider adding to the care plan of a client who is experiencing isotonic dehydration?
   1. Assisting with activities of daily living
   2. Ensuring that the client has access to an emesis basin
   3. Frequently applying lotion to manage dry skin
   4. Offering sodium-fortified beverages on a regular basis
5. Which client is at the greatest risk for a fluid volume deficit?
   1. 2-year-old with a low-grade fever
   2. 55-year-old adult who is taking a prescribed diuretic medication
   3. 14-year-old teenager with a compound fracture of the left femur
   4. 25-year-old young adult with an NG tube after abdominal surgery
6. To distinguish between dehydration and hypovolemia, on which of the following should the nurse concentrate?
   1. Heart rate
   2. Degree of thirst
   3. Speed of capillary refill
   4. Dryness of mucous membranes

See Answers on pages 62–64.

Nursing Care of the Client With Fluid Volume Deficit

- Dehydration
  - Assessment
    - Assess for changes in mental status, which can lead to seizures and coma and should be treated as a medical emergency.
    - Check for thirst.
    - Assess temperature.
    - Observe the client's skin and mucous membranes.
    - Assess skin turgor.
      - Can be unreliable in the older adult due to normal changes occurring in the aging process
    - Obtain heart rate and BP.
    - Assess color and characteristics of urine.
  - Diagnostic factors: serum osmolality greater than 300 mOsm/kg; serum sodium level greater than 145 mEq/L; elevated Hct; urine-specific gravity greater than 1.030
  - Goals of care: replace fluids; return the client to the level of functioning before becoming dehydrated
  - Treatment
    - Encourage oral fluid intake.
    - Fluids should be salt-free if sodium level is elevated.
    - Gradually administer intravenous (IV) fluids: hypotonic, low-sodium fluid; 5% dextrose in water (D_5W)
  - Complications: seizures; coma; death
  - Nursing interventions
    - Provide a safe environment.
    - Strictly monitor intake and output.
      - May require insertion of a urinary catheter to monitor output.
    - Obtain daily weights.
    - Obtain vital signs at regular intervals.
    - Closely monitor IV fluids.
    - Monitor laboratory values.

- Closely observe the client for changes in his or her level of consciousness.
- Provide adequate oral care.
- Nurses should be alert to symptoms of dehydration in all older clients, which may begin with confusion, below normal temperature, and increased heart rate.
  - Prevention
    - Educate at-risk clients and their families about dehydration.
    - Teach clients to take medications as prescribed to and monitor for side effects.
- Hypovolemia
  - Assessment
    - Assess history for probable cause of fluid volume deficit.
    - Assess for medication use including dosages and times.
    - Assess weight.
      - Evaluate weight in relation to nutritional status.
      - Assess for recent weight changes.
    - Assess BP.
      - Assess for orthostatic hypotension by performing BP while the client is lying, sitting, and standing. Record changes in pressure.
    - Monitor heart rate.
    - Monitor for changes in the level of consciousness.
      - Because of the effects of aging, older clients should be closely monitored for changes in behavior and level of consciousness, as these may be early signs of a fluid volume deficit.
    - Assess intake and output.
      - The nurse should perform a functional ability assessment of clients to determine their cognitive and physical ability to obtain adequate food and water.
    - Assess urine amount and characteristics.
      - Assess need for the placement of a urinary catheter.
    - Monitor hemodynamic values, and evaluate for changes.
  - Diagnostic factors: increased urine specific gravity; increased serum osmolality; decreased Hgb and Hct with hemorrhage; increased blood urea nitrogen (BUN) and creatinine ratio
  - Goals of care
    - Identify and correct the underlying cause of hypovolemia.
    - Replace lost fluids.
    - Normalize blood volume and vital signs.
      - Heart rate between 60 and 100 beats per minute (bpm)
      - Normal systolic BP greater than or equal to 90 mm Hg
      - Absence of orthostatic hypotension
    - Normal skin turgor
    - Urine output at least 30 mL/hr
  - Treatment
    - Aggressiveness of treatment depends on the cause and severity of hypovolemia.
    - If the client is able to tolerate oral fluids and the severity is deemed mild, rehydrate with oral rehydration solutions, which will provide essential electrolytes, fluid, and glucose.
      - Administer isotonic IV fluids.
      - Types of rehydration solutions: Elite; Cytomax; lactated Ringer (LR) solution; normal saline (NS) (0.45% dextrose in NS [D_5 ½NS] after the client has BP stabilization)
    - Rate of IV fluid infusions are dependent on severity of hypovolemia.
      - May require numerous boluses of IV fluids

- May require administration of IV albumin or blood transfusion
- Administer medications such as dopamine to normalize BP, if necessary.
- Complications
  - Hypovolemic shock
    - When at least 40% of the vascular volume is lost
    - Dramatic decrease in cardiac output
    - Urine output less than 10 mL/hr
    - Tachycardia
    - Severe hypotension
    - Cyanosis
    - Loss of consciousness
- Nursing interventions
  - Encourage oral fluid intake, if possible.
  - Obtain and maintain IV access.
  - Administer and monitor IV fluids.
  - Monitor for mental status changes.
  - Frequently obtain vital signs.
  - Maintain patent airway.
  - Administer oxygen therapy as ordered.
  - Conduct hemodynamic monitoring.
    - CVP
    - Pulmonary artery pressure (PAP)
    - PAWP
  - Monitor cardiac output.
  - Document telemetry findings.
  - Monitor skin temperature and changes in peripheral pulses.
  - Monitor laboratory values.
  - May need blood type and crossmatching to prepare for blood transfusion.
  - Teach clients to change positions slowly to prevent falls from orthostatic hypotension.
  - Closely observe for the development of complications.
  - Document all findings and client responses to interventions.
- Prevention
  - Educate high-risk clients and families on the causes of hypovolemia.
  - Encourage clients to drink adequate amounts of fluids.
  - Teach clients to take prescribed medications as directed and to report side effects.
  - Thoroughly explain to clients how certain medications can cause an increased need for fluids.
  - Teach clients to monitor their BP and pulse.

APPLICATION AND REVIEW

7. Which diagnostic laboratory result, compared with the client's baseline, supports the diagnosis of hypovolemia over that of dehydration?
   1. Increase in serum osmolality
   2. Decrease in serum hematocrit
   3. Increase in serum sodium
   4. Urine-specific gravity greater than 1.030

8. The nurse caring for a client with stabilized BP and who is being treated for hypovolemia should question the prescription for which IV solution?
    1. D_5W
    2. NS
    3. LR solution
    4. $D_5 \frac{1}{2}NS$
9. Hypovolemia shock is triggered by at least what amount of vascular volume loss?
    1. 20%
    2. 30%
    3. 40%
    4. 50%
10. All the following clients have been diagnosed with hypovolemic shock. Which assessment data are directly associated with this condition? *(Select all that apply.)*
    1. 16-year old teenager with a current BP of 110/72 mm Hg
    2. 34-year old woman with a urinary output of 15 mL/hr
    3. 46-year old man experiencing a heart rate of 124 bpm
    4. 57-year old man experiencing postsurgical delirium
    5. 60-year old woman with cyanotic nail beds
11. The nurse demonstrates an understanding of the pathophysiological cause of hypovolemic shock when prioritizing which prescribed treatment?
    1. Monitoring laboratory results
    2. Securing IV access
    3. Observing for signs of complications
    4. Monitoring mental status changes
12. Which is the **priority** preventive information that should be stressed when educating a client who is at risk for a fluid volume deficit?
    1. Regularly monitor BP and pulse.
    2. Know the early signs and symptoms of flu.
    3. Drink adequate amounts of fluids.
    4. Take medications as prescribed.

See Answers on pages 62–64.

Fluid Volume Excess

Pathophysiological Factors of Fluid Volume Excess

- Hypervolemia
  - Amount of isotonic fluid is increased in the ECF compartment.
  - An irregular collection of sodium and water causes an isotonic fluid increase of the ECF.
  - It is usually a secondary condition.
  - Sodium levels usually remain normal due to the accompaniment of water in the ECF.
  - An excess of isotonic fluid in the extracellular compartment causes the body to compensate by adjusting levels of atrial natriuretic peptide (ANP), antidiuretic hormone (ADH), and aldosterone. This adjustment causes the kidneys to release excess sodium and water from the body.
  - ADH promotes reabsorption of water into the blood from the tubules of the kidneys. Reabsorption controls the amount of fluid leaving the body via the renal system.
  - Aldosterone controls sodium and water reabsorption from the kidneys.
  - ANP works in both the kidney and the heart. ANP can increase the rate of glomerular filtration in hypervolemia and control the workload of the heart.
  - Compensatory mechanisms can become overwhelmed in hypervolemia, resulting in excess fluid being pushed from the vessels into the interstitial spaces and causing edema in the tissues.

- This displacement of fluid eventually leads to pulmonary edema and heart failure if not treated and corrected.
  - Causes: heart failure; renal failure; fluid overload from IV fluid administration; corticosteroid therapy; increased sodium intake orally or by IV fluid administration; low albumin levels; hyperaldosteronism; liver failure
- Water intoxication
  - Sodium level drops in response to rapid or overhydration.
  - Causes: syndrome of inappropriate antidiuretic hormone (SIADH); excessive water intake; psychological condition known as psychogenic polydipsia; use of tap water as fluid for irrigation of NG or PEG tubes; rapid IV infusion of hypotonic solutions
  - Because of the sodium imbalance, fluid shifts into the cells, which causes the cells to swell.
  - Increased permeability of the capillary membranes or decreased colloid osmotic pressure allows fluid to ooze from the vessels and into these third spaces.
  - Intracranial pressure increases in response to swelling of the brain cells.
- Third-spacing
  - Fluid moves out of the intravascular space into the interstitial tissue or the open cavities of the body, such as the abdomen.
  - Fluid in the interstitial tissue or in a body cavity is not able to function as circulating fluid.
  - Causes: low albumin levels; liver failure; peritonitis; heart failure; burns or crushing types of injury that destroy cell walls; pleural effusion; IV fluids

Signs and Symptoms of Fluid Volume Excess

- Hypervolemia
  - Signs and symptoms: rapid, bounding pulse; elevated BP; third heart sound (S_3, also known as a gallop); distended jugular and hand veins; crackles heard when auscultating lung fields; dyspnea; productive cough with pink, frothy sputum; edema
    - Causes of edema: increased capillary hydrostatic pressure; loss of plasma proteins (albumin); obstruction of lymphatic circulation; increased capillary permeability; anasarca (generalized edema), attributable to the progression of the fluid volume excess
- Water intoxication
  - Signs and symptoms: personality changes; headache; bradycardia; widened pulse pressure; altered level of consciousness; irritability; lethargy; cramps; muscle weakness; pupil changes due to increased intracranial pressure; weight gain
- Third-spacing
  - Signs and symptoms: fluid volume excess in the interstitial spaces; hypovolemia due to the loss of fluid from the intravascular space; decreased urine output is an early sign of third-spacing, despite adequate fluid intake.

APPLICATION AND REVIEW

13. Which information should be included in a discussion of the pathophysiological causes of fluid volume excess? *(Select all that apply.)*
    1. The condition is a result of an increase of ECF.
    2. Sodium levels usually increase dramatically in the ECF.
    3. The body attempts to regulate the problem by adjusting the levels of aldosterone.
    4. To manage the problem, the kidneys retain water in the form of urine.
    5. When improperly managed, the excess fluid is pushed into the interstitial spaces.

14. Which condition is the cause of third-spacing?
    1. Peritonitis
    2. Liver failure
    3. Intracranial pressure
    4. Heart failure
    5. Burns
15. What assessment data support the diagnosis of hypervolemia?
    1. BP of 190/96 mm Hg
    2. Distended jugular veins
    3. Dry, unproductive cough
    4. S_3
    5. Weak, thready pulse of 120 bpm
16. Which sign should alert the nurse to a burned client's early development of third-spacing?
    1. Decreased urine output
    2. Personality changes
    3. Pupil changes
    4. Irritability

See Answers on pages 62–64.

Nursing Care of the Client With Fluid Volume Excess

- Hypervolemia
    - Assessment
        - Assess for signs of increased cardiac output.
        - Assess laboratory values.
        - Evaluate protein intake.
        - Assess for the presence of chronic renal failure.
        - Assess for the development of dependent edema.
        - Check the client for the presence of pulmonary edema.
    - Diagnostic factors
        - Most laboratory values will be decreased due to hemodilution.
            - Decreased BUN, potassium, serum osmolality, and hematocrit
        - Sodium levels may remain normal due to the affinity of sodium to follow water concentrations.
        - Chest x-ray image may show pulmonary edema.
        - Oxygen levels may be decreased.
    - Goals of care
        - Restore normal fluid balance.
        - Restore normal cardiac output.
        - Return client to the level of functioning before the development of fluid volume excess.
    - Treatment
        - Determine and treat the underlying cause of fluid volume excess.
        - Provide pharmacological therapy.
            - Diuretic medication; type is prescribed on the basis of the severity of hypervolemia.
            - Electrolyte replacement
                - Potassium, sodium, and magnesium may be administered to replace electrolytes lost with the use of diuretics.
            - Digoxin, to strengthen heart contractions
            - Antihypertensive medications
            - Limited salt intake
                - Normal diet contains 6 to 15 g of salt daily.
                - Recommend a decrease down to 250 mg sodium per day.
                - Salt substitutes contain increased potassium; use caution with renal impairment.
        - Measures to maintain airway and breathing assistance may be required.

- Pulmonary edema may require treatment with morphine and nitroglycerin.
- May require hemodialysis.
- Nursing interventions
  - Strictly monitor the intake and output of fluids.
  - Obtain and maintain IV access.
  - Closely monitor IV fluid administration to prevent fluid volume overload from worsening.
  - Restrict fluids.
  - Obtain daily weights.
  - Monitor for the development of edema in the extremities.
  - Teach the client to recognize the symptoms of edema, which can affect the skin and circulation.
  - Perform thorough assessments to ensure proper circulation of affected extremities.
  - May need to apply antiembolism stockings.
  - Elevate extremities with edema.
  - Elevate the head of the bed.
  - Monitor laboratory values.
  - Obtain vital signs at frequent intervals.
  - Perform regular respiratory assessments to monitor for the development of crackles in the lung fields.
  - Provide oral care.
  - Administer diuretics as prescribed.
  - Document nursing care provided and the client's response to treatment.
- Prevention
  - Teach high-risk clients and their caregivers the symptoms of fluid volume overload.
  - Educate clients on the proper medication regimen and reportable side effects.
  - Teach clients to weigh themselves daily and to report weight gain as directed by their primary care provider.
  - Teach clients to monitor their BP and heart rate.
  - Educate clients and their families about the importance of compliance with fluid restrictions.
  - Teach clients to limit sodium in their diet.
  - Clients may need a referral to a nutritionist to help with diet planning.
- Water intoxication
  - Assessment
    - Assess for neurological changes.
    - Assess sodium level.
    - Assess vital signs.
  - Diagnostic factors
    - Serum osmolality less than 280 mOsm/kg
    - Serum sodium level less than 125 mEq/L
  - Goals of care
    - Find and treat the cause of water intoxication.
    - Return the serum sodium level to between 135 and 145 mEq/L.
    - Return the serum osmolality to between 280 and 295 mOsm/kg.
    - Observe no signs or symptoms of increased intracranial pressure.
    - Vital signs are within normal limits.
    - Client returns to premorbid level of functioning.

- Treatment
    - Restrict the intake of oral fluids.
    - Stop all IV fluids.
    - Severe cases may require the use of hypertonic solutions to decrease swelling of the cells.
    - Osmotic diuretics, such as mannitol, may be used to decrease intracranial pressure.
- Complications: seizures; coma
- Nursing interventions
    - Monitor the intake and output of fluids.
    - Monitor laboratory values.
    - Maintain fluid restrictions to prevent further sodium dilution.
    - Educate the client and caregivers on the purpose and parameters of fluid restriction.
    - Obtain IV access, and closely monitor all IV infusions.
    - Weigh the client daily.
    - Frequently perform neurological assessments.
    - Start seizure precautions.
    - Document interventions and the client's response to treatments.
- Prevention
    - Educate clients and caregivers on the cause of water intoxication.
    - Teach clients and caregivers to report the signs and symptoms of the development of water intoxication.
    - Encourage clients to weigh daily and to report their weight gain as ordered by the primary care provider.
    - Teach clients and caregivers the importance of maintaining fluid restrictions as ordered.
    - Advise clients to take medications as prescribed.

Intravenous Fluids Used to Treat Fluid Volume Deficit

- Purpose of IV fluids
    - To provide fluids and electrolytes
    - To administer blood and blood products
    - To determine the method for medication administration
    - To provide some nutritional support in compromised clients
- Types of IV fluids
    - Crystalloids
        - Contain smaller molecules than colloids
        - Effortlessly flow into cells and tissues from the bloodstream
        - Have varying levels of osmolality
        - Normal Saline, Lactate Ringers, Dextrose 5%
    - Colloids
        - Plasma expanders
        - Used when crystalloid solutions fail
        - Affect clotting by decreasing the ability of the platelets to clot
        - Remain in the circulation for up to 24 hours
        - Pull fluids into the bloodstream
        - Clients receiving colloids require close monitoring for the development of fluid volume overload and pulmonary edema.
        - Dextran
            - Higher in molecular weight than hetastarch

- Hetastarch (Hespan)
  - Similar to albumin
- Albumin
- Isotonic fluids
  - Have the same solute concentration as blood and body fluids
  - Have an osmolality between 240 and 340 mOsm/kg
  - Allow fluid replacement without pushing fluids into or outside of the body cells
  - Used to treat hypovolemia
  - Expand the ECF volume
  - Used in cardiopulmonary resuscitation
  - No swelling or shrinking of cells occurs with the introduction of isotonic fluid into the body.
    - 0.9% dextrose in NS
    - LR solution
    - D_5W
  - Large amounts of D_5W may cause hyperglycemia.
  - Administration of excess isotonic fluid can result in hypervolemia.
  - Isotonic fluids can cause hyperchloremic acidosis.
  - NS is the only fluid recommended to be administered with blood and blood products.
- Hypotonic fluid
  - Contains fewer solutes than blood.
  - Has an osmolality less than 240 mOsm/kg.
  - Provides free water, sodium, and chloride.
  - Is used to treat hypertonic dehydration.
  - May be administered to clients with gastric fluid loss.
  - Causes water to move from the intravascular space into the cell.
  - Cells swell when exposed to hypotonic fluid.
    - Can cause vascular depletion, affect the cardiac system, and increase in intracranial pressure.
    - Is contraindicated in clients with head injury, stroke, signs of increased intracranial pressure, or neurosurgery.
    - Caution should be used when administering this type of solution to clients with third-spacing issues. Hypotonic fluids are not the first choice for clients with third-spacing.
      - D_5 ½NS
- Hypertonic fluid
  - Contains more solutes than blood
  - Used to increase ECF volume and decrease swelling of the cells
  - Has an osmolality greater than 340 mOsm/kg
  - Causes water to move from the cell into the intravascular space
  - Cells shrink when exposed to hypertonic fluids.
  - Hypertonic fluid must be administered slowly.
  - Clients receiving hypertonic fluids should be closely monitored for pulmonary edema and fluid volume overload.
  - Examples: 10% dextrose in water ($D_{10}W$); 3% saline
  - Used only in critical situations to treat severe hyponatremia
  - 5% dextrose in NS (D_5NS)
  - Fluids with high concentrations of dextrose, such as 50%, and with extremely high tonicity must be administered through a central vein.

- Total parenteral nutrition (TPN)
  - Highly concentrated hypertonic solution administered to nutritionally compromised clients through a central venous line
  - Recommended for clients who are unable to sustain normal nutritional intake for a period of time
  - Client's receiving TPN should be weighed daily and frequently assessed for complications.
  - Serum glucose levels should be closely monitored.
  - Contains electrolytes, vitamins, and minerals.
  - Amino acids and lipids may be added to TPN solutions.
  - TPN mixtures can be customized to meet the client's nutritional needs.
  - Lipid emulsions to supply calories and fatty acids may be administered.
  - TPN must be infused through a central vein.
  - TPN must be infused using tubing with a filter.
  - Bags of TPN must be changed a minimum of every 24 hours.
  - Serum laboratory values must be closely monitored in clients receiving TPN.
  - Clients should be weaned off TPN, but infusion should not be suddenly discontinued.
  - Complications of TPN: infection; anaphylactic reactions; electrolyte imbalances; alterations in serum pH levels; pulmonary edema; heart failure; hyperglycemia; refeeding syndrome
- Delivery methods of IV fluids
  - Selection of the delivery method depends on the client's age, diagnosis, duration of therapy, condition of veins, purpose, and health history.
  - Central or peripheral veins may be used.
  - Peripheral lines
    - Used for short-term therapy
    - May be placed in the arm, hand, foot, or leg
    - Risk of complications when using the legs and feet of adults
    - Basilic, cephalic, or metacarpal veins used most often
  - Antecubital site
    - May be used to gain fast venous access in emergencies
    - The antecubital site is not recommended for mobile clients because of movement and distal occlusion of the IV line.
  - Guidelines
    - Veins of the head, neck, and lower extremities may be used in children and infants.
    - Avoid using veins over joints for catheter placement.
    - Avoid placing IV catheters in the feet of children able to ambulate.
    - Best practice is to place IV catheter in the hand or lower forearm and move upward as needed.
    - Avoid placing IV catheters where an injury is present or where there is a history of injury. IV catheters should not be placed in the same side as a mastectomy, lumpectomy, or the side affected by a stroke.
    - IV catheters should not be placed on or near the site of arteriovenous fistulas placed in the arm for dialysis.
  - Central lines
    - May be used for clients with inadequate peripheral veins
    - Inserted in a central vein
    - More commonly placed in the intrajugular or subclavian vein
    - Occasionally placed in the femoral vein

- Primary care providers may choose to place a central line if the client requires large volumes of fluid, TPN, nutritional supplementation, or frequent blood sampling.
- Central venous access devices
  - Central venous catheter
    - Used for short-term therapy
    - Usually placed by a surgeon or certified primary care provider
    - Provides several lumens using a single insertion site
  - Peripherally inserted central catheter (PICC)
    - Can be inserted by a certified nurse
    - Inserted using the antecubital, cephalic, basilic, or brachial vein and threaded to the subclavian vein
    - Fewer side effects than traditional central lines
    - Used for caustic antibiotics and chemotherapy
    - Can be used for several months
    - Vascular access port
      - Implanted underneath the skin of the chest
      - Used for long-term therapy
      - Accessed with a specially designed needle

Types of Intravenous Catheters

- Regular plastic catheters
  - More commonly used with central venous infusions
  - Longer than other catheters
  - Inserted through a hollow needle
- Indwelling catheters
  - More comfortable for client
  - Easily inserted over a steel needle
  - Decreased chance of infiltration
- Steel-winged infusion catheters
  - Easy insertion
  - Small, nonflexible
  - Usually reserved for clients with small or inadequate veins when other catheter insertions have failed
  - Used for short-term therapy
  - Infiltration is common.

Intravenous Administration and Associated Complications

- IV administration
  - Verify order for IV therapy.
  - Check the label of the IV solution for correct formulation and expiration date.
  - Collect supplies, including the selection of an appropriate IV cannula or catheter, and inspect carefully.
  - Cannula size should be suitable for both site, purpose, and duration of infusion.
  - The smallest gauge and length necessary to deliver prescribed therapy should be chosen.
  - Prepare the equipment by connecting the infusion bag and tubing.
  - Prime the tubing to displace air by allowing the solution to flow to the end of the tubing.
  - Replace the cap on the end of the tubing, maintaining sterility of the tubing.
  - Carry all supplies, IV tubing, IV infusion pump, and fluid to the client's room.

- Identify the client using two identifiers per agency policy.
- Check for allergies.
- Clients should be carefully screened for allergies to iodine, latex, adhesives, skin solutions and adhesives, and medications to reduce the risk of an allergic reaction.
- Explain the procedure to the client.
- Perform hand hygiene to prevent infection.
- Wear gloves to prevent exposure to blood and body fluids.
- Nonlatex gloves should be worn if the client has an allergy to latex.
- Identify a vein for insertion, and apply a tourniquet or BP cuff 4 to 6 inches above the chosen site for IV catheter insertion to distend the veins and allow visualization.
- Use of the distal veins of the forearm is recommended first to maintain patency of the proximal veins.
- Veins of the feet and lower extremities should be avoided due to the risk of thrombophlebitis. Follow agency policy when choosing appropriate IV sites.
- Raise the bed to a comfortable working height and position for the nurse.
- Position the client's arm below heart level to encourage capillary filling.
- Palpate for a pulse distal to the tourniquet.
- The client may be asked to open and close the fist several times or to position the arm in a dependent position to distend a vein.
- Warm packs can be applied for 10 to 20 minutes prior to venipuncture to promote vasodilation.
- The tourniquet should never be tight enough to occlude arterial flow. If a radial pulse cannot be palpated distal to the tourniquet, then it is too tight.
- Prepare the site by following agency protocol. Most recommend cleaning the insertion site with alcohol, chlorhexidine gluconate, or povidone-iodine swabs for 2 to 3 minutes in a circular motion and moving outward from the intended site of insertion.
- Nurses must practice and find an IV insertion technique that works for the individual nurse and client. The following are recommended steps:
    - Using the nondominant hand, hold the client's arm and use the finger or thumb to pull the skin taut over the vein to stabilize the vessel.
    - With the dominant hand, hold the needle bevel up and at 5- to 25-degree angle, depending on the depth of the vein; pierce the skin to reach but not penetrate the vein.
    - Decrease the angle of needle further until nearly parallel with the skin, then enter the vein either directly above or parallel to the vein.
    - If there is no flashback of blood in the catheter or if the attempt fails, the IV catheter should not be reinserted because of risk of damage to the catheter.
    - If backflow of blood is visible, straighten the angle and advance the needle slightly to ensure the catheter has entered the vein.
    - The next steps depend on the type of IV catheter used. Follow the manufacturer instructions.
        - Hold the needle hub, and slide the catheter over the needle into the vein.
        - Remove the needle while applying slight pressure on the skin over the catheter tip to the hub in place.
        - Release the tourniquet, and attach the IV tubing.
        - Open the clamp on the tubing to allow the fluid to drip.
        - Cover the insertion site, following agency protocol, with a transparent dressing or sterile gauze.
        - Use tape to secure the IV catheter and anchor the tubing.
        - Label the IV site with the type and length of the cannula, date, time, and initials.

- How to calculate IV flow rate
  - IV fluid must be given at a specific rate.
  - Administering fluids too slow can affect the rate of medication absorption.
  - Administering fluids too fast can cause adverse effects, including medication reactions and fluid volume overload.
  - Rates can be measured as milliliters per hour (mL/hr), liters per hour (L/hr), or drops per minute (gtt/min).
  - To control or adjust the flow rate, only drops per minute are used.
  - Each IV tubing package contains a plastic drip chamber that controls the drops per minute.
  - The packaging indicates the number of drops per milliliter (the drop factor). A number of different drop factors are available and are determined by the length and diameter of the needle.
- Common drop factors
  - 10 drops/mL (blood set)
  - 15 drops /mL (regular set)
  - 60 drops /mL (microdrop)
  - To measure the rate, the nurse must know the number of drops and the time in minutes.
- Flow rate formula

$$\frac{\text{Volume (mL)} \times \text{drop factor (gtt/mL)}}{\text{time (in minutes)}} = \text{gtt/min (flow rate)}$$

  - Example: 1200 mL IV NS is ordered over 12 hours. Using a drop factor of 60 drops/mL, how many drops per minute need to be delivered?

$$\frac{1200\,(\text{mL}) \times 60\,(\text{gtt/mL})}{12 \times 60\,(\text{total minutes})} = 100\,\text{gtt/min}$$

- Mechanical factors affecting flow rate
  - IV infusion pumps force fluid into the veins. Pumps allow medications and fluids to flow into the vein despite the height of the fluid bag. Pumps are designed to prevent complications by sounding alarms to notify the nurse of infusion problems.
  - Size of the IV cannula can limit the infusion rate. Large-bore cannulas are able to deliver more viscous fluids at a higher rate of flow. Small-bore cannulas are designed for less viscous fluids with smaller maximum infusion rates.
  - Without a pump, the IV infusion is dependent on gravity; the bag of IV fluid should be placed above the level of the client's heart.
  - The more distal from the heart, the slower the infusion rate will be.
  - IV catheters placed in the hands and arms may cause intermittent interruptions in infusion due to mobility, bending, and occlusion of the catheter.
  - IV catheters may push against the walls or valves in a vein, impeding the flow of the IV fluid.
  - Central lines placed in the subclavian vein can handle higher infusion rates than IVs in the peripheral veins.
  - Disease processes such as heart failure and renal failure limit the amount of fluid the client can safely receive.
  - Some medications have restrictions on the time frames they can be safely administered to avoid adverse effects.
- Adjusting flow rate
  - For a manual IV setup (no pump), measure the rate by counting the number of drops that fall in the drip chamber each minute (gtt/min).

- Opening and closing the roller clamp on the IV tubing and counting the drops per minute in the drip chamber can adjust the flow rate accordingly.
- For an IV setup on a pump or other electronic infusion devices, enter the flow rate measured in milliliters per hour following the manufacturer instructions. The device is able to calculate and deliver the necessary drops per minute.
- To adjust the flow rate on an IV pump, follow the manufacturer instructions for programming the flow rate into the machine.
- Complications of IV therapy
  - Infection
    - Bacteria in the infusion set, administration set, IV start kit, or around the site of IV insertion can cause infection.
    - Widespread systemic infection can start with an IV-related infection.
  - Phlebitis
    - Is defined as inflammation of the vein.
    - May be classified as bacterial, mechanical, or chemical phlebitis.
      - Chemical phlebitis is caused by medication incompatibility, rapid infusion of solutions, or highly irritating medications.
      - Mechanical phlebitis results from IV catheters being in the vein for long periods, catheters in joint or bending area of the body, poorly anchored IV catheters, and too large IV catheters.
      - Bacterial phlebitis can develop from poor aseptic technique and the failure to intervene with early signs of phlebitis.
  - Thrombophlebitis
    - Is defined as the formation of a blood clot within the vein accompanied by inflammation.
    - A blood clot blocks a vein.
  - Infiltration
    - IV fluid leaks from a vein into the surrounding tissues.
    - Is caused by IV migrating outside of a vein.
  - Extravasation
    - Medications leak into the surrounding tissues, causing blistering and necrosis of the tissue.
    - More often, infiltration is caused by vasopressors, calcium, chemotherapy drugs, and potassium.
  - Allergic reaction
    - Allergic reactions to catheters, latex, fluids, or medications can develop.
    - Stop the IV, and notify the primary care provider if the client develops streaking (a red line near the site of the IV), itching, shortness of breath, or wheezing.
    - Be prepared to administer oxygen and to follow agency protocol for managing anaphylaxis.
  - Air embolism
    - Is a rare complication of IV therapy.
    - Is most often associated with central line placement.
    - Air embolism can be prevented from occurring by completely priming the IV tubing and using an electronic infusion pump with the capability of detecting air in the line.
    - Locking adapters should be used on all IV lines and catheters.
  - Hematoma
    - Develops when blood leaks into the tissues surrounding the IV insertion site.
    - Clients with bleeding disorders or on antiplatelet therapy are at an increased risk for developing hematomas.

- Fluid volume overload
  - Develops if IV fluids are administered too fast or if the client has circulatory or cardiac issues that prevent the body from managing the fluid.
  - An infusion pump should be used to decrease the likelihood of developing fluid volume overload.
  - Clients with liver, cardiac, or renal disease should be carefully monitored for symptoms of fluid volume overload.
  - Older adult clients are at an increased risk of developing fluid volume overload.
  - Heart failure and pulmonary edema can result from fluid volume overload.
- Symptoms of IV complications
  - Infection: elevated temperature, often with an abrupt onset after infusion starts; backache; headache; respiratory rate; increased heart rate; nausea and vomiting; chills; tenderness at site of insertion; induration around site of insertion; IV with a sluggish flow; drainage at the site of catheter insertion; redness; warmth; hard feeling around the site of insertion
  - Phlebitis: warmth and redness; fever
  - Thrombophlebitis: coolness at the site; edema around the insertion site; pain at the insertion site; leaking around the catheter; no blood return; sluggish flow
  - Infiltration: burning or pain at the IV site; lack of blood return in IV; edema at the site with blanching
  - Extravasation: burning and stinging pain; redness, blistering, tissue necrosis, and ulceration
  - Allergic reaction: heart palpitations; drop in BP; increased heart rate; pain in chest, back, and/or shoulders; difficulty breathing; wheezing; jugular vein distention; altered mental status
    - If left untreated, an allergic reaction can progress to increased intracranial pressure, coma, and death.
  - Air embolism: difficulty breathing; respiratory failure; chest pain; heart failure; muscle and joint pain; stroke; confusion, loss of consciousness; bradycardia; cyanosis
  - Hematoma: swelling occurs immediately during IV catheter insertion; ecchymosis; blood oozing from insertion site
  - Fluid volume overload: edema; weight gain; neck-vein dissention; increased BP; increased respiratory rate; dyspnea; crackles in lung fields; cough

APPLICATION AND REVIEW

17. Which nursing intervention should the nurse consider as being uniquely appropriate for a client diagnosed with water intoxication?
    1. Strictly monitor the intake and output of fluids.
    2. Obtain and document daily weight.
    3. Monitor for the development of edema.
    4. Frequently perform neurological assessments.
18. Which is the common drop factor for a blood delivery set?
    1. 5 gtt/mL
    2. 10 gtt/mL
    3. 15 gtt/mL
    4. 60 gtt/mL
19. Which condition is the cause of an extravasation?
    1. Clogged vein
    2. Inflammation of the vein
    3. Allergic response to latex
    4. Medication leaking into the surrounding tissue

See Answers on pages 62–64.

Nursing Care of the Client With Intravenous Therapy

- Nursing care
  - Assessment
    - Frequently assess IV site per facility policy.
    - Assess for skin blanching, erythema, and edema.
    - Assess skin temperature.
    - Check for leaking at the IV site.
    - Assess the presence of pain at the IV site.
    - Assess the extremity that has the IV for circulation.
    - Check for the signs and symptoms of an allergic reaction, including itching and rash.
    - Assess all clients receiving IV fluids for symptoms of fluid volume overload.
  - Diagnostic factors
    - Depend on the type of IV complication encountered
    - Blood cultures
    - Radiographic images
- Magnetic resonance imaging
  - Goals of care
    - To identify the underlying cause of the IV complication
    - To maintain client comfort and safety
  - Treatment
    - Infection
      - Notify the primary care provider.
      - Remove the IV catheter.
      - Obtain cultures from the IV site.
      - Monitor the vital signs.
    - Phlebitis
      - Apply warm soaks.
    - Thrombophlebitis
      - Discontinue the IV.
      - Apply a cold compress, followed by a warm compress.
      - Elevate the extremity.
      - Restart the IV in the opposite extremity.
      - Avoid flushing the IV line if a clot is suspected.
      - Obtain cultures of the catheter and the insertion site.
      - Anticoagulant medications may be prescribed to dissolve a clot.
    - Infiltration
      - Prevent infiltration by using a small catheter.
      - Avoid placing catheters over the joints.
      - Use tape to anchor the IV catheters to prevent pulling and dangling that can dislodge the catheter from the vein.
      - Immediately stop the infusion at signs of infiltration.
      - Remove the IV catheter.
      - Elevate the affected extremity.
      - Apply warm soaks to the site of infiltration (if not contraindicated).
      - Restart a new IV on the opposite extremity, if at all possible.
    - Extravasation
      - Prevent extravasation by carefully reading medication labels for the possibility of necrosis.

- Follow agency policies when administering IV medications.
- Frequently check for blood return when administering highly potent medications.
- Be prepared to administer antidotes for toxic medications.
- Notify the primary care provider if infiltration occurs since infiltration can lead to extravasation.
- Immediately notify the primary care provider if signs of extravasation are detected.
- Assess capillary refill, pulses, color and neurological function of affected extremity.
- Elevate the extremity; apply ice, followed by warm soaks.

■ Allergic reaction
- Stop the IV.
- Administer antihistamines and antiinflammatory medications, as ordered.
- Administer oxygen.
- Elevate the head of the bead.
- Apply cool compresses to the irritated skin.

■ Air embolism
- An air embolism is a medical emergency.
- Clamp the IV tubing.
- Place the client on the left side in the Trendelenburg position.
- It is recommended to place the client on the left side to disperse the air to the right atrium.
- Administer oxygen.
- Notify the primary care provider.

■ Hematoma
- Remove the needle and/or cannula.
- Apply gentle pressure with sterile gauze.
- Cover with a dry dressing.
- Ice may be applied for the first 24 hours.
- Elevate the extremity.
- Assess for neurological function and circulatory function of extremity.

■ Fluid volume overload
- Slow the rate of fluid to a keep the vein open rate between 20 and 30 mL/hr.
- Monitor vital signs.
- Elevate the head of the bed to the high Fowler position.
- Administer oxygen.
- Assess breath sounds.
- Immediately notify the primary care provider.
- Administer diuretics as ordered.

- Prevention of IV complications
  - The nurse should perform thorough hand hygiene before touching the client or any component of the IV.
  - Strict aseptic technique should be used when starting an IV.
  - IV components should be assessed for the expiration date and any signs of contamination.
  - IV solutions should be checked for expiration dates and any signs of cloudiness or contamination before administering the IV solution to the client.
  - IV cannulas should be anchored with tape or a catheter stabilization device to prevent excessive movement at the insertion site.

- Administration sets with a twist-lock design help decrease infection.
- The IV site should be frequently assessed.
- Contaminated dressings at or around the insertion sites should be cleaned and replaced.
- 2% tincture of iodine, 10% povidone-iodine, alcohol, or chlorhexidine gluconate can be used to clean around the IV site.
- All IV ports should be cleaned with alcohol or an agency-approved antimicrobial solution before and after each access.
- IVs should be removed immediately if signs and symptoms of infection are discovered at the site.
- Change the IV sites tubing and solution as per recommended agency policy.
- All medications and medication bags should be discarded after 24 hours from the time of infusion.
- Filters should be placed at the proximal end of the IV tubing for any fluid requiring a filter.
- Nurses should always follow the guidelines of the Nurse Practice Act and agency policy when performing venipuncture and administering IV fluid and medication therapy.
- Verify the order from the primary care provider for IV insertion, medication, and fluids.
- Clarify any incomplete orders for IV therapy or medications.
- Evaluate the client for site placement, considering the history, mobility status, condition of veins, and estimated duration of the IV therapy.
- Document the time, date, size, and location of the IV catheter inserted. Note the appearance of the site after insertion.
- Document client teaching and understanding of IV therapy. Teaching should include activity restrictions and/or expectations during infusions, signs and symptoms of complications, and how to report changes.
- Infuse IV fluids with a pump or volume control device to prevent fluid volume overload, especially for pediatric clients.
- Frequently monitor the IV site.
- Assess the IV for signs of complications at regular intervals.
- Follow agency policy for changing IV tubing, catheters, and performing dressing changes.
- Regularly document the type and amount of fluid infusing and the client's response to therapy.
- Assess intake and output of fluids, and obtain daily weights.
- Always assess compatibility of medications and fluids being administered using the same IV tubing and/or catheter; solutes and crystallization can form if the fluids and medications are incompatible.
- Nurses should educate clients in the home setting regarding the care of IVs.
- A licensed nurse may supervise home infusion therapies.
- Provide written instructions.
- Perform a demonstration.
- Allow for the return demonstration, if possible.
- Educate the client and caregiver regarding needed laboratory specimens.
- Teach the client and caregiver to report any side effects of infusion.
- Teach the client and caregiver to identify and report any signs of IV complications, including infiltration, fluid volume overload, and phlebitis, among others.
- The nurse should perform a thorough assessment of the client, IV site, and infusion equipment with each visit.

APPLICATION AND REVIEW

20. Which interventions should the nurse implement when it is been confirmed that a client is experiencing thrombophlebitis at an IV access site? *(Select all that apply.)*
    1. Elevate the extremity.
    2. Initially apply warm compresses.
    3. Obtain a culture of the insertion site.
    4. Culture the catheter tip.
    5. Flush the line before its removal.

See Answer on pages 62–64.

ANSWER KEY: REVIEW QUESTIONS

1. **1 Insensible fluid loss cannot be accurately measured and comes from sources that include sweat and the process of respiration.**

   2, 3, 4 Stools, urine, and emesis are examples of measurable fluid loss referred to as sensible loss.
   Client Need: Physiological Integrity; **Cognitive Level:** Analysis; **Nursing Process:** Implementation

2. **1 An arterial line is inserted into an artery to allow for continuous BP monitoring while providing access for arterial blood samples.**

   2 A central venous catheter is inserted and positioned in the superior vena cava; it is not generally used to access blood samples. **3** The pulmonary artery catheter is positioned just inside the pulmonary artery; it is not generally used to access blood samples. **4** An electronic sphygmomanometer is an external device to access BP on an intermittent basis. It does not allow for blood samples to be accessed.
   Client Need: Physiological Integrity; **Cognitive Level:** Understanding; **Integrated Process:** Teaching and Learning

3. **4 Dehydration is a deficit of fluid volume or a loss of water from the body's cells (intracellular).**

   1 Hypovolemia can occur when fluids and solutes are lost from the extracellular space. **2** Hypovolemia can occur when the output of fluid exceeds the intake of fluid. **3** The decreased circulating fluid volume noted with hypovolemia can also develop from third-space fluid shifts.
   Client Need: Physiological Integrity; **Cognitive Level:** Understanding; **Integrated Process:** Teaching and Learning

4. **2 Isotonic dehydration is generally caused by either vomiting and/or diarrhea. The emesis basin is appropriate for measuring and containing vomitus.**

   1 Although a client may be fatigued because of dehydration, assistance with care is not focused on a direct symptom of the dehydration process; rather, its focus is the outcome of the dehydration. **3** Dry skin is a sign of fluid volume deficit; lotion would have little effect on the cause of the problem. **4** Isotonic dehydration does not involve a loss of sodium.
   Client Need: Physiological Integrity; **Cognitive Level:** Applying; **Nursing Process:** Planning

5. **3 A compound fracture of the femur places the 14-year-old client at risk for active bleeding and is therefore the greatest risk for fluid volume deficit.**

   1 Although a fever is a cause of fluid loss, the amount of loss associated with a low-grade fever does not present the risk associated with bleeding. **2** Although ill-managed diuretic therapy can result in a fluid volume deficit, this situation does not present the risk that active bleeding creates. **4** Although an NG tube can cause a fluid volume deficit, this situation does not present the risk that active bleeding creates.
   Client Need: Physiological Integrity; **Cognitive Level:** Analysis; **Nursing Process:** Assessment

6. **3 Capillary refill is dependent on blood volume and circulation; these factors are compromised when the client is experiencing hypovolemia.**

   1, 2, 4 Tachycardia, thirst, and dry mucous membranes are associated with both dehydration and hypovolemia.
   Client Need: Physiological Integrity; **Cognitive Level:** Application; **Nursing Process:** Assessment

7. **2 A decrease in serum hematocrit is consistent with blood loss and the resulting hypovolemia.**

   1 An increase in serum osmolality is noted. **3** An increase in serum sodium is associated with dehydration. **4** An increase in urine-specific gravity is noted.

   Client Need: Physiological Integrity; **Cognitive Level:** Analysis; **Nursing Process:** Assessment

8. **1 D_5W is a hypotonic solution that will draw water into the dehydrated cells.**

   2, 3, 4 NS, D_5 ½ NS, and LR solution are all isotonic solutions that will stay in the vascular system and reverse the hypovolemic condition.

   Client Need: Physical Integrity; **Cognitive Level:** Applying; **Nursing Process:** Evaluation

9. **3 Hypovolemic shock occurs when at least 40% of the vascular volume is lost.**

   1, 2 Although serious, 20% to 30% blood loss is not generally a trigger for hypovolemic shock. **4** 50% blood is 10% more than sufficient blood loss to trigger hypovolemic shock.

   Client Need: Physiological Integrity; **Cognitive Level:** Knowing; **Integrated Process:** Learning and Teaching

10. **3 Tachycardia is associated with the heart's attempt to improve circulation that is impaired by hypovolemic shock. 5 Cyanosis is an outcome of impaired circulation of oxygenated blood that is a result of hypovolemic shock.**

    1 Severe hypotension is associated with hypovolemic shock. **2** Urinary output below 10 mL/hr is associated with hypovolemic shock. **4** Postsurgical delirium is not associated with hypovolemic shock.

    Client Need: Physiological Integrity; **Cognitive Level:** Analysis; **Nursing Process:** Evaluation

11. **2 Hypovolemic shock is triggered by a fluid loss, often in the form of hemorrhage. Appropriately replacing the fluids is vital, and IV access is critical to accomplishing this goal.**

    1 Although appropriate and necessary for the evaluation of treatment, monitoring laboratory results is not directed toward correcting the initial problem of hypovolemia. **3** Although appropriate and necessary for the assessment of the client and for the evaluation of treatment, observing for signs of complications is not directed toward correcting the initial problem of hypovolemia. **4** Although appropriate and necessary for the assessment of the client and for the evaluation of treatment, monitoring mental status changes is not directed toward correcting the initial problem of hypovolemia.

    Client Need: Physiological Integrity; **Cognitive Level:** Analysis; **Nursing Process:** Planning

12. **3 The priority preventive intervention regarding a fluid volume deficit is to regularly and sufficiently hydrate the client.**

    1 Although appropriate, monitoring the client's BP and pulse rate allows for early detection, not the prevention, of a fluid deficit. **2** Although appropriate, recognizing the early signs and symptoms of flu allows for early treatment, not prevention, of a fluid deficit. **4** Although appropriate, taking medications as prescribed does not have the same affect as a client being sufficiently hydrated to prevent a fluid deficit.

    Client Need: Health Promotion and Maintenance; **Cognitive Level:** Analysis; **Integrated Process:** Teaching and Learning

13. **Answers: 1, 3, 5**

    1 Hypervolemia is an increase in the amount of isotonic fluid in the ECF compartments. **3** An excess of isotonic fluid in the ECF compartments causes the body to compensate by adjusting the levels of ANP, ADH, and aldosterone. **5** Compensatory mechanisms can become overwhelmed in hypervolemia, resulting in excess fluid being pushed from the vessels into the interstitial spaces, which causes edema in the tissues.

    2 Sodium levels usually remain normal because of the accompaniment of water in the ECF compartments. **4** The compensatory mechanism causes the kidneys to release excess sodium and water from the body.

    Client Need: Physiological Integrity; **Cognitive Level:** Understanding; **Integrated Process:** Teaching and Learning

14. **Answers: 1, 2, 4, 5**

    Causes of third-spacing include situations that cause fluid to move out of the intravascular space into the interstitial tissue or open cavities such as peritonitis, liver failure, heart failure, and burns.

    3 Increased intracranial pressure is an outcome associated with water intoxication.

    Client Need: Physiological Integrity; **Cognitive Level:** Understanding; **Integrated Process:** Teaching and Learning

15. **Answers: 1, 2, 4**

    Assessment data typical of hypervolemia include hypertension, distended jugular veins, and auscultation of S_3.

    3 A productive cough with pink, frothy sputum is characteristic of hypervolemia. **5** A rapid, bounding pulse is characteristic of hypervolemia.

    Client Need: Physiological Integrity; **Cognitive Level:** Applying; **Nursing Process:** Assessment

16. **1 Because of the shifting of fluids into the interstitial spaces, decreased urine output, despite adequate fluid intake, is an early sign of third-spacing.**

    2, 3, 4 Personality changes, pupil changes, and irritability are all signs of water intoxication.

    Client Need: Physiological Integrity; **Cognitive Level:** Applying; **Nursing Process:** Assessment

17. **4 With the association of increased intracranial pressure, frequent neurological assessment is uniquely important to the care of a client experiencing water intoxication.**

    1, 2 Strict monitoring of intake and output of fluids, as well as monitoring and documenting daily weights, are equally important to both the management of hypervolemia and water intoxication. **3** Edema is an outcome associated with hypervolemia, not water intoxication.

    Client Need: Physiological Integrity; **Cognitive Level:** Applying; **Nursing Process:** Planning

18. **2 The drop factor for a typical blood delivery set is 10 gtt/mL.**

    1 5 gtt/mL is not a common drop factor for any IV blood delivery set. **3** 15 gtt/mL is the drop factor for a regular delivery set. **4** The drop factor for a microdrop set is 60 gtt/mL.

    Client Need: Physiological Integrity; **Cognitive Level:** Understanding; **Integrated Process:** Teaching and Learning

19. **4 An extravasation is damage caused by the medication leaking into the surrounding tissue.**

    1 A clogged vein results in thrombophlebitis. **2** Phlebitis is inflammation of the vein. **3** An allergic reaction results from a sensitivity to latex.

    Client Need: Physiological Integrity; **Cognitive Level:** Understanding; **Integrated Process:** Teaching and Learning

20. **Answer: 1, 3, 4**

    Appropriate nursing interventions when a client develops a thrombophlebitis at an IV site include elevating the extremity to help manage the edema and obtaining cultures of the insertion site and of the catheter tip to determine appropriate antibiotic therapy.

    2 Cold therapy should be initiated first, followed by warm compresses. **5** The IV line should not be flushed until it is determined that there is no clot.

    Client Need: Physiological Integrity; **Cognitive Level:** Analysis; **Nursing Process:** Planning

Concepts of Acid-Base Balance 4

ACID-BASE BALANCE OVERVIEW

Hydrogen Ion Concentration

- The chemical symbol representing hydrogen ion is H^+.
  - Hydrogen has an atomic weight of 1.
  - Hydrogen is not only the smallest ion, but its concentration in body fluids is very small in relation to other elements.
- Hydrogen plays an important role in promoting the production of adenosine triphosphate (ATP).
  - The proton's electrical charge is critical and matters more than the concentration of the ion.
- Body fluids are described and compared based on the proportion of hydrogen ion present, .e pH level, the proportion of hydrogen ions in the body that needs to remain in a specific ge, and the concentration of hydrogen in body fluids, which is very small.
- Rising concentration of hydrogen
  - Binds to compounds (proteins)
  - Changes charge, shape, and function
  - The bicarbonate (HCO_3^-) buffer system is the removal process for hydroge
    - Low partial pressure of carbon dioxide ($PaCO_2$) has hydrogen react w HCO_3^-.
    - High hydrogen stimulates breathing, resulting in low $PaCO_2$.

Acids and Bases

- An acid is a mixture of two or more elements that can give up a hy gen ion.
  - Acids can give up hydrogen ions when dispersed into water (H   ).
- A base is a mixture of two or more elements that can accept a b rogen ion.
  - Bases can accept hydrogen ions when dispersed into H_2O.
- The pH is affected by acids and bases by influencing hydroge on production and elimination.
- Buffer is a substance that can act as a base or an acid.
- Minor changes in the pH of body fluids can cause majo roblems. (Figure 4.1)
- Normal serum pH levels
  - Arterial blood: between 7.35 and 7.45
  - Venous blood: between 7.32 and 7.42
  - Normal blood pH: between 7.35 and 7.45
    - A lower pH level and acidosis occur attr atable to excess hydrogen ions.
    - A higher pH level and alkalosis occ attributable to a decreased concentration of hydrogen ions.
  - The body maintains hemostasis, de te acids being added through the metabolism of ingested foods and fluids.
  - Acid and bases are continually be g added to maintain pH balance.
- Small changes in the pH level can srupt many physiological functions: hormones; electrolytes; electrical impulses of the heart; gastrointestinal functioning.
- Increased pH levels (increased alkalinity or a decrease of hydrogen ion concentration) can be caused by pneumonia, dehydration, infection, and renal diseases.

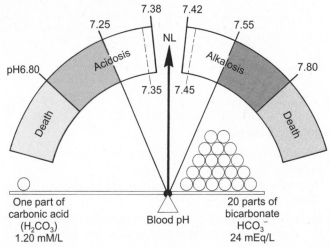

FIGURE 4.1   Normal blood pH is 7.40 ± 0.02 (one standard deviation [SD]) or ± 0.05 (two SDs). Acid-base balance occurs when the ratio of bicarbonate (HCO_3^-) to carbonic acid (H_2CO_3) is 20:1. Any change in this ratio tips the balance and swings the pointer to the acidosis or alkalosis side. pH levels below 7.25 and above 7.55 are both life threatening, and the extremes of 6.8 or 7.8 cause death. (From Price, S. A., & Wilson, L. M. [2012]. *Pathophysiology: Clinical concepts of disease processes*, [6th ed.]. St. Louis: Mosby–Elsevier.)

- Decreased pH levels (increased acidity or an increase of hydrogen ion concentration) can be caused by overhydration, heart failure, and medications (thiazide loop diuretics, digitalis, insulin, antibiotics, chemotherapy).
- Critical (fatal) serum pH levels are less than 6.9 or more than 7.8. With increases in hydrogen ions, the pH level decreases.

APPLICATION AND REVIEW

1. Which ion plays an important role in the body's ability to produce the component needed to create ATP?
   1. Carbonic acid (H_2CO_3)
   2. HCO_3^-
   3. Carbon dioxide (CO_2)
   4. Hydrogen
2. What reaction should the nurse expect in a client experiencing an increased concentration of hydrogen?
   1. Increased $PaCO_2$
   2. Increased respiratory rate
   3. Hydrogen will lose its positive electrical charge.
   4. Blood pH level will be between 7.35 and 7.45.
3. What characteristic is uniquely observed in a buffer substance?
   1. It is created by ingested foods and fluids.
   2. It can function as either a base or an acid.
   3. It is comprised of two elements that give up an hydrogen ion.
   4. Its normal blood pH level is between 7.35 and 7.45.

4. A client's pH is 7.35. What action should the nurse take to minimize client risk?
   1. Assess for renal failure.
   2. Monitor cardiac rate and rhythm.
   3. Educate the client on the importance of iron supplements.
   4. Implement standard precautions to manage infection risks.
5. What intervention should the nurse implement when noting a client's pH is 7.46?
   1. Review the client's prescription for a loop diuretic.
   2. Monitor the rate of the client's intravenous (IV) fluids.
   3. Assess the client's blood pressure.
   4. Assess the client's temperature.

See Answers on pages 84–86.

Defense Mechanisms

- Three lines of defense provide hemostasis of the body's pH level to maintain a normal hydrogen ion concentration.
  - Buffer system: responds immediately (in seconds) to minimize large changes in the hydrogen ion concentration
  - Respiratory system: responds within minutes after a substantial change in the hydrogen ion concentration
  - Renal system: is the most powerful at maintaining stability with acid-base balance, and responds in over hours to days to restabilize the hydrogen ion concentration after a sudden shift

Buffer System

- The buffer system is analogous to a chemical sponge.
  - Excess hydrogen ions are absorbed.
  - Needed hydrogen ions are released.
- The by-products of regular metabolism produce acids.
  - In the breakdown of glucose, CO_2 is released and eliminated by exhalation from the lungs.
  - The metabolism of fats yields fatty acids and keto acids.
  - The metabolism of proteins yields sulfuric acid.
  - The anaerobic metabolism of glucose yields lactic acid.
  - Destruction of cells results in the liberation of intracellular acids into the extracellular fluid (ECF).
- Substances that accept hydrogen ions are potential sources of bases: sodium hydroxide (NaOH); ammonia (NH_3); aluminum hydroxide ($Al[OH]_3$); HCO_3^-.
- The ECF has a narrow range for pH. There are three body-regulating mechanisms: chemical buffers, respiration, and the kidneys.
- Chemical buffers are constantly present in body fluids and therefore are the first line of defense.
  - Four primary buffer systems in the body help stabilize the pH: the HCO_3^- (H_2CO_3) system, phosphate system, protein system, and hemoglobin system.
- HCO_3^- is found in intracellular fluids (ICFs) and ECFs.
  - Controls small changes in the pH
  - Responds immediately to changes in the pH
  - Administered intravenously in cases of emergencies

- Unique because each of the two elements can be regulated
    - CO_2 content is adjusted by the respiratory system.
    - HCO_3^- ion content is adjusted by the renal system.
  - HCO_3^- (H_2CO_3) is the most important buffer system in the body.
- Phosphate buffers are located in the ICF, similar to HCO_3^-, and respond quickly to changes in the pH.
- Proteins are located in the ICF as hemoglobin and in the ECF as albumin and globulins and also rapidly respond to fluctuations in the pH.
- The HCO_3^- (H_2CO_3) system (also called the carbonate system) is comprised of a mixture of H_2CO_3 and sodium bicarbonate ($NaHCO_3$), with both in the same solution.
- H_2CO_3 is an extremely weak acid. In solution, H_2CO_3 separates into CO_2 and H_2O.
- Hydrolysis of HCO_3^- in a solution yields
  - Hydroxyl ion
  - Increase in alkalinity in the solution
  - Ratio of H_2CO_3 to base HCO_3^-: 1:20 to maintain a normal pH between 7.35 and 7.45
  - Small amounts of potassium HCO_3^-, calcium HCO_3^-, and magnesium HCO_3^- in the body
- Primary buffer system in the human body is the carbonate system.
- When hydrochloric acid (HCl), a strong acid, is added to a solution with $NaHCO_3$, the reaction is $HCl + NaHCO_3 \rightarrow NaHCO_3 + H_2O$.
  - Hydroxyl ion of the NaOH combines with the hydrogen ion from the H_2CO_3 to form H_2O and $NaHCO_3$.
  - $NaHCO_3$ is a weak base.
  - Adding a strong base to a buffer solution, the pH will increase only slightly.

Respiratory System

- The second line of defense in changes in the pH are respiratory mechanisms.
  - CO_2 is constantly formed in the body through intracellular metabolic processes.
    - Carbon in foods is oxidized to form CO_2.
    - CO_2 moves out of the cells and into interstitial fluids and then into intravascular fluids.
    - CO_2 is transported to the lungs, diffuses into alveoli, and is exhaled.
  - CO_2 responds to acute and sudden changes in the pH when chemical buffers can no longer restore pH levels to normal.
  - $PaCO_2$ has a direct association with pH.
    - In the arterial blood, catalyzed by carbonic anhydrase, CO_2 reacts with H_2O to form H_2CO_3.
    - The H_2CO_3 rapidly separates into a hydrogen ion and an HCO_3^- ion.
    - When the respiratory rate increases, the CO_2 levels decrease.
    - When the respiratory rate decreases, the CO_2 levels increase.
    - When the rate of metabolic CO_2 formation is increased, the concentration in the ECF also increases.
  - The breathing mechanism is controlled by unique receptors in the brain and to changes in CO_2 levels.
  - Clients with chronic obstructive pulmonary disease (COPD) who receive too much oxygen show a decreased respiratory rate, resulting in the retention of CO_2, which can lead to acidosis.
  - If the respiratory rate is decreased, the amount of CO_2 in the ECF will increase.

- The respiratory system acts as in two ways to control the hydrogen ion concentration.
  - The feedback system responds to the hydrogen ion concentration.
    - Hydrogen ion concentration increases (acidosis) in the ECF.
      - The respiratory system increases in rate and depth.
      - Additional CO_2 is exhaled.
    - Changes in respiratory rate can transform the hydrogen concentration in the body fluids.
      - CO_2 concentration in the ECF decreases.
      - With additional CO_2 removed, less is available to mix with H_2O to form H_2CO_3.
      - Less H_2CO_3 is formed when less CO_2 is available.
      - The pH does not lower as it would if more H_2CO_3 were available in the ECF.
  - The respiratory system that regulates the hydrogen ion concentration works at 50% to 75% efficiency.
    - If the pH drops quickly from 7.4 to 7.0, the respiratory system can restore it to 7.2 to 7.3 in approximately 1 minute.
    - Initially, as the hydrogen ion concentration approaches a normal range, the stimulus to the respiratory system ceases.
    - The chemical buffering system will finish restoring the pH to normal levels.

APPLICATION AND REVIEW

6. Which defense mechanism will respond most quickly to a significant change in body pH?
   1. Cardiovascular system
   2. Respiratory system
   3. Buffer system
   4. Renal system
7. Which buffering system is considered the most important to the stabilization of the pH?
   1. HCO_3^- (H_2CO_3) system
   2. Phosphate system
   3. Protein system
   4. Hemoglobin system
8. Which buffer system is found in both the ICF and the ECF in a single form?
   1. HCO_3^-
   2. Phosphate
   3. Proteins
   4. Hemoglobin
9. The brain controls breathing in response to what trigger?
   1. Increase in respiratory rate
   2. Changes in the CO_2 levels
   3. Action of one of the buffer systems
   4. Increase of hydrogen ions in the ECF
10. What response should the nurse expect when a patient who is diagnosed with COPD receives a high rate of supplemental oxygen?
    1. Decrease in respiratory rate
    2. Development of respiratory alkalosis
    3. Normalization of respiratory rate and depth
    4. Release of CO_2 ions from the vascular system

See Answers on pages 84–86.

Renal System

- The third line of defense against fluctuations in the pH is the renal mechanisms.
  - Most powerful regulating system for acid-base balance
  - Longer process to restore acid-base balance
  - The renal system controls the pH by excreting different amounts of acid or base.

- Three primary renal mechanisms for compensating for imbalances with acid-base balance: tubular kidney movement of HCO_3^-; kidney tubule formation of acids; formation of ammonium (NH_4^+) from amino acid catabolism
- In normal metabolism, the body has an abundance of extra acids.
  - To maintain balance, the kidneys excrete more hydrogen ions in the urine.
  - Urine is normally acidic.
- HCO_3^- is made in other areas of the body, such as in the pancreas or kidneys.
  - HCO_3^- can move from the kidneys back into the blood when blood hydrogen ions are high.
  - HCO_3^- can be excreted from the kidneys into the urine when blood hydrogen ions are low.
    - When HCO_3^- ions are excreted, the urine becomes more alkaline.
  - When HCO_3^- is reabsorbed back into the blood
    - The kidneys have an excess of negatively charged ion-phosphate.
    - Due to this negative charge
      - Hydrogen ions are drawn into the urine to combine with dihydrogen phosphate (H_2PO_4) to produce an acid termed phosphoric acid (H_3PO_4).
      - Ion-phosphate is excreted in the urine.
    - Normal breakdown of amino acids produces NH_3.
      - Normal amino acids associate with hydrogen ions to form NH_4^+.
      - NH_4^+ is excreted in urine.
      - The net loss of hydrogen ions results in an increase in blood pH.
- Unlike the respiratory system, the renal system continues to react until the extracellular pH is normal.
  - Older adults have less nephrons in the kidneys.
  - Response time to the renal system may be extended.
    - Younger adults require 6 to 10 hours to achieve acid-base balance.
    - Older adults (or anyone with fewer nephrons) may require 18 to 48 hours to achieve acid-base balance.
- The respiratory system that maintains acid-base balance is approximately 50% to 75% efficient.
- The renal system can partially or completely neutralize the excess acid or alkali in body fluids.
- Through returning and excreting substances from body fluids, the renal system can compensate for hours from deviations from normal concentrations of acid or base.
  - When the pH or ECF lowers, the renal system eliminates more hydrogen or ions to return to a balance.
  - When the pH or ECF rises, renal system eliminates more HCO_3^- ions to return to a balance.

Summary of Regulatory Systems for Acid-Base Balance

- Chemical mechanisms: protein buffers; extracellular (albumin, globulins); intracellular (hemoglobin)
  - Chemical buffers: extracellular (HCO_3^-); intracellular (phosphate, HCO_3^-)
  - Action: very rapid; immediately responds to changes in acid-base conditions; manages small fluctuations in hydrogen ion production and elimination under normal metabolic and health conditions
- Respiratory mechanisms
  - Increased hydrogen ions: assist when fluctuations of hydrogen ion concentration are acute
  - Increased CO_2: stimulates central respiratory neurons; increases respiratory rate and depth; results in a loss of CO_2 and hydrogen ion concentration

- Decreased hydrogen ions and CO_2: inhibits central respiratory neurons; decreases respiratory rate and depth; results in the retention of CO_2; increases in hydrogen ion concentration
- Renal mechanisms
  - Mechanism to decrease the pH: increases renal excretion of HCO_3^-; increases renal reabsorption of hydrogen ions
  - Mechanism to increase pH: decreases renal excretion of HCO_3^-; decreases renal reabsorption of hydrogen ions
  - Action: most powerful regulator of acid-base balance; responds to large or chronic changes in hydrogen ion production or elimination; requires more time than other systems but is more efficient

Acidosis

- Acidosis is a result of a surplus of hydrogen ions.
  - Arterial pH less than 7.35
- Surplus of hydrogen ions
  - Excess of acids releases hydrogen ions.
  - Reduction in the elimination of acids results in the retention of hydrogen ions.
- Positively charged hydrogen ions are in abundance.
  - Results in an imbalance of other electrolytes, specifically, the other positive ion electrolytes: potassium; calcium; sodium
  - Can lead to disturbances in function of the following systems: cardiac; central nervous; neuromuscular; respiratory
- Acidotic pH results from a cascade of events.
  - Incomplete exchange of oxygen and CO_2
  - Retention of CO_2
  - Excess CO_2 forms H_2CO_3
  - H_2CO_3 splits into two ions: hydrogen ions; HCO_3^-
  - Chemical formula of changes that result in acidotic pH
    - $H_2O + CO_2 + H_2CO_3 \rightarrow H^+ + HCO_3^-$
    - Free hydrogen ions in the blood result in acidosis.
  - Causative or contributory factors for acidosis: respiratory depression; poisoning; cerebral edema; myasthenia gravis; obesity; asthma; cancer; thrombus; pneumonia; tuberculosis; adult respiratory distress syndrome (ARDS); emphysema; cystic fibrosis; spinal cord injuries

Respiratory Acidosis

- Any clinical situation (acute or chronic) that interferes with the following:
  - Respiratory functions
    - Ventilation
    - Perfusion
    - Pulmonary gas exchange
  - Retention of CO_2
    - Increases blood H_2CO_3
    - Results in respiratory acidosis
  - Disruption of normal balance of H_2CO_3 and base HCO_3^-
    - CO_2 is retained.
      - H_2CO_3 in the ECF is increased.
      - The pH level drops below the normal range.

- Kidneys attempt to compensate.
  - Retain HCO_3^- (base) to try to increase the pH level
  - Excrete hydrogen ions
- If the body's regulatory system is able to maintain balance, the acidosis will be compensated (corrected).
- Clients with chronic lung disease have chronic respiratory acidosis.
  - In chronic conditions, the kidneys have time to compensate for acidosis.
  - In acute conditions, the kidneys do not have the time to compensate for acidosis, which usually takes hours or days to compensate for the imbalance.
    - Therefore medical intervention is required if the imbalance is not corrected by the regulatory mechanisms of the body.
- Treatment of respiratory acidosis requires identifying the type—acute or chronic.
  - Correct the acidity.
    - Medical intervention includes the administration of IV medication with HCO_3^-.
    - Administer sodium lactate.
      - Lactate oxidizes to H_2CO_3.
      - Sodium reacts with H_2CO_3 to form $NaHCO_3$.
- Airway obstruction caused by lung cancer or other tumors, poor gas exchange in the capillaries, or retention of CO_2 and resulting acidosis
- Capillary diffusion interference
  - Lowers gas exchange between the alveoli and capillary membranes in the lung
  - CO_2 builds up and is retained.
  - Poor chest expansion results in poor gas exchange and the retention of CO_2 (emphysema).
- Respiratory depression
  - Causes include chemical or physical mechanisms.
  - Brainstem stimulation can affect inhalation and exhalation.
    - Causes insufficient exchange of oxygen and CO_2.
- Respiratory conditions can decrease chest expansion and increase the risk for respiratory acidosis: emphysema; ankylosing spondylitis; pleural effusion; pneumothorax; pneumonia.
- Nursing considerations
  - Assess for airway obstruction: foreign body; lymph node enlargement; tight clothing; constriction of bronchioles; asthma; emphysema; lung cancer; excess mucus production
  - Assess for conditions related to poor alveolar-capillary diffusion: aspiration of fluids; emphysema; ARDS; COPD; lung cancer; tuberculosis; pulmonary embolism; pulmonary edema; chest trauma
  - Assess for poor chest expansion: respiratory muscle weakness; trauma
  - Assess for chest deformities: broken ribs; flail chest; muscular dystrophy; rhabdomyosarcoma; ascites; hemothorax; severe obesity; abdominal tumors
  - Assess for chemical causes of respiratory depression: anesthetics; opioids; poisons
  - Assess for electrolyte imbalances: hyponatremia; hyperkalemia; hypercalcemia
- Nursing assessment by systems for the causes of acidosis
  - Cardiovascular system: bradycardia; tall T wave on electrocardiogram (ECG); widened QRS complex on ECG; prolonged PR interval on ECG; hypotension; thready peripheral pulses
  - Central nervous system (CNS): confusion; lethargy; stupor; coma
  - Neuromuscular system: bilateral flaccid paralysis; hyporeflexia; weakness
  - Respiratory system: abnormal rate; abnormal intensity; Kussmaul respirations; Cheyne-Stokes respirations; apnea followed by deep breaths

- Integumentary (skin) system: dry; flushed; pale; warm; cyanotic
- Psychosocial-related causes: any change in behavior; recent uncooperative behavior; unable to recognize family or other individuals
- Nursing assessment for the physical causes of respiratory depression
  - Head or spinal cord trauma
  - Cerebral edema
  - Cerebral aneurysm
  - Cerebrovascular accident
  - Overhydration
  - Arterial blood gases (ABGs): pH less than 7.35; CO_2 concentration greater than 45 mm Hg
  - Monitor respirations every hour: rate; depth; pattern
- Additional nursing assessments
  - Monitor serum electrolytes daily: sodium; potassium; calcium.
  - Provide pulmonary toilet or hygiene.
    - Use physical therapy.
    - Increase respiratory diffusion.
    - Decrease airway obstruction.
  - Administer medications that raise alveolar-capillary diffusion: metaproterenol sulfate (Alupent); albuterol sulfate (Ventolin); salmeterol xinafoate (Serevent); pirbuterol acetate (Maxair)
  - Administer the following as prescribed: oxygen therapy; chemotherapy; radiation therapy
  - Administer bronchial smooth muscle relaxants medications: albuterol sulfate (Ventolin); ephedrine (Akovaz); isoproterenol (Isuprel); terbutaline (Bronclyn); atropine (Atropine); aminophylline (Phyllocontin); theophylline (Elixophyllin)
  - Administer bronchial mucolytic medications to dilute secretions.
    - Acetylcysteine sodium: Mucomyst; Mucosil

Metabolic Acidosis

- pH level lower than 7.35
- Loss of HCO_3^- from the ECF or accumulation of acids
- Excess acid and a deficit in base are the causes of metabolic acidosis.
  - Overproduction of hydrogen ions: carbon monoxide poisoning; diabetic ketoacido starvation; fever; hypoxia; ethanol ingestion; salicylate toxicity; sepsis
  - Failure to eliminate hydrogen ions: renal failure
  - Underproduction of HCO_3^- ions: renal failure; pancreatitis; liver failure; dehydra n; uremia
  - Elimination of HCO_3^- ions: diarrhea; vomiting
- The acidotic pH is a result of excessive breakdown of fatty acids, associated with ex ive exercising, seizures, and a hypermetabolic state (lactic acidosis attributable to diabeti to-acidosis and starvation).
- Forty percent of newly diagnosed children with insulin-dependent diabetes mellitus (DM) have metabolic acidosis.
- Two causes of metabolic acidosis: lack of HCO_3^- and excessive acid production by th ody
- Metabolic acidosis can occur after the ingestion of substances that are very acidic in ture.
  - ethyl alcohol
  - methyl alcohol poisoning
  - acetylsalicylic acid (aspirin) toxicity

- Renal failure can result in metabolic acidosis.
  - Renal tubules cannot transport the hydrogen ions in the urine.
  - Results in an accumulation of hydrogen ions
  - HCO_3^- is produced in the kidney tubules and pancreas.
    - Diseases of the kidneys result in an HCO_3^- deficit.
    - Normal production of hydrogen ions leads to an excess accumulation.
- Vomiting or diarrhea can result in an excess elimination of HCO_3^-.
  - pH levels are within normal limits.
  - Excess is proportional to HCO_3^-.
- Nursing assessments
  - Skin turgor for dehydration
  - Alcohol or aspirin ingestion
  - Serum creatinine to assess renal function
  - Serum amylase to assess for pancreatitis or pancreatic cancer
  - ABG for pH <7.35; HCO_3^- level <24 mEq/L
  - History of seizures, heavy exercise, starvation, and diarrhea
  - Temperature every 4 hours for fever
  - IV hydration to treat dehydration
  - Monitoring of ECG and serum potassium levels
    - Potassium can become elevated as hydrogen ions move into the cells and displace potassium.
  - Metabolic acidosis is considered a medical emergency.
    - Presentation of metabolic disorders are not as apparent as respiratory disorders.
    - Nurses have to be aware of clients at high risk for metabolic acidosis and make appropriate assessments.
  - Medications to address acidosis
    - Often with metabolic acidosis, the ECF volume deficit needs to be corrected with parenteral fluids.
    - Insulin levels should be assessed if acidosis is due to diabetic ketoacidosis.
      - Carbohydrates and insulin must be supplied.
    - Antidiarrheal medications and rehydration therapy are needed to treat diarrhea.
    - Antiemetic medications and rehydration therapy are needed to treat diarrhea.
    - IV solutions of HCO_3^- or lactate are needed to support base HCO_3^-.
      - Administer IV HCO_3^- if venous plasma HCO_3^- level is <20 mmol/L (mEq/L) or the arterial level is <20 mmol/L (mEq/L).
    - Fluid replacement and dialysis are needed for clients with renal failure.

Alkalosis

- Alkalosis results from an excess of base (principally HCO_3^-) in the ECF.
  - Increased pH level >7.45
- Alkalosis is caused by respiratory or metabolic conditions or both.
- Clinical signs and symptoms are similar, regardless of whether the cause of alkalosis is metabolic or respiratory in nature.
- The primary side effect of alkalosis on the body is overstimulation of the CNS.
  - The CNS and peripheral nervous system are affected, but alkalosis often first starts with the peripheral nerves.
  - Muscles go into tetany (tonic spasm).
  - Other symptoms are nervousness and convulsions.
  - Alkalosis can impact the respiratory muscles and cause death.

- HCO_3^- is usually the cause for an overproduction of base or the lack of clearance.
- Treatment of alkalosis is to manage the underlying condition(s).
- Systems affected by alkalosis: central nervous; cardiovascular; muscular
- Symptoms of alkalosis are related to hypocalcemia and hypokalemia.

Respiratory Alkalosis

- Excessive reduction of CO_2 through accelerated respirations (hyperventilation)
  - Results from a lack of H_2CO_3.
  - Decrease in $PaCO_2$ results in an increase in pH.
    - Alkalosis results
  - With excessive amounts of CO_2 exhaled, the H_2CO_3 decreases in the ECF.
- Incidence of respiratory alkalosis is not as prevalent as respiratory acidosis.
- If the body's regulatory mechanisms are inadequate to correct the imbalance, the underlying causes are treated.
  - For fever, use antipyretic medications.
  - Treat anxiety with sedatives.
  - For hyperventilation, ask the client to breathe into a paper bag to rebreathe exhaled CO_2.
  - The settings on the mechanical ventilator are improper.
  - The CNS develops tumors or lesions.
  - Medications can be an underlying cause: progesterone; aspirin; catecholamine (e.g., isoproterenol, epinephrine)
- Goal is to treat the respiratory alkalosis by increasing the amount of CO_2 in the body.

Metabolic Alkalosis

- Causes of metabolic alkalosis
  - Ingestion of large amounts of $NaHCO_3$ or the loss of acid through vomiting or gastric suctioning
    - Loss of hydrogen ions (occurring with hypokalemia) as the kidneys attempt to conserve potassium and excrete acids
  - Increase in base excess or decrease in acid components (acid deficit)
  - Causes of excess base: ingestion of HCO_3^-; acetates; citrate; lactates from oral antibiotics (HCO_3^- intake); blood transfusion (citrate intake); total parenteral nutrition (TPN); hyperalimentation lactate intake; treatment of diabetic ketoacidosis or lactic acidosis (IV administration of HCO_3^-)
- Causes of a lowering of acid components: prolonged vomiting; nasogastric (NG) suctioning; Cushing syndrome (hypercortisolism); hyperaldosteronism; adrenal tumor; sepsis; postoperative status; overhydration with IV fluids (lactated Ringer solution); hypoproteinemia; licorice ingestion
  - Medications
    - Thiazide
    - Diuretics
      - Especially thiazide and loop diuretics result in a potassium, chloride, and hydrogen loss
      - Loss of hydrogen ions occurs with hypokalemia.
      - Kidneys conserve potassium and excrete acids.
    - Steroids
    - High-dose carbenicillin and penicillin
- Symptoms related to the cardiovascular system: tachycardia; hypovolemia; hypotension; hypokalemia; potential for digitalis toxicity (myocardium becomes more sensitive to digitalis and an alkalosis state)

- Symptoms related to the CNS: agitation; confusion; lightheadedness; tingling of mouth and toes (paresthesias); seizures; hyperreflexia
- Symptoms related to the musculoskeletal system: cramps; muscle spasms in the legs; continuous spasms (tetany); decrease in hand strength; loss of ability to stand and support body weight
- Metabolic and respiratory alkalosis; the serum pH lowers as the body attempts to regain electroneutrality
  - Metabolic acidosis: pH <7.35; HCO_3^- <24 mEq/L
  - Respiratory acidosis: pH <7.35; $PaCO_2$ >45 mm Hg
  - Metabolic alkalosis: pH >7.45; HCO_3^- >28 mEq/L
  - Respiratory alkalosis: pH >7.45; $PaCO_2$ <35 mm Hg
- Assessments
  - pH of ABGs
    - Metabolic or respiratory alkalosis: pH >7.45
    - Metabolic alkalosis: higher HCO_3^- level (>29 mEq/L)
    - Respiratory alkalosis: lower HCO_3^- level (<22 mEq/L)
  - Assess serum hypocalcemia <8.5 mg/dL and positive Chvostek-Weiss and Trousseau signs.
    - Positive Chvostek-Weiss sign: The front of the tragus and facial muscles contract when pressure is applied.
    - Positive Trousseau sign: If the inflated blood pressure cuff is greater than the systolic pressure and is held for 1 to 4 minutes, the client's hands and fingers spasm with palmar flexion.
    - Conduct a daily review for hypokalemia by serum blood levels <3.5 mEq/L.
  - Assess for weakness using touch, push and pull, and grasps.
  - Assess for elevated heart rate and decreased blood pressure, which are signs of alkalosis.
  - Assess for an elevated respiratory rate in respiratory alkalosis or metabolic acidosis.
  - Assess serum digoxin levels for potential toxicity. Toxicity level is a value greater than 2.4 ng/mL.
  - Assess for hyperreflexia with a reflex hammer at the patella tendon.
  - Administer fluids and electrolytes (orally or IV) as prescribed.
  - Administer an antiemetic medication to alleviate nausea and vomiting.

Summary of Acid-Base Imbalances (Table 4.1)

- Respiratory acidosis (excess H_2CO_3)
  - Causes: chronic lung disease; surgery; airway obstruction; pneumonia
  - Compensation mechanism: buffer system; renal system (more hydrogen ions are excreted)
- Respiratory alkalosis (H_2CO_3 deficit)
  - Causes: increased pulmonary ventilation; encephalitis; hypoxia; fever; salicylate poisoning; asthma; anxiety
  - Compensation mechanism: buffer system; renal system (excrete more HCO_3^-)
- Metabolic acidosis (base deficit)
  - Causes: diabetic ketoacidosis; uremic acidosis; diarrhea; starvation; renal failure
  - Compensation mechanism: buffer system; respiratory system (rapid and deep breathing); renal system (excrete more hydrogen; retain more HCO_3^-)
- Metabolic alkalosis (base excess)
  - Causes: excessive ingestion of base (acids); vomiting; gastric suctioning; excess aldosterone; steroids; diuretics
  - Compensation mechanism: buffer system; respiratory system; slow and shallow breathing; renal system (retain more hydrogen; excrete more HCO_3^-)

TABLE 4.1	Simple Acid-Base Disorders			
			BICARBONATE–CARBONIC ACID RATIO	
Acid-Base Disorder	**Cause**	**20:1**	**Compensation**	
Respiratory acidosis	Hypoventilation (retained carbon dioxide [CO_2])	Ratio <20:1	Renal: Retention of HCO_3^-; excretion of acid salts; increased ammonia (NH_3) formation	
Respiratory alkalosis	Hyperventilation (excessive loss of CO_2)	Ratio >20:1	Renal: Excretion of HCO_3^-; retention of acid salts; decreased NH_3 formation	
Metabolic acidosis	Retention of fixed acids Loss of base bicarbonate (HCO_3^-)	Ratio <20:1	Lungs: Hyperventilation Renal: As in respiratory acidosis	
Metabolic alkalosis	Loss of fixed acids Gain of base HCO_3^- Potassium (K^+) depletion	Ratio >20:1	Lungs: Hypoventilation Renal: As in respiratory alkalosis	

From Price S. A., & Wilson, L. M. (2012). *Pathophysiology: Clinical concepts of disease processes*, (6th ed.). St. Louis: Mosby–Elsevier.

NORMAL BLOOD GASES

Adults

- ABGs have similar normal values in children and adults. However, the values in infants are slightly lower.
  - Newborn ABG values are lower than the values in a child or adult.
  - Older adults have a normal partial pressure of arterial oxygen (PaO_2); it is lower than that of a child or younger adult.
- Arterial blood
  - Acid-base (pH): between 7.35 and 7.45
    - Key indicator to detect acidosis or alkalosis
  - $PaCO_2$: between 35 and 45 mm Hg
    - Measurement of adequate ventilation and respiratory portion of acid-base imbalance
    - H_2CO_3 cannot be directly measured in a hospital laboratory. H_2CO_3 concentration is proportional to the $PaCO_2$, which can be evaluated.
    - Average arterial $PaCO_2$ is 40 mm Hg; the average venous $PaCO_2$ is 46 mm Hg.
    - If $PaCO_2$ is elevated, then more CO_2 is being retained. A high $PaCO_2$ indicates respiratory acidosis.
    - If $PaCO_2$ is lower, then more CO_2 is being exhaled.
    - $PaCO_2$ with respiratory acidosis will be above normal.
  - HCO_3^-: between 22 and 26 mEq/L
    - Measurement of the metabolic assistance to acid-base deviations (metabolic acidosis)
    - Calculated from pH and $PaCO_2$
  - Base excess: between -2 and $+2$
    - Indication of a deviation of HCO_3^- concentration from the normal range
    - Base excess compares the actual HCO_3^- level with the normal level. Results range between -2 and $+2$.
    - A low value indicates acidosis, and a high value indicates alkalosis.

- Po$_2$ at sea level: between 80 and 100 mm Hg
  - Demonstrates pressure that causes oxyhemoglobin binding
  - Dependent on barometric pressure
- Saturation of hemoglobin with oxygen (SaO$_2$): between 96% and 98%
  - Reflects differences of oxyhemoglobin
  - Measured or calculated from PaCO$_2$, pH, and body temperature
- Concentration of hemoglobin in serum: 15 g/dL
  - Identifies the changes of gas transport attributable to anemia
- Mixed venous blood
  - Acid-base (pH): between 7.33 and 7.43
    - Detection of acidosis or alkalosis
  - PaCO$_2$: between 41 and 57 mm Hg
    - Measurement of adequate ventilation and respiratory portion of acid-base imbalance
  - HCO$_3^-$: between 24 and 28 mEq/L
    - Measurement of metabolic assistance to acid-base deviations (metabolic acidosis)
    - Calculated from pH and PaCO$_2$
  - Base excess: between 0 and +4
    - Indication of deviation of HCO$_3^-$ concentration from the normal range
  - Po$_2$ at sea level: between 35 and 40 mm Hg
    - Demonstrates pressure that causes oxyhemoglobin binding
    - Dependent on barometric pressure
  - SaO$_2$: between 70% and 75%
    - Reflection of the differences of oxyhemoglobin
    - Measured or calculated from PaCO$_2$, pH, and body temperature
  - Concentration of hemoglobin in serum: 15 g/dL
    - Identification of the changes of gas transport attributable to anemia
  - For clients who are critically ill and/or undergoing cardiac catheterization, obtaining arterial blood samples may not be possible.
  - Mixed venous blood gas analysis in association with arterial analysis is a good indicator of adequacy of tissue oxygenation and cardiac output (Table 4.2).

Older Adults (Geriatric Population)

- Changes in the physiological structures of the pulmonary system can affect diagnostic laboratory tests.
- Age-associated changes can be identified in results of ABGs, pulse oximetry, and pulmonary function studies.
- Age-appropriate norms need to be incorporated into the interpretation of diagnostic tests.
- Pulmonary aging reduces vital capacity and expiratory flow rates, and it lowers the PaO$_2$.
- PaO$_2$ declines with age (up to age 75 years and then increases).
  - Mean PaO$_2$ for adults older than 75 years is approximately 83 to 85 mm Hg.
  - Although PaO$_2$ lowers with aging, tissue profusion is adequate.
- Multiple factors can account for the changes in laboratory values for older adults.
  - Diet
  - Exercise
  - Multisystem diseases
  - Physiological and structural age-related changes
  - There is a ±2 standard deviation (CD) in the normal laboratory test based on healthy individuals.

TABLE 4.2	Arterial Blood Parameters Used for the Analysis of Acid-Base Status	
Parameter	**Normal Value**	**Definition and Implications**

Partial pressure of arterial oxygen (PaO$_2$)	80–100 mm Hg	PaO$_2$ in arterial blood decreases with age.
		In adults <60 years of age:
		  60–80 mm Hg: mild hypoxemia
		  40–60 mm Hg: moderate hypoxemia
		  <40 mm Hg: severe hypoxemia

pH	7.40 (±0.05); two standard deviations (SDs)
	7.40 (±0.05); one SD
		Identifies whether there is acidemia or alkalemia; the value using two SDs from the mean is the common clinical value
		  pH <7.35: acidosis
		  pH >7.45: alkalosis

Hydrogen (H$^+$)	40 (±2) nmol/L or mEq/L	The hydrogen ion concentration may be used instead of the pH.
Partial pressure of arterial carbon dioxide (PaCO$_2$)	40 (±5.0) mm Hg	PaCO$_2$ <35 mm Hg: respiratory alkalosis >45 mm Hg: respiratory acidosis
Carbon dioxide (CO$_2$) content	25.5 (±4.5) mEq/L	Is the classic method of estimating bicarbonate (HCO$_3^-$) Measures HCO$_3^-$ plus dissolved CO$_2$ The latter is generally quite small except in respiratory acidosis.
Standard HCO$_3^-$	24 (±2) mEq/L	HCO$_3^-$ concentration is estimated after fully oxygenated arterial blood has been equilibrated with CO$_2$ at a PaCO$_2$ of 40 mm Hg at 38° C, which eliminates the influence of respiration on the plasma HCO$_3^-$ concentration.

Base excess	0 (±2) mEq/L	Reflects a pure metabolic component
		Base excess = 1.2 × deviation from 0.
		  Metabolic acidosis: negative
		  Metabolic alkalosis: positive
		Is misleading in respiratory and mixed acid-base disturbances.
		Is not essential for the interpretation of acid-base disturbances.

Anion gap	12 (±4) mEq/L	Anion gap (or delta) reflects the difference between the unmeasured cations (potassium, magnesium, calcium) and unmeasured anions (albumin, organic anions, hydrogen phosphate, sulfate). Is useful in identifying types of metabolic acidosis A value of >16–20 indicates that acidosis is caused by the retention of organic acids as in diabetic ketoacidosis.

From Price S. A., & Wilson, L. M. (2012). *Pathophysiology: Clinical concepts of disease processes*, (6th ed.). St. Louis: Mosby–Elsevier.

- In the interpretation of ABG results, abnormal values do not necessarily confirm a disease or disorder.

Newborns

- Newborns and young infants have small arteries and spontaneously move, making an arterial puncture a difficult procedure.
  - Arterial damage is possible.
  - Arterial blood in infants does not necessarily reflect a resting state. Infants often cry during venipuncture. Changes during the venipuncture procedure can result in respiratory changes.
    - Hyperventilation
    - Holding breath and cessation of breathing

- Both modifications in ventilation patterns can change the values for oxygen, CO_2, and pH in the infant's blood.
- For newborns, placement of an umbilical arterial catheter provides ABG samples without any alterations.
- For older infants, capillary puncture is used to reduce the risks and technical expertise associated with ABG samples.
- Capillary samples are primarily obtained from the heel, but the fingers and earlobes can also be used.
- To obtain the best results to ensure the capillary sample closely resembles ABG levels, the sample must be obtained from a warm extremity.
  - Unreliable values will be obtained if the extremity for the sample is edematous, acrocyanotic, or not sufficiently warm because of poor peripheral circulation.
- Normal values for ABGs in infants at room air
  - pH
    - Newborn: 7.25 to 7.35
    - Age 24 hours: 7.30 to 7.40
    - Age 2 days to 1 month: 7.32 to 7.43
    - Age 1 month to 2 years: 7.34 to 7.46
  - PaO_2
    - Newborn: 50 to 70 mm Hg
    - Age 24 hours: 60 to 80 mm Hg
    - Age 2 days to 1 month: 85 to 95 mm Hg
    - Age 1 month to 2 years: 85 to 105 mm Hg
  - $PaCO_2$
    - Newborn: 26 to 40 mm Hg
    - Age 24 hours: 26 to 40 mm Hg
    - Age 2 days to 1 month: 30 to 40 mm Hg
    - Age 1 month to 2 years: 30 to 45 mm Hg
  - HCO_3^-
    - Newborn: 17 to 23 mEq/L
    - Age 24 hours: 18 to 25 mEq/L
    - Age 2 days to 1 month: 16 to 25 mEq/L
    - Age 1 month to 2 years: 20 to 28 mEq/L
  - Base excess
    - Newborn: -10 to -2 mEq/L
    - Age 24 hours: -4 to $+2$ mEq/L
    - Age 2 days to 1 month: -6 to $+1$ mEq/L
    - Age 1 month to 2 years: -4 to $+2$ mEq/L

Respiratory Origin

- Review the laboratory values, and identify an imbalance; then determine the origin of the imbalance.
- Respiratory in origin
  - Respiratory acidosis
    - If the cause is respiratory, the individual's $PaCO_2$ will be abnormal.
    - Elevated $PaCO_2$ indicates the client is retaining CO_2.
    - Decreased respiratory rate and depth will cause an increase in blood level of H_2CO_3.
    - Respiratory acidosis occurs when the pH is low and the $PaCO_2$ is high.

- Respiratory alkalosis
  - Lower $PaCO_2$ indicates the client is exhaling too much CO_2, which causes hyperventilation.
  - In respiratory alkalosis, the pH is high and the $PaCO_2$ is low.
- Treatment
  - Correct the underlying respiratory issue.
    - Lower respiratory rate
      - Oxygen therapy (nasal cannula, rebreathing mask, ventilator) depends on the severity of the imbalance.
      - Treat the underlying causes for the respiratory issue: oxygen therapy Ventilation; medications
    - Higher respiratory rate
      - Client needs to rebreathe his or her own exhaled CO_2.
      - Client can use a large paper bag or inhalation of 5% CO_2 at intervals.
  - Respiratory acidosis
    - Elevated $PaCO_2$ has to be gradually lowered.
    - Mechanical ventilation can be used.
    - Adequate ventilation is the primary treatment for the resolution of respiratory acidosis.
  - Respiratory alkalosis
    - Levels of CO_2 are increasing.
  - Oxygen therapy to clients with chronic respiratory issues (e.g., chronic retention of CO_2) should be administered titrated to achieve optimal levels for the individual clients and to achieve oxygen saturation of 88% to 92%.
  - Respiratory acidosis intervention is to increase the respiratory rate, conserve HCO_3^- ions, and excrete hydrogen ions.
  - Respiratory alkalosis intervention is to reduce the amount of CO_2 exhaled, and excrete HCO_3^- ions and conserve hydrogen ions.

Metabolic Origin

- Acid-base imbalance that is metabolic in origin will cause changes in the HCO_3^- levels.
- Metabolic in origin
  - Metabolic acidosis
    - Lower pH level at <7.35
    - Abnormal HCO_3^- level
  - Metabolic alkalosis
    - Elevated pH level at >7.45
    - Abnormal HCO_3^- level
- Metabolic acidosis
  - In mild metabolic acidosis, the client may be asymptomatic.
  - Metabolic acidosis often results from a decrease in alkali reserve.
  - Loss of HCO_3^- is from the gastrointestinal tract, kidneys, or an overproduction of acid.
  - Symptoms: general malaise; dull headache; nausea and vomiting; possible abdominal discomfort
    - With progression of acidosis (increase severity), changes in the mental state occur.
- Metabolic alkalosis
  - Results from excess base HCO_3^-
    - Can result from excessive base ingested or given parentally
    - Loss from the body through vomiting or suctioning

- Symptoms
  - CNS stimulation: paresthesias (abnormal sensations, numbness, prickling); restlessness; confusion; tetany
- Unlike the respiratory acid-base balances, metabolic HCO_3^- gains or losses are not directly visible but are exhibited through other body systems.
  - Abnormal ABGs
  - Alterations in client's CNS reactions
  - Activation of acid-base compensatory mechanisms
    - The respiratory system is the first to react.
    - Change in respiratory rate may be due to a physiological response to metabolic acidosis.
- In respiratory imbalances, the HCO_3^- level is normal.
  - Altered respiratory rate is not necessarily an indication of a respiratory imbalance.
    - ABG results for a client with a metabolic imbalance will demonstrate an abnormal HCO_3^- level.
    - A lower pH stimulates the respiratory system to exhale more CO_2 to reduce the H_2CO_3 level.
    - In metabolic acidosis, the client will have respirations that are deep and rapid.
- When compensation occurs in metabolic acidosis, the pH rises somewhat but stays below normal.
  - The $PaCO_2$ falls, attributable to hyperventilation.
  - Kidneys conserve HCO_3^- ions.
    - HCO_3^- ions rise toward normal.
    - CO_2 content also rises to normal.
  - In partial compensated metabolic acidosis, the pH, HCO_3^-, and CO_2 return to near normal levels but remain slightly below normal.

Anion Gap

- Not all ions are ordinarily measured.
  - The sum of the measured cations will be greater than the sum of anions.
  - Anion gap is the difference between cation and anion measurements.
  - Evaluation of the anion gap can assist in determining the type of metabolic acidosis.
- If the anion gap is elevated
  - Acidosis is likely due to organic acids, such as lactate and ketoacids.
  - Anion gap recognizes that there are anions in the body that are not ordinarily measured.
- Treatment
  - Correct the cause of the metabolic acidosis.
    - In severe acidosis, administer IV fluids to correct the base HCO_3^- deficit.
    - Alkalinizing solutions, such as $NaHCO_3$ or lactate-containing solutions, can be parenterally administered.
    - Complications of therapy may be hypernatremia (excess sodium) and fluid volume overload.
  - Correct the cause of the metabolic alkalosis.
    - Replace lost acid in the form of fluid or medication-containing chloride.
    - If the metabolic alkalosis is caused by vomiting, potassium levels may be lower and may need to be replaced.

APPLICATION AND REVIEW

11. On which area of instruction should a nurse focus when educating a group of older adults on the possible factors that can affect their diagnostic laboratory values? *(Select all that apply.)*
    1. Diet
    2. Exercise
    3. Presence of cognitive decline
    4. Acceptable SDs
    5. Presence of multiple chronic disorders

12. What will be the likely source for a diagnostic sample on a 24-hour-old infant needing evaluation of arterial blood?
    1. Umbilical arterial catheter
    2. ABG sample
    3. Capillary blood from the finger
    4. Capillary blood from the earlobe

13. Which newborn is demonstrating normal ABG values at birth? *(Select all that apply.)*
    1. pH: 7.28
    2. $PaCO_2$: 61 mm Hg
    3. HCO_3^-: 20 mEq/L
    4. PaO_2: 30 mm Hg
    5. $PaCO_2$: 22 mm Hg

14. A client is demonstrating the classic signs of respiratory alkalosis including tachypnea. What intervention should the nurse **initially** implement?
    1. Secure IV access.
    2. Prepare for assisted ventilation.
    3. Administer supplemental oxygen.
    4. Support the client in rebreathing methods.

15. The nurse should be concerned when a client diagnosed with COPD has what oxygen saturation? *(Select all that apply.)*
    1. 86%
    2. 88%
    3. 90%
    4. 93%
    5. 98%

16. When considering HCO_3^- levels and associated pH, which client should the nurse assess for a metabolic-related acid-base imbalance? *(Select all that apply.)*
    1. 7.30
    2. 7.34
    3. 7.40
    4. 7.45
    5. 7.47

17. A client, who has been vomiting large amounts for 48 hours and now has had an NG tube inserted is at risk for which acid-base imbalance?
    1. Respiratory alkalosis
    2. Respiratory acidosis
    3. Metabolic alkalosis
    4. Metabolic acidosis

18. When reviewing the ABG results of a client diagnosed with respiratory alkalosis, what should the nurse expect regarding the HCO_3^- level?
    1. Notable increase
    2. Slight increase
    3. Slight decrease
    4. Normal level

19. What respiratory assessment is consistent with a diagnosis of metabolic acidosis?
    1. Respiratory rate of 5 breaths per minute: deep
    2. Respiratory rate of 10 breaths per minute: normal
    3. Respiratory rate of 26 breaths per minute: deep
    4. Respiratory rate of 30 breaths per minute: shallow

20. What intervention will the nurse prioritize when managing the care of an older adult client being treated for a diagnosis of severe metabolic acidosis?
    1. Monitor the IV administration of LR solution.
    2. Frequently assess the client's apical heart rate for rate and rhythm.
    3. Institute seizure precautions according to institutional policies.
    4. Monitor the intake and output of fluids.

See Answers on pages 84–86.

Nursing Interventions

- Assess the client's level of consciousness: alert; oriented; drowsy response to stimulation
  - If restless, assess the client's respiratory level (rate and depth).
- Assess the client's skin: color changes; temperature; moist or dry
- Assess the client's vital signs: apical pulse; rate; rhythm
- With changes in the client's CNS
  - Protect the client from injury (unconscious or during convulsions).
  - In acidosis, the client may have depression of the CNS that could cause unconsciousness.
  - In alkalosis, the client may have stimulation of the CNS that could cause convulsions.
- Monitor the client's intake and output of fluids.
  - Is especially important for older adults and children

ANSWER KEY: REVIEW QUESTIONS

1. **4 The hydrogen ion plays an important role in promoting the production of ATP.**
   1 H_2CO_3 is a compound associated with the separation of H_2CO_3. **2** HCO_3^- is a primary buffer system in the human body's carbonate system. **3** CO_2 is the by-product of regular metabolism.
   Client Need: Physiological Integrity; **Cognitive Level:** Understanding; **Integrated Process:** Teaching and Learning

2. **2 High hydrogen stimulates breathing, resulting in a lower $PaCO_2$.**
   1 High hydrogen stimulates breathing, resulting in a lower $PaCO_2$. **3** The hydrogen ion will not lose it's positive electrical charge. **4** An increase in hydrogen ions will cause the blood's pH to change; between 7.35 and 7.45 is the normal range.
   Client Need: Physiological Integrity; **Cognitive Level:** Analysis; **Nursing Process:** Analysis

3. **2 A buffer is a substance that can act as a base or an acid.**
   1 The body maintains hemostasis, despite the fact that acids are added through the metabolism of ingested foods and fluids. **3** An acid is a mixture of two or more elements that can give up a hydrogen ion. **4** Normal pH is between 7.35 and 7.45.
   Client Need: Physiological Integrity; **Cognitive Level:** Understanding; **Integrated Process:** Teaching and Learning

4. **2 The client's pH is at low normal. A risk for cardiac impulse dysfunctions increases with a low pH.**
   1 Renal failure is associated in an increased pH. **3** Iron supplements are not generally associated with a low pH. **4** Infection is associated with an increase in pH.
   Client Need: Physiological Integrity; **Cognitive Level:** Applying; **Nursing Process:** Planning

5. **4 Increased pH (above 7.45) can be caused by an infection; the temperature is generally elevated in response to a bacterial infection.**
   1 Decreased pH (below 7.35) can be caused by ineffective loop diuretic therapy. **2** Decreased pH (below 7.35) can be caused by overhydration that could be triggered by too rapid of an IV infusion rate. **3** Decreased pH (below 7.35) can be caused by heart failure that would affect blood pressure.
   Client Need: Physiological Integrity; **Cognitive Level:** Analysis; **Nursing Process:** Planning

6. **3 The buffer system responds almost immediately (in seconds) to minimize large changes in the hydrogen ion concentration.**

   1 The cardiovascular system is not one of the defense mechanisms used to maintain hemostasis. **2** The respiratory system responds within minutes after a substantial change in the hydrogen ion concentration. **4** The renal system response occurs over hours to days to restabilize the hydrogen ion concentration after a sudden shift.

   Client Need: Physiological Integrity; **Cognitive Level:** Understanding; **Integrated Process:** Teaching and Learning

7. **1 The HCO_3^- (H_2CO_3) system is considered the most important.**

   2 Although the phosphate system is one of the four buffer systems, it is not considered the most important. **3** Although one of the four buffer systems, the protein system is not considered the most important. **4** Although one of the four buffer systems, the hemoglobin system is not considered the most important.

   Client Need: Physiological Integrity; **Cognitive Level:** Understanding; **Integrated Process:** Teaching and Learning

8. **1 HCO_3^- is found in both the ICFs and the ECFs.**

   2 Phosphate buffers are located in the ICF. **3** Proteins are located in the ICF as hemoglobin and in the ECF as albumin and globulins. **4** Hemoglobin is found in the ICF.

   Client Need: Physiological Integrity; **Cognitive Level:** Understanding; **Integrated Process:** Teaching and Learning

9. **2 The breathing mechanism is controlled by unique receptors in the brain and to changes in the CO_2 levels.**

   1 The rate and depth of respirations are triggered by the brain's response to the CO_2 levels. **3** The buffer system does not trigger respirations. **4** An increase of hydrogen ions in the ECF is a feedback response to hydrogen ion concentration.

   Client Need: Physiological Integrity; **Cognitive Level:** Understanding; **Integrated Process:** Teaching and Learning

10. **1 Clients diagnosed with COPD who receive too much oxygen show a decreased respiratory rate.**

    2 Clients diagnosed with COPD who receive too much oxygen are at risk for developing respiratory acidosis. **3** Clients diagnosed with COPD who receive too much oxygen show a decreased respiratory rate. **4** Clients diagnosed with COPD who receive too much oxygen show a decreased respiratory rate resulting in the retention of CO_2.

    Client Need: Physiological Integrity; **Cognitive Level:** Analysis; **Nursing Process:** Assessment

11. **Answers: 1, 2, 4, 5**

    Multiple factors, including diet, exercise, standard deviations, and multiple chronic disorders, can account for changes in laboratory values for older adults.

    3 Cognitive decline is generally not a change factor for physiological results.

    Client Need: Physiological Integrity; **Cognitive Level:** Understanding; **Nursing Process:** Analysis

12. **1 For newborns, placement of an umbilical arterial catheter provides arterial blood samples without any alterations.**

    2 Due to a variety of factors, a traditional arterial puncture is not advised. **3** For older infants, capillary puncture from the fingers is used to reduce the risks associated with arterial sampling. **4** For older infants, capillary puncture from the earlobes is used to reduce the risks associated with arterial sampling.

    Client Need: Physiological Integrity; **Cognitive Level:** Application; **Nursing Process:** Planning

13. **Answers: 1, 3**

    2, 5 Normal $PaCO_2$ in a newborn is between 26 and 40 mm Hg. **4** Normal PaO_2 in a newborn is between 50 and 70 mm Hg.

    Client Need: Physiological Integrity; **Cognitive Level:** Applying; **Nursing Process:** Evaluation

14. **4 The client needs to rebreathe his or her own exhaled CO_2; he or she can use a large paper bag or inhalation of 5% CO_2 at intervals.**

    1 Securing IV access is not directly associated with the initial intervention for respiratory alkalosis. **2** Assisted ventilation would not be an initial intervention. **3** The client needs CO_2; oxygen is not a priority.

    Client Need: Physiological Integrity; **Cognitive Level:** Application; **Nursing Process:** Planning

15. **Answers: 2, 3**

    Optimal oxygen saturation level should be between 88% and 92% for a client with respiratory issues resulting in chronic CO_2 retention.

    1, 4, 5 Optimal oxygen saturation level should be between 88% and 92% for a client with respiratory issues resulting in chronic CO_2 retention.

    Client Need: Physiological Integrity; **Cognitive Level:** Understanding; **Nursing Process:** Evaluation

16. **Answers: 1, 2, 5**

    Normal pH levels are between 7.35 and 7.45; these clients are at risk.

    3, 4 Normal pH levels are between 7.35 and 7.45; these clients are at risk.

    Client Need: Physiological Integrity; **Cognitive Level:** Applying; **Nursing Process:** Assessment

17. **3 Severe and prolonged vomiting and suctioning increase the risk for developing metabolic alkalosis.**

    1, 2 Neither vomiting nor suctioning are risks for metabolic alkalosis. **4** Due to the circumstances described, the client's gastrointestinal losses are severe enough to suggest metabolic alkalosis rather than metabolic acidosis.

    Client Need: Physiological Integrity; **Cognitive Level:** Analysis; **Integrated Process:** Teaching and Learning

18. **4 In respiratory imbalances, the HCO_3^- level is normal.**

    1, 2, 3 In respiratory imbalances, the HCO_3^- level is normal.

    Client Need: Physiological Integrity; **Cognitive Level:** Application; **Nursing Process:** Analysis

19. **3 In metabolic acidosis, the client will have respirations that are deep and rapid.**

    1, 2, 4 In metabolic acidosis, the client will have respirations that are deep and rapid.

    Client Need: Physiological Integrity; **Cognitive Level:** Application; **Nursing Process:** Analysis

20. **1 In severe metabolic acidosis, IV fluids are administered to correct the base HCO_3^- deficit. Correcting the deficit has priority.**

    2 Although appropriate, assessing the heart rate is associated with determining the effectiveness of treatment; the treatment takes priority. **3** Although appropriate, instituting seizure precaution is associated with client safety regarding adverse reactions to the deficit; the treatment takes priority. **4** Although appropriate, monitoring the intake and output of fluids is associated with determining the effectiveness of treatment; the treatment takes priority.

    Client Need: Physiological Integrity; **Cognitive Level:** Analysis; **Nursing Process:** Planning

Nursing Assessment 5

NURSING ASSESSMENT OVERVIEW

Client History

- Clinical assessment includes a client history that identifies risk factors that could contribute to fluid and electrolyte imbalance.
- Medical conditions
  - Is there a disease process that could result in a fluid and electrolyte imbalance? If so, what type of imbalance?
    - Respiratory acidosis
    - Respiratory alkalosis
    - Metabolic acidosis
    - Metabolic alkalosis
    - Hyperkalemia
    - Hypokalemia
    - Hyperphosphatemia
    - Hypocalcemia
- Risk factors
  - Age
    - The very young are likely to have clinical dehydration, extracellular volume (ECV) deficit, and/or osmolality imbalances.
    - The very old are likely to have ECV excess or deficit and osmolality imbalances.
  - Chronic disease
    - Cancer
      - Hypercalcemia
        - ○ Cancer cells secrete chemicals that cause calcium to enter the bone.
      - Hyperkalemia, hypocalcemia, and hyperphosphatemia result directly from tumor lysis syndrome.
      - The resulting hyperkalemia, hypocalcemia, and hyperphosphatemia depend on the side effects of therapy and other imbalances.
        - ○ Anorexia
        - ○ Diarrhea
    - Chronic diarrhea
      - Crohn disease
      - Irritable bowel syndrome
      - Celiac disease
      - Can result in an ECV deficit, clinical dehydration, hypokalemia, hypocalcemia, chronic hypomagnesemia, and/or metabolic acidosis
    - Heart failure
      - Diminished cardiac output reduces perfusion of the kidneys.
      - Heart failure activates the renin-angiotensin-aldosterone system (RAAS).
      - The aldosterone effect on the kidneys results in ECV excess and the risk for hypokalemia.

- Diuretic agents increase the risk for hypokalemia.
- Dietary sodium is restricted because sodium holds water in the extracellular fluid (ECF), resulting in greater ECV excess.
- Oliguria and renal disease
  - Kidneys have a reduced ability to make urine.
  - Acute nephritis causes a sudden onset of oliguria.
  - Chronic kidney disease can result in oliguria.
  - Renal disease and the resulting oliguria prevent the normal excretion of fluid, resulting in ECV excess, hyperkalemia, hypermagnesemia, hyperphosphatemia, or metabolic acidosis.
  - Severity of electrolyte and/or fluid imbalance mirrors the severity of the kidney disease.
- Respiratory disease
  - Many acute and chronic respiratory disorders can result in respiratory acidosis.
  - Impaired gas exchange results in retained carbon dioxide (CO_2), which results in higher partial pressure of CO_2 ($PaCO_2$), and respiratory acidosis.
  - Respiratory conditions include such diseases as chronic obstructive pulmonary disease (COPD), cystic fibrosis, and asthma, among others.
- Burns
  - Clients with burns are at a high risk for an ECV deficit.
  - Plasma shifts to interstitial fluid.
  - Increased evaporation and exudate output increases.
  - Service area of the burn correlates to fluid loss.
  - Increased cellular metabolism can result in metabolic acidosis.
- Trauma
  - Hemorrhage can result is an ECV deficit with the loss of blood.
  - Crushing injuries can result in hyperkalemia.
    - Cells are damaged, and a massive amount of intracellular potassium is released into the blood.
  - Head injury can change antidiuretic hormone (ADH) secretion.
    - Too little ADH can result in diabetes insipidus.
    - Clients excrete large amounts of urine.
  - Head injury can result in excess secretion of ADH, resulting in hyponatremia, and/or retained water and concentrated urine.
- Environment
  - Does the client work, live, or exercise in a hot environment?
    - Fluid and electrolytes are lost through sweating.
    - Excessive sweating without adequate fluid and sodium replacement can lead to ECV deficit, hypernatremia, and clinical dehydration.
- Nutrition
  - Anorexia, bulimia, starvation diets, or high fat–no carbohydrate diets can lead to metabolic acidosis.
- Emotional conditions
  - Psychiatric conditions could result in the ingestion of excessive fluids or an insufficient intake of fluids.
    - Clients with schizophrenia and who go untreated could be concerned that their food and/or water has been tampered with and, consequently, refuse to eat or drink.
    - Clients with bipolar disorder who go untreated could limit their intake of food and drink.

- Depression, if not identified and treated, could lead to a decrease in fluids and an imbalanced nutritional diet.
- Socioeconomic conditions
  - Living conditions
    - Excessive heat in the summer attributable to a lack of fans and air conditioning
    - Access to fluids at home and work
    - Dietary intake of salt, fluids, and foods rich in potassium, calcium, and magnesium
    - Client's ability to chew (dental disease) and swallow
      - Alterations can result in inadequate intake of electrolyte-rich foods and fluids.
  - Alcohol consumption
    - How much and what type of alcohol does the client consume in a day and in a week?
- Cultural and religious beliefs
  - Can influence dietary and fluid intake and how clients communicate their needs
  - May cause an individual to refuse treatment
  - An older adult in the family may be the person to whom explanations are given and health care decisions are made instead of the client.
    - Hot and cold health beliefs may cause a client to refuse cold oral fluids because they believe hot foods will restore the body into balance.
    - Clients may need to kneel on the floor to pray several times each day.
  - Seek the client and family values and preferences in the history interview.
  - Ask about preferences for fluid temperatures and food preferences.
  - Determine the appropriate length of intravenous (IV) tubing if the client needs to kneel on a floor prayer mat.
  - Seek the client's acceptance or abstinence from therapeutic regimens.
    - Respect the client and family member's decisions.
  - Some clients refuse whole blood because of religious or personal beliefs.
    - Explore other body products or alternatives.
  - With naturally dark skin tones, carefully assess for subtle changes in skin color.
  - Communicate client and family values and choices to all members of the health care team.
- Medications
  - Obtain a complete list of the client's medications including prescription, over-the-counter, and herbal medications.
  - Check each drug with a drug reference database to assess the risk for potential alterations.
    - Fluids and electrolytes
    - Acid-base balance
  - Discuss the use of antacid drugs.
    - Baking soda can cause ECV excess because of its high sodium content.
    - Excessive use of calcium carbonate can affect electrolyte balance.
  - Laxatives and enemas
    - Routine use of laxative and enemas can remove fluids and electrolytes from the body.
  - Diuretics
    - Clients with heart disease or hypertension who use diuretic medications need to be monitored on a regular basis.
  - Is there any medication or treatment that could affect the person's fluid and electrolyte balance?
    - Review current and past prescription medications.
      - For example, a diuretic medication could result in hypokalemia.
    - Review current and past over-the-counter medications.
    - Review current and past herbal medications.

- What are the unusual losses of body fluids and their sources?
  - Vomiting
  - Diarrhea
  - Wound drainage
- Are there any dietary restrictions concerning food or fluids that are associated with the loss of body fluids?
- What is the volume of fluids and nutrients that the client has received both orally and parenterally?
- What is the balance between fluid intake versus output?
  - Urine
  - Stool
  - Wound drainage
  - Emesis

APPLICATION AND REVIEW

1. Which of the following clients demonstrate a potential risk factor for a fluid and electrolyte imbalance? *(Select all that apply.)*
   1. 6-month-old infant
   2. Cold-packing plant employee
   3. Client diagnosed with asthma
   4. Client prescribed with a loop diuretic medication
   5. Client diagnosed with Crohn disease
2. Which assessment will help determine the risk for an ECV deficit for a client who has experienced a second-degree burn?
   1. Source of the burn
   2. Respiratory rate and rhythm
   3. Amount of service area burned
   4. History of long-term diuretic therapy
3. A client has sustained a crushing injury to both legs. The nurse will monitor serum laboratory results for an increase in which component?
   1. Sodium
   2. Potassium
   3. Magnesium
   4. CO_2
4. A client has developed a comorbid condition associated with a head injury. Which assessment information supports the existence of an excess of ADH?
   1. Diaphoresis
   2. Dilated pupils
   3. Hypotension
   4. Concentrated urine
5. Which client is at an increased risk for developing metabolic acidosis?
   1. Man diagnosed with exercise-induced asthma
   2. Man on a high protein–no carbohydrate diet
   3. Woman who has heavy menstrual periods
   4. Woman diagnosed with diabetes insipidus
6. A practicing Muslim client is admitted for a metabolic imbalance. The nurse demonstrates the greatest degree of cultural and religious sensitivity when implementing which one of the following interventions?
   1. Assessing the client for acceptance of prescribed therapies
   2. Discussing the client's food and fluid preferences
   3. Supporting religious practices such as praying
   4. Completing a medication history

See Answers on pages 107–110.

PHYSICAL ASSESSMENT

Head, Ears, Eyes, Nose, and Throat (HEENT)

- Facial
  - Severe fluid volume deficit (FVD)
    - Thin and pale facial expression
    - Eyes sunken and soft to palpation
- Oral cavity
  - Dry mouth
    - Thirst
      - Thirst is a subjective experience.
      - Water pulled from cells results in stimulation of the thirst center.
      - Any situation causing intracellular dehydration results in the thirst sensation.
      - The purpose of the thirst sensation is to stimulate fluid intake.
      - Dilute ECFs.
      - Hypercalcemia, hyperglycemia, fever, and an increase of 2 mEq/L of serum sodium are circumstances that cause intracellular dehydration result in thirst.
      - Is protective of the normal serum sodium level.
      - Hypernatremia seldom occurs unless thirst is inhibited or the thirst sensation is ineffective as a result of being unconscious or a lack of water.
      - Sense of thirst is diminished in older adults.
      - Lower level of consciousness may reduce fluid intake.
      - Sudden lower blood volume attributable to hemorrhage can increase thirst levels.
- Tearing of eyes
  - In clients with FVD, eye tearing is reduced.
  - The presence of crying is a good indicator of fluid volume balance in infants and children.

Integumentary System

- Skin turgor
  - Pinched skin should return to a normal position when released.
  - Elasticity of skin is related to the interstitial fluid volume (IFV).
  - In a client with FVD, the skin slowly returns to normal and may take seconds to do so.
  - In addition, skin turgor testing (pinching of the skin) can determine the characteristics of skin elasticity (Figure 5.1).
  - Individuals 55 years of age or older have less elasticity to their skin. Alternate sites for performing a skin turgor assessment include the forehead and sternum for older adults and the abdomen and thighs (medial aspects) for children.
  - Skin turgor lowers after losing 3% to 5% of body weight.
  - Infants who are obese may have misleading normal skin turgor.
  - With hypernatremia, infants may have a thickness of skin.
- Tongue turgor
  - Tongue tissue associated with FVD: tongue is smaller; exhibits longitudinal furrows; is not affected by age
- Capillary refill
  - Often used with children (Figure 5.2)
    - Technique to measure capillary refill
      - Apply pressure to a fingernail for 5 seconds.
      - Release the pressure.

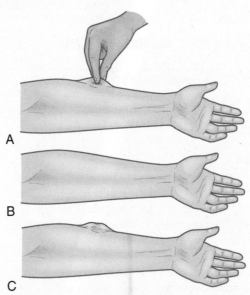

FIGURE 5.1   Skin turgor assessment. **A.** Pinch the skin to assess turgor. **B.** The skin returns to its original position when hydrated. **C.** The skin remains raised when dehydration is present. (From Lewis, S. L., Bucher, L., Heitkemper, M. M., Harding, M. M., Kwong, J., & Roberts, D. [2017]. *Medical-surgical nursing: Assessment and management of clinical problems*, [10th ed.]. St. Louis: Elsevier.)

Capillary refill time

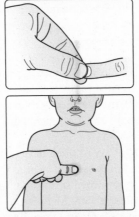

Press on the skin of the sternum or a digit at the level of the heart
Apply blanching pressure for 5 s
Measure time for blush to return
Prolonged capillary refill if >2 s

FIGURE 5.2   Measuring capillary refill time. (From Lissauer, T., & Carroll, W. [2018]. *Illustrated textbook of paediatrics*, [5th ed.]. Philadelphia: Elsevier.)

- Note the time for the normal color of the nail to return.
- A change should be noticed in less than 1 to 2 seconds under normal conditions.
  - A slower capillary refill can be due to
    - Lower peripheral perfusion attributable to FVD
    - Constriction of peripheral vessels: lower cardiac output; anemia
    - Slower capillary refill attributable to smoking
    - Capillary refill time longer than 4½ seconds (associated with severe organ failure)
- Edema
  - Accumulation of interstitial fluid
  - Apparent, once interstitial fluid volume (IFV) is greater than 2.5 to 3.0 liters
  - Edema is attributed to
    - Greater capillary permeability
      - Fluid leaks into the interstitium after trauma or burns.
    - Greater capillary hydraulic pressure
      - Fluid is forced into the interstitium.
      - Occurs with heart failure and venous obstruction
    - Lower plasma oncotic pressure
  - Occurs with hypoalbuminemia (encourages transfer of fluid to the interstitium)
  - Lymphatic blockage
    - Permits lymphedema
    - Can be attributable to enlarged lymph nodes in clients with cancer, blocked lymph nodes, removal of lymph nodes
  - Edema classification
    - Localized edema with thrombophlebitis
    - Generalized edema with heart or renal failure
      - Spreads throughout the body
      - Accumulates in the periorbital and scrotal areas as a result of lower tissue hydrostatic pressure
      - Attributable to salt retention, normally resulting in pitting
        - Press a finger on soft tissue, preferably over a bone.
        - After removing the pressure, the "pit" disappears.
    - Dependent edema
    - Peripheral edema
      - Subjective measure
      - Rated by a plus signs' range from 1+ to 4+
      - Measured in the extremity with a millimeter tape, in the same area each day (a more objective measure) and at the same time each day
      - Low or no peripheral edema associated with water retention (due to excessive secretion of ADH)

APPLICATION AND REVIEW

7. Which assessment information suggests a client may be experiencing a severe FVD?
   1. Excessive tearing
   2. Bloodshot eyes
   3. Sunken eyes
   4. Itchy eyes
8. Which notation related to an older adult's skin assessment suggests a possible FVD?
   1. Minor bruising is noted.
   2. Skin appears redden but dry.
   3. Normal turgor appears within 2 seconds.
   4. Several skin tears are noted on the arms.

9. When assessing capillary refill, a nurse demonstrates the technique by applying pressure to the nail bed for what amount of time?
   1. 2 seconds
   2. 4 seconds
   3. 5 seconds
   4. 7 seconds
10. Which assessment question should the nurse ask a client whose normal capillary refill returns in 3 seconds?
    1. "Are you being treated for asthma?"
    2. "Do you smoke any tobacco products?"
    3. "Have you ever spontaneously fainted?"
    4. "How much iron do you consume weekly?"

See Answers on pages 107–110.

Thorax and Lungs

- Pulmonary edema
  - Results from extra shifting of fluid from vascular spaces to the pulmonary interstitium and air spaces
  - Cardiogenic pulmonary edema
    - Pulmonary capillary pressure is greater than the force that keeps fluid within the vascular space.
    - Forces include serum oncotic pressure and interstitial hydrostatic pressure.
    - Collection of extravascular lung water affects pulmonary function and gas exchange. Symptoms include dyspnea, anxiety, expectoration of pink fluid, and use of accessory respiratory muscles.

Neurological System

- Neuromuscular irritability
  - Important for assessing calcium, sodium, and magnesium deficits
  - Assessments include deep-tendon reflexes.
    - Chvostek-Weiss sign (Figure 5.3)
      - Facial nerve tapped (2 cm anterior to earlobe)
      - Positive response: unilateral twitching of the facial muscles affecting the eyelid and lips (usually 25% of individuals have a positive response)
      - Can indicate hypocalcemia or hypomagnesemia (not specific)
    - Trousseau sign (Figure 5.4)
      - Inflate a blood pressure cuff 20 mm Hg above systolic pressure for 3 minutes.
      - Cramping of the hand is a positive response.
        - Thumb and fifth finger come together.
        - Second and fourth fingers extend.
        - The Trousseau sign is more specific to hypocalcemia than the Chvostek-Weiss sign.
        - Usually 1% to 4% of individuals have a positive response.
- Deep-tendon reflexes
  - Common reflexes include biceps, triceps, brachioradialis, patellar, and Achilles.
  - Deep-tendon reflexes are triggered by quickly tapping a semistretched tendon with a percussion hammer.
    - Response is a spontaneous contraction.
    - Reflexes may be hyperactive attributable to hypocalcemia, hypomagnesemia, or alkalosis.

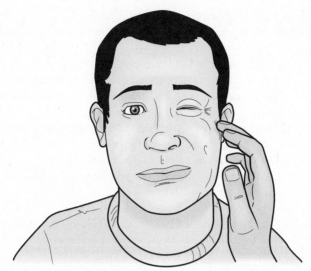

FIGURE 5.3 Facial muscle response, indicating a positive Chvostek-Weiss sign. (From Ignatavicius, D. D., & Workman, M. L. [2010]. *Medical-surgical nursing: Critical thinking for collaborative care*, [6th ed.]. Philadelphia: Saunders–Elsevier.)

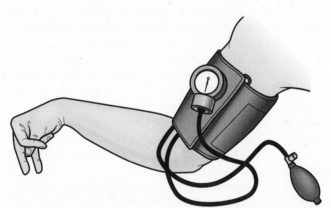

FIGURE 5.4 Muscle contraction and flexion, indicating a positive Trousseau sign. (From Ignatavicius, D. D., & Workman, M. L. [2010]. *Medical-surgical nursing: Critical thinking for collaborative care*, [6th ed.]. Philadelphia: Saunders–Elsevier.)

- ▪ Reflexes may be hypoactive attributable to hypercalcemia, hypermagnesemia, or acidosis.
- ▪ Other factors can affect deep-tendon reflexes.

Vital Signs

- Temperature
  - Rise in body temperature in the client with hypernatremia
    - ▪ Can be due to excessive water loss
    - ▪ Potential cause: lack of fluid for sweating
    - ▪ Dehydration affecting the hypothalamus, which regulates body heat

- Lower body temperatures with isotonic FVD
  - Probably due to decreased basal metabolic rate as a result of an FVD
- Fever
  - Can be the cause of fluid imbalance
  - Higher metabolic rate, resulting in more metabolic waste
    - Fluid is needed to make a solution for excretion through the renal system.
    - Result is an increased loss of fluid.
  - Can be the cause of hyperpnea (faster respiratory rate)
    - Loss of water vapor by the lungs
  - Can be the cause of a loss of body fluids
    - Each 1° increase of body temperature over 37° Celsius is a 10% increase in the water requirement.
- Pulse rate
  - One of the early signs of FVD is tachycardia (an elevated pulse rate).
  - Pulse may feel weak with decreased fluid volume.
  - Pulse may feel bounding with excess fluid volume.
- Respiratory rate
  - Rapid and deep respiratory rate can occur as a method of compensation in the presence of FVE and FVD.
    - Can be attributable to metabolic acidosis
    - Can also be the cause of respiratory alkalosis and respiratory acidosis
  - Shallow and slow respiratory rate can occur as another method of compensation.
    - Can be attributable to metabolic alkalosis
    - May be the primary reason for respiratory acidosis
  - Respiratory muscle weakness or paralysis can be a result of the following:
    - Severe hypokalemia
    - Hyperkalemia in severe hypermagnesemia
      - Respiratory center can be paralyzed with a magnesium level of 10 to 15 mEq/L.
    - Fluid volume excess
      - Auscultate moist rales without accompanied cardiopulmonary disease
- Blood pressure
  - Signifies the force that the circulating blood exerts on the blood vessels
  - Increased in FVE and decreased in FVD
  - Measured by
    - Directly by indwelling arterial catheter
    - Indirectly by a sphygmomanometer (blood pressure cuff)
      - Cuff needs to fit the client's arm.
        - Too narrow cuff can give false high readings.
        - Too wide cuff can give false low readings.
        - Width of cuff should approximate 40% of the circumference of the upper arm of an adult.
  - Adult (over age 18 years)
    - Normal systolic blood pressure less than 120 mm Hg
    - Normal diastolic blood pressure less than 80 mm Hg
    - Hypotension is systolic pressure less than 90 mm Hg
- Pulse pressure
  - Defined as the difference between the systolic blood pressure and the diastolic blood pressure

- Pulse pressure lower than 30 mm Hg occurs in clients with FVD.
  - Client with hypovolemia and a narrow pulse pressure
    - Indicates decreased cardiac output (descending systolic blood pressure) and increased peripheral vascular resistance (ascending diastolic blood pressure)
    - Body attempts to maintain sufficient blood pressure with vasoconstriction.
    - Measurement is useful when monitoring fluid volume replacement.
- Mean arterial pressure (MAP)
  - MAP is the best method to assess clients with unstable pressure.
  - The MAP that is needed to maintain adequate tissue perfusion in the coronary arteries, brain, and kidneys is 60 mm Hg.
    - Typical MAP range: between 70 and 110 mm Hg
    - Calculation for MAP
      - $[(2 \times \text{diastolic}) + \text{systolic}] \div 3$
      - If the diastolic pressure is 80 mm Hg and systolic pressure is 140 mm Hg, the MAP is approximately 100 mm Hg.
- Orthostatic blood pressure
  - Procedure for detecting hypovolemia
    - Blood pressure and pulse rate are measured while the client is lying flat and then after transitioning to a standing posture.
    - Transitioning from lying to standing causes an abrupt drop in venous return. Normally, such transitions are mediated and compensated by the cardiovascular system.
    - A healthy individual's cardiac return is stabilized by the increased peripheral resistance and a slight increase in heart rate. Systolic pressure decreases slightly, and diastolic pressure may rise slightly.
  - A lowering of systolic pressure greater than 20 mm Hg, accompanied by the symptoms of tachycardia and/or light-headedness, may indicate orthostatic hypotension attributable to intravascular volume deficit.
  - To be specific for hypovolemia, the increase in pulse rate must be 20 to 10 beats per minute (bpm) when transitioning from a lying position to a standing position.
  - Other conditions that can result in orthostatic hypotension include autonomic neuropathy (diabetes) and sympatholytic antihypertensive medications.
- Central venous pressure (CVP)
  - Describes the pressure in the right atrium or vena cava
  - Provides information regarding blood volume, effectiveness of the heart's pumping ability, and vascular tone
  - Measured with a water manometer
    - Pressure in the right atrium: from 0 to 4 cm of water
    - Pressure in vena cava: approximately 4 to 11 cm of water
  - Measured with a transducer system
    - Normal range: between 0 and 7 mm Hg.
  - CVP value below the range may indicate decreased blood volume, vasodilation, and/or any condition that decreases venous return to the heart.
  - CVP value above the range may indicate increased fluid volume, vasoconstriction, and/or heart failure.
  - Trends are more informative than simply absolute values.
    - Upward and downward trends can be identified through frequent measurement readings.

- Evaluation of the CVP reading in relation to other clinical data: blood pressure; fluid intake (oral, IV); urinary output
  - For example, an increase in CVP with an increase in blood pressure could indicate adequate fluid replacement.
  - With normal cardiac and pulmonary function, the CVP value is a good guide to evaluating blood volume.
- Pulmonary artery pressure
  - CVP may not provide a complete assessment for clients who are critically ill.
  - Pulmonary artery catheter is an invasive hemodynamic method of assessment.
  - Use of the pulmonary artery catheter gives direct measurement from the right atrium, right ventricle, pulmonary arteries, and pulmonary capillary wedge pressure.
  - Assess fluid balance in clients with complex clinical presentations.
    - Assessment is especially important for clients whose fluid and drug management could have a major impact on their condition; consequently, close fluid monitoring is indicated.
- Urine volume
  - Adult urine output averages 1 mL/kg body weight per hour.
  - The range for adult urine output averages between 0.5 and 2 mL/kg/hr.
  - Average adult urine output: 1500 mL/day
    - Range: between 1000 and 2000 mL/day
    - Equal to between 40 and 80 mL/hr for adults
  - Pediatric urine output parameters depend on age and weight.
  - With stress, the 24-hour urine volume in adults decreases.
    - Range: between 750 and 1200 mL/day
    - Equal to between 30 and 50 mL/hr
      - When the body is under stress, the production of stress hormones (aldosterone and ADH) increases.
  - Lower urine output suggests FVD.
  - Higher urine output suggests fluid volume excess.
  - The assumption is that the kidneys are functioning normally and able to respond to both an increased and decreased fluid volume.
  - Factors that affect urine volume
    - Amount of fluid intake
      - An increase in the amount of fluid intake can result in an increase in fluid output.
      - A decrease in the amount of fluid intake can result in a decrease in fluid output.
      - A normally functioning kidney excretes 500 mL of concentrated urine when fluids are severely restricted.
      - If large amounts of body fluids are lost through the skin, lungs, and gastrointestinal (GI) tract, the urine volume will be decreased.
      - If a large amount of waste products are to be excreted, such as high solute loads, diabetes, high protein tube feedings, thyrotoxicosis, and/or fever may be indicated.
      - If the kidneys lose the ability to concentrate urine, the volume of urine produced will be decreased, which is common in the older adult population and those clients with diabetes insipidus.
      - Blood volume can affect urine output in normally functioning kidneys.
        - Hypovolemia will be associated with lower urine output.
        - Hypervolemia will be associated with higher urine output.

- Hormonal influences
  - ○ If aldosterone and ADH production is increased, the urine output will be lower (retention of sodium and water).
  - ○ Absence of ADH can result in large output of urine, such as neurogenic diabetes insipidus.

Urine Volume and Concentration

- Urine concentration
  - Kidneys are constantly altering the concentration of electrolytes and other elements to help the body achieve and maintain hemostasis.
  - Two tests measure the kidneys' ability to perform the balancing of electrolytes.
    - Urine-specific gravity (SG)
      - Is measured with a reagent strip or urinometer or refractometer
      - Denotes the proportion of solids that have gone into the solution per the total volume of the solution
      - Large molecules (e.g., albumin, glucose, radioactive contrast dyes) hinder the accuracy of the urine SG when testing is performed with a urinometer or refractometer, but not a reagent strip.
      - When measuring urine concentration in a client known to have proteinuria (abnormal quantities of protein in the urine) or glucosuria (glucose in the urine), a urine SG reagent strip is used.
      - Urine SG test is frequently used in clinical sites.
      - Urine SG test compares the density of a urine specimen with distilled water (1.000).
    - Urine osmolality
      - Is measured in a laboratory test
      - Denotes the amount of particles per unit of the solution
      - Large molecules, such as albumin, glucose, and radioactive contrast dyes, do not hinder the osmolarity test results.
      - When measuring urine concentration with a client known to have proteinuria or glucosuria, the osmolarity test is used.
  - Sodium chloride, sulfate, phosphate, and urea in urine raise the urine SG level greater than 1.000 (range is between 1.003 and 1.035).
  - Normal renal concentration is indicated by a urine SG of 1.023 or higher (random sample).
  - A healthy adult with normal fluid intake produces urine with osmolality between 500 and 859 mOsm/kg.
  - A dehydrated individual has an elevated osmolality up to 1400 mOsm/kg.
  - A water-overloaded individual has a lowered osmolality down to 40 mOsm/kg.
  - Significance of osmolality and urine SG
    - Depends on the client's clinical status
    - An elevated urine SG and osmolality is consistent with FVD.
      - Normal kidney function tries to retain fluid.
      - Less solutes are excreted.
      - Postdehydration urine osmolality can be three times greater than plasma osmolality.
    - Clients with neurogenic diabetes insipidus have a low urine SG.
      - Individuals excrete a large volume of water attributable to the absence of ADH.
    - Fixed low urine SG 1.000 is present in the individual with isosthenuria.
      - Serious kidney disease occurs when a loss in the ability to concentrate the urine is present.
      - Urine is excreted with unchanged filtrate.

Fluid Intake and Output

- Client fluid intake and output (I&O)
  - Careful monitoring of a client's fluid I&O can alert and prevent fluid balance issues.
  - Accurate fluid I&O needs to be recorded in the client's record.
  - Standard of care includes an I&O assessment on any client with a condition or disease that increases his or her risk for a fluid volume overload or deficit.
    - Evaluate fluid I&O during every shift and assess over a 24-hour period.
  - Vigilance is important in clients with an electrolyte imbalance.
  - Compare fluid I&O gains and/or losses during every shift and over time for trends.
  - Clients who are critically ill will need hourly monitoring of their fluid I&O.
  - Stable clients will require I&O monitoring every 8 or 12 hours.
  - Full clinical picture is gained by comparing and contrasting fluid I&O per shift and daily changes.
- Positive and negative fluid balance
  - Positive fluid balance: intake exceeds output
  - Negative fluid balance: output exceeds intake
  - Based on the client's condition, it may become temporarily necessary to cause a positive or negative fluid balance.
    - Positive fluid balance may be necessary for the client with a severe fluid volume deficit or when aggressive fluid replacement therapy is indicated.
    - Positive fluid balance is contraindicated for clients with renal failure (consumes more fluid than excreted by diseased kidneys).
    - Negative fluid balance may be necessary for the short term when IV diuretic medications are being administered, for example, to the client with heart failure and/or pulmonary edema.
    - Negative fluid balance can be dangerous for a client with severe GI disorder (vomiting and diarrhea), which requires aggressive fluid and electrolyte replacement.
- Important considerations for fluid I&O measurement
  - Measure and document all fluids taken into the body from multiple sources.
    - Oral liquids (volume documented in milliliters)
      - Foods that return to liquid at room temperature: Jell-O; ice cream; popsicles
      - Foods that are liquid at room temperature: soup broth; syrup
      - Ice chips: recorded as one-half the volume (100 mL of ice chips is recorded as 50 mL of water)
    - IV fluids: small bags (medication and secondary infusion); large bags (primary infusion); blood products
    - Fluid and water administered through GI feedings
    - Fluid(s) used to flush enteral feeding tubes
    - Fluid(s) used to flush nasogastric drainage tubes
    - Enema solutions
  - Measure and document all fluids excreted or lost from the body from multiple sources: urine; vomit; liquid stool; drainage from gastric suction tubes; drainage from chest tubes; drainage from wound drainage collection devices (Jackson-Pratt [JP] drain, vacuum-assisted [wound VAC] closure).
  - Estimated loss from sources that cannot be directly measured
    - Sweat: quantified as mild, moderate, or severe
    - Hyperventilation
      - Results in the loss of water vapor

- Normally, the source of the average loss of 300 mL of water vapor is through the respiratory route.
- Drainage from large wounds on a dressing is quantified as mild, moderate, or severe.
- Educate all personnel for accurate I&O measurements and the importance of accurately recording all I&O findings.
- Educate the client and family members about the importance of strict I&O and the definition of fluids.
  - Provide the client and family with a conversion table from English/household measurement to metric.
    - One teaspoon equals 5 mL
    - One tablespoon equals 15 mL
    - One fluid ounce equals 30 mL
    - One cup (8 ounces) equals 240 mL
    - One pint (16 ounces) equals 480 mL (0.5 L)
    - One quart (32 ounces) equals 960 mL (1 L)

Body Weight Measurement

- Daily weights are important for clients with current or possible fluid balance difficulties.
- Accurate body weight is usually easier to obtain than obtaining ongoing I&O measurements.
- Rapid variations in weight can accurately detail changes in body fluid volume for most clients.
  - Rapid weight gain or loss of 1 kg (2.2 pounds) is approximately the gain or loss of 1 L of fluid.
    - Direct fluid increases and decreases in the body are reflected in body weight changes.
    - A fluid shift attributable to tissue damage and associated bloodstream loss (e.g., burns, trauma) will have the same weight as before the shift in fluid.
      - Body weight is not helpful in assessing fluid volume status.
  - Using body weight as an indicator of fluid balance assumes that the client's dry weight is stable over time.
    - This assumption holds for short (hour-to-hour) periods.
    - Changes in body weight are related to body fluid volume versus tissue mass changes.
    - For discrete hourly changes of fluid volume, using metabolic scales are recommended.
  - Loss of body weight occurs when total fluid output exceeds total fluid intake.
    - Rapid loss of body fluid differs for adults and children.
      - Children with a rapid loss of 5% of total body weight indicates mild FVD.
      - Children with a rapid loss of 6% to 10% of total body weight indicates moderate FVD.
      - Children with a rapid loss of more than 10% of total body weight indicates severe FVD.
  - On the contrary, a rapid gain of body weight occurs when total fluid output is less than total fluid intake.
    - Long-term (day-to-day) changes in body weight are indicative of changes in tissue mass, as well as body fluid volume.
      - Factors affecting tissue mass that have to be assessed include caloric intake and metabolic status.
    - A reduction of approximately 3400 calories is required to lose 1 pound of tissue mass. The reason for this change could include lower caloric intake, increased metabolic rate, and a combination of lower caloric intake and increased metabolic rate.

- Procedure for weighing clients
  - Use the same scale each time; variations between scales can cause different readings.
  - Measure the weight at a consistent time each day and in the morning after the first void.
  - The client needs to wear similar clothing, and the clothing needs to be dry.
  - If the client is unable to stand for weighing, alternative methods can be used: small portable scale; sling-type scale; hospital bed with built-in weight scale; wheelchair scale.
- Ensure that the scales are accurate and calibrated. Establish a schedule for periodically assessing the accuracy of scales and recalibrating.

APPLICATION AND REVIEW

11. A nurse, counseling a client about weight loss, answers the client's question, "How many calories must be eliminated to lose 1 pound of body tissue?"
    1. 900
    2. 1200
    3. 3400
    4. 5200

See Answer on pages 107–110.

Specimen Collection to Evaluate Fluid Status

- Blood specimens
  - Frequent phlebotomy procedures for withdrawing a blood sample can contribute to anemia.
    - Taking more blood than required for analysis can occur with frequent testing.
    - Within the first 2 weeks of hospitalization in an intensive care unit (ICU), more than 50% of clients developed iron-deficiency anemia.
    - The amount of blood drawn daily from clients who are critically ill is often triple the amount for a general client.
  - Prevention of hemolysis of a blood specimen
    - Hemolysis of peripheral or central line blood specimens can give erroneous results from analysis of hemolyzed blood.
    - Hemolysis of blood may damage red blood cells, causing hemoglobin to enter the plasma, producing a pink-to-red tinge in the plasma when the blood is centrifuged.
    - Rupture of red blood cells results in the electrolytes (potassium, phosphate, magnesium) flowing into the plasma, resulting in false high levels for the major cellular ions.
    - Prevalence of hemolyzed blood specimens can be as high as 3.3% of all routine specimens; five times higher than other causes for unsuitable laboratory blood specimens.
  - Primary causes of hemolysis of blood specimens can include
    - Delay in transporting for testing
    - Use of a syringe with excessive suction applied
      - Hemolysis is less likely if blood is collected with evacuated tubes versus syringes.
    - Blood drawn through a small needle or catheter
      - Rupture of red blood cells
      - Excessive shaking of the collection tube to mix the blood with the anticoagulant
  - Obtain peripheral venous blood samples.
    - Avoid drawing blood samples if the site is above an infusing IV line.
    - Blood for serum biochemical and hematological profiles should be drawn from the opposite arm.

- Avoid clenched fist and the prolonged use of a tourniquet when blood is being drawn for potassium levels.
  - Can cause an erroneous elevation, as much as 1 mEq/L, in the potassium level.
- Obtain central and arterial blood samples.
  - Frequently used in ICUs to collect blood samples
  - Reduces the need for multiple peripheral venipunctures
  - Convenient site for obtaining blood specimens for clients who are critically ill
  - Useful for collecting samples for arterial blood gases for clients with acute metabolic or respiratory issues
  - Sources of error with collecting an arterial blood specimen
    - Blood specimens can be contaminated by recently infused IV fluids.
    - Accidental heparin (flushes) can be introduced into the blood sample and alter the partial thromboplastin time results.
    - Sodium citrate in flush solutions can mix with the sample, resulting in hypocalcemia and low pH.
    - Due to convenience, collecting arterial blood specimens can result in more frequent blood draws.
    - Facility protocol is recommended for blood tests to minimize the amount of blood drawn.
- Urine specimens
  - Single specimen is recommended at first void due to greater concentration.
    - To avoid false readings, collect specimen in a sterile container.
    - Deliver a fresh specimen within 1 hour of collection.
  - 24-hour specimen
    - A 24-hour specimen is used to measure the amount of electrolytes excreted.
    - Laboratory collection container needs to have a preservative.
    - Failure to collect all urine in a 24-hour period could affect the accuracy of the test results.
    - Enlist the client and family members to save all urine.
    - The laboratory will have specific directions; the specimen may need to be refrigerated.
    - Follow specific directions from the laboratory for the specimen.
    - Record start and stop times for the 24-hour urine specimen.

Changes in Fluid Balance Related to the Client's Age (Older Adults)

- Skin: loss of elasticity; decreased skin turgor; decreased oil production; poor indicator of fluid status, especially the back of the hand; dry and easily damages
- Kidneys: lower glomerular filtration; lower concentrating capacity; poor excretion of waste products; increased risk for water loss and increased risk of dehydration
- Muscular: lower muscle mass; greater risk for dehydration
- Neurological considerations: diminished thirst reflex; lower fluid intake; greater risk for dehydration
- Endocrine: adrenal atrophy; poor regulation of sodium and potassium; greater risk for hyponatremia; greater risk for hyperkalemia

Sources of Fluid Ingestion and Elimination

- Measured intake: oral fluids; parenteral fluids; irrigation fluids; enemas
- Not measured intake: solid foods; metabolism
- Measured output: urine; emesis; fecal; drainage from body sources (vagina, wounds)
- Not measured output: perspiration; vapors from lungs through respiration

Common Sources of Fluid Imbalances

- Dehydration: blood loss and hemorrhage; emesis (vomiting); urine; diarrhea; profound salivation; burns; large wounds; long-term restriction or lack of oral fluids; diuretic therapy; prolonged GI suctioning; hyperventilation; diabetes insipidus; impaired swallowing; inhibition of thirst reflex; level of consciousness–unconscious; fever; inhibited motor function
- Fluid overload: aggressive fluid replacement; late-stage kidney failure; cardiac conditions—heart failure; extended corticosteroidal medication; syndrome of inappropriate antidiuretic hormone (SIADH); psychiatric disorders that include polydipsia (excessive thirst); water intoxication that can result from IV fluid therapy

APPLICATION AND REVIEW

12. Which factors will the nurse measure when calculating a client's fluid output? *(Select all that apply.)*
    1. Urine
    2. Menses
    3. Emesis
    4. Perspiration
    5. Wound drainage
13. Which client is at risk for developing dehydration? *(Select all that apply.)*
    1. Client experiencing acute heart failure
    2. Client diagnosed with diabetes insipidus
    3. Client diagnosed with late-stage kidney failure
    4. Client with second-degree burns over 40% of the body
    5. Client who is both bed-bound and cognitively impaired

See Answers on pages 107–110.

Nursing Assessment of Blood Test for Primary Electrolytes

- Serum sodium is represented by the chemical symbol Na^+.
  - Major cation (positively charged particle) in the ECF
  - Obtained by the body through the ingestion of foods and fluids
    - Foods high in sodium content include seasonings, canned, smoked, pickled, and processed foods.
    - Despite ingestion of foods high in sodium, the blood level of sodium is balanced and regulated by the kidneys.
  - Low sodium levels inhibit the secretion of ADH and natriuretic peptide (NP) and trigger aldosterone secretion.
  - High sodium levels inhibit aldosterone secretion and directly stimulate the secretion of ADH and NP.
  - Hyponatremia
    - Serum sodium level: below 136 mEq/L
    - Cerebral changes attributable to excitability of the central nervous system (CNS) and increased intracranial pressure
    - Careful assessment of the client, including level of consciousness and mental status
    - Neuromuscular changes such as muscle weakness
      - Diminished tendon reflexes
      - Test both arm and leg strength; muscle weakness is more pronounced in the extremities.

- Hypernatremia
  - Serum sodium level: above 145 mEq/L
  - More sodium is available to move rapidly through the cell membranes during depolarization, making tissues excited and over-responding to stimulation.
    - Cellular dehydration with cellular shrinkage occurs.
    - Eventually, the dehydrated excitable tissue will not respond to stimuli.
  - Cognitive and neuromuscular changes
  - Intestinal changes
    - Increased motility, resulting in nausea, vomiting, and diarrhea
    - Hyperactive bowel sounds
    - Frequent and watery stools
  - Cardiovascular changes
    - Hypovolemia with decreased plasma volume
    - Rapid, weak, and thready pulse
    - Difficulty palpating peripheral pulses
    - Lower blood pressure and central venous pressure
    - Dizziness and light-headedness attributable to hypovolemia
- Serum potassium is represented by the chemical symbol K^+ (Table 5.1).
  - Potassium is a major cation of the intracellular fluid (ICF).
  - Concentration results can be falsely elevated attributable to the following:
    - Blood sample left at room temperature (blood hemolyzes and releases potassium)
    - Tourniquet used to obtain a blood sample was applied for an extended period
  - With acidosis, serum potassium is elevated.
    - Potassium shifts from the cells to the plasma.
  - With alkalosis, serum potassium is decreased.
    - Potassium shifts into the cells from the plasma.
  - Hypokalemia
    - Serum potassium level: below 3.5 mEq/L
    - Most of the total body's potassium is inside the cells, therefore minimal changes cause major cell membrane excitability.
    - Muscle weakness attributable to a stronger stimulus is needed to contract muscles.
    - Cardiovascular changes, including weak, slow, and thready pulse; irregular heart rate; and postural hypotension, can occur.
      - Significant electrocardiographic (ECG) changes and dysrhythmias occur.
    - Neurological changes: altered mental status; irritability and anxiety
    - Intestinal changes: hypoactive bowel sounds; abdominal distention; vomiting and constipation
  - Hyperkalemia
    - Serum potassium level: above 5.0 mEq/L
    - Excitable tissues, especially cardiac
    - Cardiac changes: Heart is extremely sensitive to serum potassium increases, which can lead to heart block and ventricular fibrillation
    - Neuromuscular changes: skeletal muscles twitch (initial change); tingling or a burning sensation; numbness in extremities; flaccid muscles, resulting in respiratory depression (if hyperkalemia worsens)
    - Intestinal changes: increased motility; diarrhea and hyperactive bowel sounds
    - Intestinal changes rarely occur in individuals with normal renal function; most cases occur in the hospital in those undergoing medical treatment.

TABLE 5.1 Potassium Imbalances: Causes and Manifestations

Hyperkalemia	Hypokalemia
(Potassium >5.0 mEq/L [mmol/L])	(Potassium <3.5 mEq/L [mmol/L])

Causes

Hyperkalemia	Hypokalemia
Excess Potassium Intake	*Potassium Loss*
• Excessive or rapid parenteral administration • Potassium-containing drugs (e.g., potassium penicillin) • Potassium-containing salt substitute	• *Gastrointestinal losses:* diarrhea, vomiting, fistulas, nasogastric suction, ileostomy drainage • *Renal losses:* diuretic medications, hyperaldosteronism, magnesium depletion • *Skin losses:* diaphoresis • Dialysis
Shift of Potassium Out of Cells	*Shift of Potassium Into Cells*
• Acidosis • Tissue catabolism (e.g., fever, crush injury, sepsis, burns) • Intense exercise • Tumor lysis syndrome	• Increased insulin release (e.g., intravenous dextrose load) • Insulin therapy (e.g., with diabetic ketoacidosis) • Alkalosis • Increased dose of epinephrine (e.g., stress)
Failure to Eliminate Potassium	*Lack of Potassium Intake*
• Renal disease • Adrenal insufficiency • *Medications:* Angiotensin II receptor blockers, ACE inhibitors, heparin, potassium-sparing diuretic agents, NSAIDs	• Starvation • Diet low in potassium • Failure to include potassium in parenteral fluids, if NPO

Clinical Manifestations

Hyperkalemia	Hypokalemia
• Fatigue, irritability • Muscle weakness, cramps • Loss of muscle tone • Paresthesias, decreased reflexes • Abdominal cramping, diarrhea, vomiting • Confusion • Irregular pulse • Tetany	• Fatigue • Muscle weakness, leg cramps • Soft, flabby muscles • Paresthesias, decreased reflexes • Constipation, nausea, paralytic ileus • Shallow respirations • Weak, irregular pulse • Hyperglycemia
Electrocardiographic Changes	*Electrocardiographic Changes*
• Tall, peaked T wave • Prolonged PR interval • ST segment depression • Widening QRS • Loss of P wave • Ventricular fibrillation • Ventricular standstill	• Flattened T wave • Presence of U wave • ST segment depression • Prolonged QRS • Peaked P wave • Ventricular dysrhythmias • First- and second-degree heart block

ACE, Angiotensin-converting enzyme; *NPO,* nothing by mouth (*nil per os*); *NSAIDs,* nonsteriodal antiinflammatory drugs.
From Lewis, S. L., Bucher, L., Heitkemper, M. M., Harding, M. M., Kwong, J., & Roberts, D. (2017). *Medical-surgical nursing: Assessment and management of clinical problems,* (10th ed.). St. Louis: Elsevier.

APPLICATION AND REVIEW

14. Which preexisting condition places a client at risk for a sodium imbalance?
    1. 12-year-old boy experiencing an asthma attack
    2. 25-year-old adult who smokes two packs of cigarettes a day
    3. 45-year old man who has sustained a concussion
    4. 70-year-old woman who has been diagnosed with renal failure
15. A client has a serum sodium level of 134 mEq/L. Assessment of which system should the nurse make a **priority** when providing for client safety?
    1. Cardiac
    2. Cognitive
    3. Respiratory
    4. GI
16. Which assessment information is most reliable in confirming a diagnosis of hypernatremia?
    1. Three watery stools within an 8-hour period
    2. Reports of dizziness upon standing
    3. Serum sodium level of 149 mEq/L
    4. Hyperactive bowel sounds
17. A client's serum potassium level is unexpectedly elevated. Which question should the nurse ask regarding possible causes for false results?
    1. "Was the sample promptly refrigerated?"
    2. "What time of day was the sample drawn?"
    3. "Does the client have a history of smoking?"
    4. "What was the client's cardiac rate at the time?"
18. Which assessment data would support the possibility of a diagnosis of hypokalemia? *(Select all that apply.)*
    1. Serum potassium level of 3.8 mEq/L
    2. Hypoactive bowel sounds
    3. Altered mental state
    4. Irregular heartbeat
    5. Diarrhea
19. Which serum potassium level would be used as the criterion for diagnosing a client with hyperkalemia?
    1. Greater than 3.0 mEq/L
    2. Greater than 4.0 mEq/L
    3. Greater than 5.0 mEq/L
    4. Greater than 6.0 mEq/L
20. Which organ tissue is most affected by changes in serum potassium levels?
    1. Nerve
    2. Kidney
    3. Muscle
    4. Cardiac

ANSWER KEY: REVIEW QUESTIONS

1. **Answers: 1, 3, 4, 5**
   2 People who work, live, or exercise in a hot environment, not cold, are at risk for increased sweating, resulting in fluid and electrolyte loss.
   Client Need: Physiological Integrity; **Cognitive Level:** Analysis; **Nursing Process:** Assessment
2. **3 Burns place a client at high risk for an ECV deficit. The extent of the surface area of the burn correlates to the amount of fluid loss, resulting in a plasma-to-interstitial fluid shift.**
   1 The source of the burn is not a factor in determining the risk for an ECV deficit. **2** Although the respiratory rate and rhythm can be factors in the development of respiratory acidosis, they are not major risk

factors associated with burns. **4** Although diuretic therapy can result in hypokalemia, it is not a major risk factor associated with burns.
Client Need: Physiological Integrity; **Cognitive Level:** Application; **Nursing Process:** Assessment

3. **2 Crushing injuries can result in hyperkalemia; cells are damaged, and a massive amount of intracellular potassium is released into the blood.**
   1 Excessive sweating without adequate fluids and sodium replacement can lead to hypernatremia. **3** Renal disease and the resulting oliguria prevent normal excretion of fluids, resulting in hypermagnesemia. **4** Impaired gas exchange results in retained CO_2 (higher $PaCO_2$) and respiratory acidosis.
   Client Need: Physiological Integrity; **Cognitive Level:** Application; **Nursing Process:** Assessment

4. **4 Vasopressin, also named ADH, is a hormone synthesized as a peptide prohormone in neurons in the hypothalamus. A head injury can result in an excess secretion of ADH, resulting in hyponatremia, which is triggered by the retaining of water and concentrated urine.**
   1 Diaphoresis (excessive sweating) causes a loss of fluids, but it is not associated with a head injury. **2** Although dilated pupils are associated with some forms of head injury, this condition is not associated with an excess of ADH. **3** Hypotension is not associated with ADH levels.
   Client Need: Physiological Integrity; **Cognitive Level:** Application; **Nursing Process:** Assessment

5. **2 Anorexia, bulimia, starvation diets, or high fat–no carbohydrate diets can lead to metabolic acidosis.**
   1 Respiratory conditions, such as asthma, can result in respiratory acidosis. **3** Heavy menstrual periods can result in iron-deficiency anemia. **4** Diabetes insipidus is associated with ADH secretion and can result in an imbalance of sodium.
   Client Need: Physiological Integrity; **Cognitive Level:** Analysis; **Nursing Process:** Assessment

6. **1 Determining the client's acceptance or rejection of therapeutic therapies is important for the nurse to ensure adherence to the treatment.**
   2 Although an appropriate intervention, food and fluid preferences can be addressed after assessing for an acceptance of the treatment. **3** Although an appropriate intervention, supporting religious practices has less priority than understanding the client's feelings concerning the treatment and accepting that treatment. **4** Although an appropriate intervention, completing a medication history is standard when caring for all clients; it is not necessarily related to cultural or religious sensitivity.
   Client Need: Psychosocial Integrity; **Cognitive Level:** Applications; **Nursing Process:** Assessment

7. **3 Sunken eyes that feel soft to palpation is a symptom of severe FVD.**
   1 Excessive tearing is not a sign of FVD but possibly a sign of allergies. **2** Bloodshot eyes are not a sign of FVD but possibly a sign of allergies or an infection. **4** Itchy eyes are not a sign of FVD but possibly a sign of allergies.
   Client Need: Physiological Integrity; **Cognitive Level:** Application; **Nursing Process:** Assessment

8. **3 In a situation with FVD, the skin slowly returns to normal, and it may take seconds to do so.**
   1 Minor bruising is not directly related to fluid volume, but it may relate to a possible coagulation issue. **2** FVDs do not exhibit dry, redden skin. **4** Skin tears are not directly related to fluid volume, but they may indicate a possible age-related skin change.
   Client Need: Physiological Integrity; **Cognitive Level:** Analysis; **Nursing Process:** Evaluation

9. **3 The technique to measure capillary refill requires initially applying pressure to a nail bed for 5 seconds.**
   1 Applying pressure for 2 seconds is insufficient when assessing capillary refill. **2** Applying pressure for 4 seconds is insufficient when assessing capillary refill. **4** Applying pressure for 7 seconds is overly aggressive when assessing capillary refill.
   Client Need: Physiological Integrity; **Cognitive Level:** Application; **Nursing Process:** Evaluation

10. **2 A slower capillary refill can be due to the constriction of peripheral vessels. Smokers will have a slower capillary refill because of the effects of nicotine.**
    1 Asthma does not directly produce peripheral vessel constriction. **3** Fainting does not directly produce peripheral vessel constriction, but it may be caused by poor perfusion of the brain. **4** Iron

does not directly produce peripheral vessel constriction; it would be a possible concern in diagnosing anemia.

Client Need: Physiological Integrity; **Cognitive Level:** Application; **Nursing Process:** Assessment

11. **3 A reduction of approximately 3400 calories is required to lose 1 pound of tissue mass.**

    1 A reduction of 900 calories would be insufficient for the loss of 1 pound of tissue weight since such a loss requires a reduction of 3400 calories. **2** A reduction of 1200 calories would be insufficient for the loss of 1 pound of tissue weight since such a loss requires a reduction of 3400 calories. **4** A reduction of 5200 calories would be more than sufficient for the loss of 1 pound of tissue weight since such a loss requires a reduction of only 3400 calories.

    Client Need: Health Promotion and Maintenance; **Cognitive Level:** Understanding; **Integrated Process:** Teaching and Learning

12. **Answers: 1, 2, 3, 5**

    Measurable sources of output include urine, body drainage such as menses and wound drainage, and emesis. **4** Perspiration is not measured but may be estimated in extreme cases.

    Client Need: Physiological Integrity; **Cognitive Level:** Understanding; **Nursing Process:** Planning

13. **Answers: 2, 4, 5**

    Conditions that increase the risk for dehydration include diabetes insipidus, burns, and cognitive impairment with inhibited motor function.

    1, 3 Both acute heart failure and late-stage kidney failure are risk factors for fluid overload.

    Client Need: Physiological Integrity; **Cognitive Level:** Analysis; **Nursing Process:** Assessment

14. **4 Despite ingestion of food high in sodium, the blood level of sodium is balanced and regulated by the kidneys. Impaired kidney function would increase the risk for hypernatremia.**

    1 Neither age nor asthma are risk factors for a sodium imbalance. **2** Although smoking is a general health risk, it is not a specific factor for the development of a sodium imbalance. **3** A head injury is not generally considered a risk factor for the development of a sodium imbalance.

    Client Need: Physiological Integrity; **Cognitive Level:** Analysis; **Nursing Process:** Assessment

15. **2 Hyponatremia exists when the serum sodium level is below 136 mEq/L. Cerebral changes due to excitability of the CNS and increased intracranial pressure make it important to provide careful assessment of the client's level of consciousness and mental status.**

    1 Hyponatremia exists when the serum sodium level is below 136 mEq/L. Cardiac changes are not generally the primary changes associated with hyponatremia. **3** Hyponatremia exists when the serum sodium level is below 136 mEq/L. Respiratory changes are not the primary changes associated with hyponatremia. **4** Hyponatremia exists when a serum sodium level is below 136 mEq/L. GI changes are not the primary changes associated with hyponatremia.

    Client Need: Physiological Integrity; **Cognitive Level:** Application; **Nursing Process:** Assessment

16. **3 A serum sodium level over 145 mEq/L is the accepted criterion for a diagnosis of hypernatremia.**

    1 Although diarrhea is associated with hypernatremia, there are other possible causes. **2** Although dizziness is associated with hypernatremia, there are other possible causes. **4** Although hyperactive bowel sounds are associated with hypernatremia, there are other possible causes.

    Client Need: Physiological Integrity; **Cognitive Level:** Analysis; **Nursing Process:** Assessment

17. **1 Serum potassium level can be falsely elevated as a result of the blood sample being left at room temperature, since blood hemolyzes and releases potassium.**

    2 The time of day is not relevant to a falsely elevated serum potassium level. **3** Smoking is not relevant to a falsely elevated serum potassium level, but it would affect capillary refill time. **4** Cardiac rate is affected by potassium levels, but it is not relevant to a falsely elevated serum potassium level.

    Client Need: Physiological Integrity; **Cognitive Level:** Analysis; **Nursing Process:** Assessment

18. **Answers: 2, 3, 4**

    Hypoactive bowel sounds, altered mental state, and an irregular heartbeat are symptoms and signs associated with hypokalemia.

1 A serum potassium level of 3.8 mEq/L is within the normal range. **5** Constipation, rather than diarrhea, is associated with hypokalemia.

Client Need: Physiological Integrity; **Cognitive Level:** Application; **Nursing Process:** Assessment

19. **3 The normal potassium level in the blood is between 3.5 and 5.0 mEq/L. A serum potassium level greater than 5.0 mEq/L is considered hyperkalemia.**

    1 The normal serum potassium level in the blood is between 3.5 and 5.0 mEq/L; 3.0 mEq/L is considered hypokalemic. **2** The normal serum potassium level in the blood is between 3.5 and 5.0 mEq/L; 4.0 mEq/L is within the normal range. **4** The normal serum potassium level in the blood is between 3.5 and 5.0 mEq/L; 6.0 mEq/L is well above the criteria for diagnosing hyperkalemia.

    Client Need: Physiological Integrity; **Cognitive Level:** Understanding; **Integrated Process:** Teaching and Learning

20. **4 The tissue most excited by potassium is cardiac tissue. The heart is extremely sensitive to serum potassium increases, which can lead to heart block and ventricular fibrillation.**

    1 Nerve tissue is excited by potassium, but it is not as sensitive nor as dramatically affected by these changes as is cardiac tissue. **2** Normal kidney tissue is not as sensitive to potassium as is cardiac tissue. **3** Muscle tissue is excited by potassium, but it is not as sensitive nor as dramatically affected by these changes as is cardiac tissue.

    Client Need: Physiological Integrity; **Cognitive Level:** Understanding; **Integrated Process:** Teaching and Learning

Sodium Imbalance 6

SODIUM IMBALANCE OVERVIEW

Significance of Sodium

- Sodium is the most plentiful solute in the extracellular fluid (ECF) and comprises 90% of ECF cations.
  - Serum sodium is represented by the chemical symbol Na^+.
  - Sodium is the principle electrolyte.
  - Sodium is measured in serum levels.
  - Primary determinate of the osmolarity of the ECF
    - Normal osmolarity: between 275 and 300 mOsm/kg
  - Normal range of serum sodium: between 135 and 145 mEq/L
  - The amount of sodium inside the cell is approximately 10 mEq/L.
  - Sodium must be constantly pumped out of the cells into the bloodstream by the sodium-potassium pump.
  - Sodium attracts fluid to help maintain the ECF volume and fluid balance of the body.
    - Controls the distribution of water
    - Contributes to osmotic pressure
  - Sodium levels should be interpreted based on fluid status.
    - Dehydration can lead to an increase in serum sodium levels attributable to blood concentration.
    - Fluid excess can dilute sodium in the blood, resulting in decreased serum sodium levels.
  - Sodium is necessary for the transmission of nerve impulses.
    - An electrical charge is created by the movement of the sodium-potassium pump within the cells, which allows transmission of neuromuscular impulses.
  - Cerebral cells are highly sensitive to changes in the sodium level and fluid volume.
    - Brain cells swell with hyponatremia.
    - Brain cells shrink with hypernatremia.
    - Both changes can result in seizures, coma, and death.
  - Sodium combines with bicarbonate and chloride to maintain acid-base balance.

Control of Sodium

- Dietary ingestion of sodium and intestinal absorption of electrolytes determine the serum sodium level.
- Sodium requirements vary according to age and size.
- A person should ingest at least 0.5 to 2.7 grams of sodium per day.
- Due to imbalanced nutrition and poor dietary intake, people tend to ingest approximately 6 grams of sodium per day.
- Thirst
  - Thirst is the desire to drink fluid and is triggered by the thirst center, which is located in the anterior hypothalamus.
  - Osmoreceptors respond to changes in fluid osmolarity and fluid volume of the blood.

- An increase in blood osmolarity or the sodium levels causes a shift of fluid from the intracellular fluid (ICF) compartment to the ECF compartment, which causes cells to shrink.
- The shrinking cells stimulate the thirst mechanism.
- The thirst mechanism transmits signals to the cerebral cortex of the brain, increasing the desire to consume fluids.
- By drinking fluids, the ECF volume is increased, reducing osmolarity.
- Hemorrhage and trauma can also trigger the thirst mechanism.
- Kidney function
  - The kidneys work to excrete excess amounts of sodium in the blood.
  - Hormonal regulatory mechanisms in the body help control and maintain sodium levels by influencing the concentration of sodium in the blood through kidney function.
  - Aldosterone, from the adrenal gland, and antidiuretic hormone (ADH), or vasopressin, from the pituitary gland, adjust the way the kidneys respond with water and sodium to maintain the appropriate total amount of sodium and water in the body.
- Gastrointestinal (GI) tract
  - The rate of sodium absorbed from the GI tract is proportional to intake.
  - Sodium is excreted with waste products from the GI tract.
  - Clients with stomach and bowel disorders may have more problems with electrolyte absorption and excretion.
  - Clients with suction are at risk for sodium imbalances.
- Skin
  - Sodium is excreted through the skin with perspiration.
  - Diaphoresis increases the amount of sodium excreted.
  - Clients with increased temperature should be monitored for increased loss of water through the skin.
  - Strenuous activity increases the amount of perspiration produced.
  - Hot and humid climates may increase the amount of sodium and water lost through the skin.
  - Respirations
  - Normal breathing results in total body water loss each day.
  - Increased respirations can result in increased amounts of water lost and can affect electrolyte balance.
  - Clients experiencing pain and anxiety may have increased respirations, which can result in excess water loss.
- Renin-angiotensin-aldosterone system (RAAS)
  - RAAS is triggered by decreased renal perfusion.
  - RAAS is caused by low fluid volume, low blood pressure, dehydration, and low cardiac output.
  - Low renal perfusion stimulates renin secretion by the kidney's juxtaglomerular mechanism.
  - Renin begins the RAAS to increase blood volume and blood pressure.
  - Renin converts angiotensin to angiotensin I.
  - Angiotensin-converting enzymes (ACE) in the lungs change angiotensin I into angiotensin II.
  - Angiotensin II is a vasoconstrictor.
  - Angiotensin II binds to receptors in the adrenal cortex to cause the manufacture and release of aldosterone.
- Hormones
  - Increased sodium levels trigger the thirst mechanism, and the posterior pituitary gland releases the ADH.

- In response to the ADH, the kidneys retain water to help dilute the blood volume and restore normal osmolality.
- As the sodium level decreases, osmolality decreases, thirst and ADH are stopped, and the kidneys begin to excrete more water.
- Aldosterone uses a feedback loop to regulate sodium.
  - Aldosterone is a steroidal hormone produced in the adrenal cortex in the adrenal gland.
  - Aldosterone is necessary for sodium conservation.
  - It works to conserve sodium in the sweat glands, colon, kidneys, and salivary glands.
  - Aldosterone manages homeostatic regulation of sodium, potassium, and blood pressure.
  - Aldosterone acts on the mineralocorticoid receptors of the distal tubules in the kidneys and in the ducts of the nephrons.
  - Aldosterone affects the reabsorption of sodium and the excretion of potassium from the kidneys.
  - This reabsorption affects water retention, water excretion, blood volume, and blood pressure.
  - Antihypertensive drugs can interfere with the action and production of aldosterone.
- Natriuretic peptides
  - Natriuretic peptides initiate the process of natural diuresis by the body.
  - Three major peptides
    - Atrial natriuretic peptide (ANP)
      - Produced by the atria of the heart
      - Secreted when excess fluid volume expands the chambers of the atria
      - Stimulates natriuresis at the glomerulus
      - Increases glomerular filtration rate
    - Brain natriuretic peptide (BNP)
      - Produced by the ventricles of the heart
      - Excreted in response to ventricles being stretched by fluid volume overload
      - Stimulates natriuresis at the glomerulus
      - Increases glomerular filtration rate
    - C-type natriuretic peptide (CNP)
      - Produced by endothelial cells of the arteries
      - Produced by the ventricular cells of the heart
      - Limited diuretic effect
- Sodium-potassium pump (Figure 6.1)
  - The sodium-potassium pump is an active transport mechanism that helps maintain stable sodium levels in the body.
  - With diffusion, sodium tends to move inward toward the cells, potassium tends to move outward toward the ECF.
  - To counteract this natural tendency, the sodium-potassium pump is at work in every cell of the body.
  - The sodium-potassium pump requires energy in the form of adenosine triphosphate (ATP).
  - ATP consists of phosphorous and magnesium.
  - Phosphorous and magnesium drive sodium out of the cell and potassium into the inside of the cell wall.
  - The sodium-potassium pump works to prevent swelling of the cells.
  - An electrical charge is created by the movement of the sodium-potassium pump, which allows transmission of neuromuscular impulses.

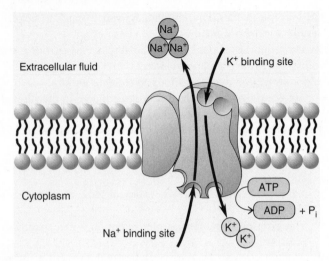

FIGURE 6.1 Schematic drawing of sodium-potassium. (From Banasik, J. L., & Copstead, L. E. C. [2019]. *Pathophysiology*, [6th ed.]. St. Louis: Elsevier.)

- Sodium has many functions.
  - Maintains blood volume
  - Maintains blood pressure
  - Necessary for the transmission of nerve impulses
  - Required for the function of the sodium-potassium pump
  - Maintains osmotic pressure
  - Maintains balance between acid and base
  - Produces muscular work and activity
  - Promotes the flow of water between sections on a cellular level

APPLICATION AND REVIEW

1. Which information accurately applies to sodium?
   1. Is the most common extracellular electrolyte.
   2. Its chemical symbol is S^+.
   3. It controls the distribution of water.
   4. Normal serum sodium levels are between 275 and 300 mEq/L.
   5. It contributes to osmotic pressure.
2. Which action places a client at risk for an increase in serum sodium levels?
   1. Drinking a 6-cup pot of caffeine coffee over 5 hours.
   2. Eating 1 cup of salty peanuts while watching television.
   3. Administering 1000 cubic centimeters (cc) of intravenous (IV) fluid over 2 hours.
   4. Running a 10-mile race on a hot August day.
3. Which human cell is most highly sensitive to sodium levels and volume fluid shifts?
   1. Cardiac
   2. Kidney
   3. Brain
   4. Skin

4. How much sodium should a nurse suggest as being an acceptable amount for daily consumption?
   1. Only 1 to 2 grams
   2. At least 0.5 to 2.7 grams
   3. Between 3 and 4 grams
   4. No more than 6 grams
5. Which effect does the anterior hypothalamus have on fluid and electrolyte balance if it is damaged?
   1. Brain cells shrink, causing a decrease in sodium levels.
   2. Serum osmolarity is increased by the need to consume fluids.
   3. ECF volume is increased, and osmolarity is decreased.
   4. The thirst center is affected, resulting in an altered need to drink fluids.
6. Which substances are influential in the regulation of the kidneys' role in sodium management? *(Select all that apply.)*
   1. Water
   2. Potassium
   3. Aldosterone
   4. Vasopressin
   5. ADH
7. Which medical condition places the client at risk for a sodium disorder?
   1. Bladder infection
   2. Red, itchy facial rash
   3. Mitral valve prolapse
   4. Irritable bowel syndrome
8. How does anxiety directly affect water loss?
   1. It increases vasoconstriction.
   2. It decreases kidney function.
   3. It increases respiratory rate.
   4. It decreases the thirst drive.
9. Which detail is the direct physiological response triggered by ADH?
   1. Thirst response
   2. Retention of fluid
   3. Conservation of serum sodium
   4. Decreased serum osmolality
10. Which physiological process counteracts the natural tendencies for the movement of sodium and potassium?
    1. Diffusion
    2. Sodium-potassium pump
    3. BNP
    4. ANP

See Answers on pages 128–130.

Sources of Sodium

- Dietary sources of sodium are primarily through the ingestion of sodium chloride with food.
  - Sources of sodium in the diet occur with the daily ingestion of sodium chloride.
  - Major dietary sources of sodium: canned soups; canned vegetables; processed meats; table salt; processed snack foods (chips, crackers); seafood; condiments, such as ketchup and soy sauce; cheese; fast food
  - Sodium may be hidden in medications for the treatment of colds and coughs.
  - Some antacids contain sodium.
  - A diet high in sodium can increase the loss of calcium in the urine.
  - Loss of calcium triggers the removal of calcium from the bones.
  - Diets consisting of 3 grams or more per day of sodium can increase the risk of stomach cancer by irritating the stomach lining.
  - Current dietary recommendations
    - Limit sodium to no more than 2300 mg a day (approximately 1 teaspoon of salt).
    - For older adults and clients with hypertension, diabetes, or chronic kidney disease, the recommendation is to consume no more than 1500 mg (approximately two-thirds of a teaspoon) of sodium each day.

- ■ Try to avoid adding table salt to foods.
- ■ Shop for fresh foods rather than processed foods that are high in sodium.
- ■ Choose fresh or frozen vegetables over canned vegetables.
- ■ Try to prepare more meals at home to limit salt from meals eaten at fast food establishments.
- ■ Season foods with herbs, spices, and natural juices.
- ■ Check the labels of all foods, spices, herbs, and seasoning blends to assess salt content.
- ■ Current guidelines recommend limiting foods with more than approximately 480 mg of sodium per serving.
- Excess sodium intake is linked to kidney disease because of its effect on blood pressure.
- Chronic high blood pressure damages organs by injuring the blood vessels that supply them, and the kidneys are particularly vulnerable to such damage.

Hyponatremia

- Serum sodium levels less than 135 mEq/L
- Common electrolyte imbalance
- Deficient sodium in relation to the proportion of water in the body
- Severe hyponatremia, less than 125 mEq/L, has a high risk of mortality.
- A serum sodium level less than 120 mEq/L is considered a medical emergency.
- Older adult clients and postoperative clients are at a greater risk of developing hyponatremia.
- Nothing by mouth (NPO) status may place clients at risk of hyponatremia.
- Onset may be sudden or gradual.
  - Sudden onset is associated with increased risk of death.
  - Rapid fall greater than 120 mEq/L in sodium levels within 48 hours can cause significant symptoms.
  - A gradual decline over days and weeks may allow sodium to fall to 110 mEq/L with few symptoms.
- Pathophysiological factors
  - The majority of clients with hyponatremia is the result of decreased kidney function.
  - The kidneys are unable to excrete enough water, which allows dilution of sodium in the vascular system.
  - Continued action of ADH or diuretics affects urinary dilution.
  - Chronic diseases that can affect ADH are renal failure, heart failure, and cirrhosis.
  - Cells swell as a result of decreased ECF osmolality (Figure 6.2).
  - Severe cellular swelling can cause seizures, loss of consciousness, and irreversible neurological damage.
  - Swelling of the brain cells can inhibit the release of ADH, which leads to excess water elimination through the kidneys in the form of diluted urine.
  - The formation of diluted urine causes the body to respond with a loss of electrolytes.
  - Kidney dysfunction can cause hyponatremia.
    - ■ Failure of the nephrons to receive and excrete appropriate amounts of water
    - ■ Failure of the nephrons to excrete excess sodium
    - ■ Failure of the nephrons to reabsorb appropriate amounts of sodium
  - A drop in serum sodium levels causes fluids to shift.
  - Fluid moves by osmosis from the ECF compartment into the ICF compartment.
  - This fluid shift causes hypovolemia and possibly cerebral edema to develop.
  - Hyponatremia can develop when the vascular volume is diluted from excess water gain.
  - Inadequate sodium intake can cause hyponatremia.

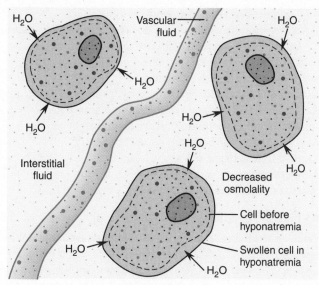

FIGURE 6.2   Cell swelling in hyponatremia. (From Banasik, J. L., & Copstead, L. E. C. [2019]. *Pathophysiology*, [6th ed.]. St. Louis: Elsevier.)

- Hyponatremia classifications
  - Depletional hyponatremia (inadequate sodium intake)
  - Hypovolemic hyponatremia
    - Sodium and water decrease in the ECF compartment.
    - Sodium loss exceeds water loss.
    - Causes: vomiting; diarrhea; gastric suctioning; excessive sweating; fistulas; burns; wound drainage; cystic fibrosis; osmotic diuresis; adrenal insufficiency; diuretic drugs; nephritis
    - Signs and symptoms: thirst; dry mouth; tachycardia; orthostatic hypotension; azotemia (abnormally high levels of urea and creatinine in the blood); oliguria (production of small amounts of concentrated urine)
- Hypervolemic hyponatremia
  - Water and sodium levels increase in the ECF compartment.
  - More water is gained than sodium.
  - Serum sodium levels become diluted in the excess water.
  - Edema develops from the excess water gain.
  - Causes: renal failure; hypotonic IV fluids; heart failure; liver failure; hyperaldosteronism (increased aldosterone production by the adrenal glands)
  - Signs and symptoms: headache; lethargy; confusion; apathy; nausea; vomiting; diarrhea; muscle cramps; muscle spasms
- Isovolemic hyponatremia
  - Sodium levels are low as a result of increased amounts of isotonic fluid in the body.
  - Clients do not have edema or other signs of hypervolemia.
  - The presentation of total serum sodium levels is normal.
  - Causes: hypothyroidism; renal failure; glucocorticoid deficiency
- Syndrome of inappropriate antidiuretic hormone (SIADH)
  - Causes increased release of ADH
  - Results in increased water retention

- Disrupts normal sodium levels by dilution
- Causes: trauma; stroke; oral antidiabetic medications; chemotherapy; diuretics; hormones; barbiturates; cancer; chronic obstructive pulmonary disease; asthma; lung tumors; psycho-active drugs
- Drugs associated with hyponatremia
  - Diuretics: bumetanide; furosemide; hydrochlorothiazide; amiloride
  - Antipsychotics: fluphenazine; thiothixene; thioridazine
  - Antidiabetics: tolbutamide; chlorpropamide
  - Anticonvulsants: carbamazepine; acetazolamide
  - Anticoagulants: heparin
  - Antineoplastics: cyclophosphamide; vincristine
  - Sedatives: morphine; barbiturates

Nursing Care of the Client With Hyponatremia

- Assessment: neurological status; level of consciousness; apical heart rate; skin turgor; mucous membranes; signs of muscle twitching; signs of neuromuscular irritability; symptoms of edema; orthostatic blood pressures; hemodynamic monitoring; serum osmolality; serum sodium levels; urine sodium levels; urine-specific gravity; hematocrit values; plasma protein levels
- Diagnostic factors: serum sodium level less than 135 mEq/L; elevated plasma protein levels; increased urine-specific gravity; elevated urine sodium levels; elevated hematocrit; urine-specific gravity less than 1.010
  - Clients with SIADH may have increased urine-specific gravity and urine sodium levels greater than 20 mEq/L.
- Signs and symptoms: headaches; shortened attention span; lethargy; confusion; disorientation; irritability; tremors; weakness; muscle weakness; stupor; delirium; ataxia; psychosis, including hallucinations; seizures; coma
  - Signs and symptoms can vary, depending on how low the sodium level drops.
  - If hyponatremia occurs with hypovolemia, symptoms may include low blood pressure, tachycardia, orthostatic hypotension, decreased central venous pressure, decreased pulmonary artery wedge pressure, and/or decreased pulmonary artery pressure.
  - Clients with accompanying hypervolemia may experience elevated hemodynamics, including central venous pressure, pulmonary artery pressure, and/or pulmonary artery wedge pressure; edema; hypertension; rapid, bounding pulse; weight gain; shortness of breath; coughing; crackles in lung fields
- Goals of care
  - Return the serum sodium level to between 135 and 145 mEq/L.
  - Client will remain free from injury.
  - Prevent neurological complications when correcting the sodium deficit.
  - Fluid volume status will return to normal; no signs and symptoms of fluid volume deficit or fluid volume excess.
- Treatment
  - Varies, based on severity and cause
  - If hyponatremia was caused by SIADH, then examine the source of ADH and restrict water intake.
  - Diuretics may be administered if hyponatremia was caused by excess water.
  - Restrict fluid intake.
  - Administer oral sodium supplements.
  - Normal saline solution may be administered intravenously.

- Severe cases may require infusion of 3% or 5% saline solution.
  - The client should be in the intensive care unit.
  - Both 3% and 5% saline solutions should be administered slowly.
  - Normal saline solution is administered in small volumes.
  - Monitor for signs of fluid volume overload: crackles; edema; shortness of breath; bulging hand veins; jugular vein distention; edema
  - Saline is usually administered in conjunction with a diuretic agent, such as furosemide.
  - Tolvaptan is administered for the treatment of hypervolemic hyponatremia with a serum sodium of 125 mEq/L or less.
- Complications: seizures; coma; permanent neurological damage
- Nursing interventions
  - Identify clients at high risk.
    - Infants
    - Young children
    - Adults older than 60 years of age
    - Clients taking medications: antibiotics; IV solutions; diuretics; corticosteroids; over-the-counter medications
  - Restrict free water as ordered.
    - Give fluids in small amounts throughout the day.
    - Administer fluids high in electrolytes.
  - Increase sodium intake.
  - Obtain weight daily.
    - Clients should be weighed at the same time each day.
    - Clients should wear the same type of clothing with each measurement of weight.
  - Obtain, measure, and record all intake and output (I&O).
    - Record fluid intake from all sources at least every 8 hours.
    - Record fluid intake from parenteral medications: IV fluids; oral intake; any IV flushes; flushes for tube feedings
      - Record ice chips as approximately one-half their volume.
    - Record amount and type of all fluids lost by the client: urine; liquid stool; emesis; drainage (chest, wounds, nasogastric tubes); any fluids aspirated out of the body
      - Subtract any fluids used in tube irrigation from the total fluid output.
    - Measure output in calibrated containers.
      - Observe the container at eye level.
      - Record the amount using the bottom of the meniscus as a guide.
    - I&O collection can be delegated to unlicensed personnel, if properly instructed.
  - Assess skin turgor.
    - Avoid using the back of the hand to obtain skin turgor measurements in older adult clients.
    - The skin of the chest and forehead are best for determining turgor.
  - Complete frequent neurological assessments.
    - Monitor level of consciousness: alert; oriented (person, place, time, situation).
    - Assess for signs of stupor or coma.
    - Assess pupils for PERRLA (pupils equal, round, react to light, and accommodation).
    - Determine if the client is alert and oriented.
    - Compare alertness and orientation to the baseline.
  - Assess orthostatic blood pressures.
    - Assess blood pressure while the client is in the lying position.
    - Assess blood pressure with the client in the sitting position.

- Assist the client to a standing position, and assess blood pressure.
- A change greater than 10 mm Hg between readings indicates postural hypotension.
- Use caution as clients may experience dizziness and light-headedness.
- Document measurements.
- Monitor cardiac status.
  - Frequently assess apical heart rate for rate and rhythm.
  - Observe for jugular vein distention.
  - Observe for peripheral edema.
  - Palpate peripheral pulses.
- Assess for muscle twitching.
  - Establish a baseline for deep tendon reflexes, muscle strength, and tone.
  - Frequently monitor for changes in baseline.
- Report any changes in the level of consciousness to the primary care provider.
- Monitor serum sodium levels.
  - Normal serum sodium: between 135 mEq/L and 145 mEq/L
- Report significant changes in sodium level to the primary care provider.
- Monitor urine-specific gravity.
  - Normal: 1.000 and 1.030
- Assess serum osmolality.
  - Less than 275 mOsm/L indicates hyponatremia.
- Administer oral sodium supplements as ordered.
- Administer medications as prescribed.
  - Client may receive acetaminophen or other nonsteriodal antiinflammatory drugs (NSAIDs) for headaches.
  - Antiemetics may be administered to treat nausea and vomiting.
  - Antiepileptics may be administered to prevent or treat seizures.
  - Corticosteroids may be administered to decrease cerebral edema.
  - Arginine vasopressin-receptor antagonists may be administered to increase water excretion without sodium loss in some clients.
- Initiate and maintain IV access.
  - Closely monitor IV site for signs of infection or infiltration: redness; swelling; sluggish flow; leaking at site
- Administer prescribed IV fluids.
  - May administer small amounts of IV hypertonic saline solutions as ordered to increase the sodium level
  - All clients receiving hypertonic solutions should be closely monitored for cardiac dysrhythmias.
  - Hypovolemic hyponatremia may be treated with normal saline administered intravenously to restore fluid and sodium balance.
- Closely monitor IV sodium administration.
  - Avoid increasing the sodium level too quickly to prevent pulmonary edema and central nervous system (CNS) irritability.
  - Monitor for signs of pulmonary edema: anxiety; shortness of breath; labored breathing; tachypnea; coughing; orthopnea; cyanosis
- Educate the client and caregiver about medications and IV fluids.
- Teach the client and caregiver about the causes of hyponatremia.
- Teach the client and caregiver about foods high in sodium.

- Assess for symptoms of fluid volume overload with IV fluid administration: crackles; enlarged neck veins; full hand veins; shortness of breath; crackles
- Educate clients about the symptoms to report.
  - Teach clients the signs of sodium deficiency and when to report.
  - Provide education about specific diagnoses and the signs of exacerbation.
- Encourage clients to drink fluids containing electrolytes to replace fluids: broth; sports drinks; Pedialyte
- Educate the client and caregiver about fluid restrictions.
  - Evenly distribute fluid throughout the day.
  - Teach the client to consume fluids in moderation.
  - Portion liquids with small cups.
  - May use ice to wet mouth. One medium ice cube is equivalent to 1 ounce of water.
  - Take medications with soft food, such as applesauce, to conserve liquids.
  - Gum and sugar-free hard candy can stimulate salivary glands.
  - Be aware of hidden fluid in food: Jell-O; yogurt; fruit; vegetables; meat cooked in heavy liquids and gravies; any food that dissolves to liquid when warm
- Provide a safe environment.
  - Limit visitors.
  - Provide decreased stimuli.
  - Place the call light within reach.
- Reorient confused clients.
- Implement fall precautions.
  - Assess the risk for falls; clients with orthostatic hypotension are at a greater risk of falling.
  - Place the bed in the low position.
  - Lock the wheels of the bed.
  - Clear pathways.
  - Use nightlights.
  - Place assistive devices within reach of the client.
  - Place necessary items, such as water, telephone, and remote controls, in reach of the client.
  - Have the call light within reach.
  - Instruct the client to call for help with ambulating.
  - Encourage the family to sit with the client, if needed.
- Prepare for seizures.
  - Oxygen that is easily accessible
  - Suction equipment at the bedside
  - Padded side rails
  - Preparation for intubation
  - Preparation for cardiac defibrillation
- Documentation: neurological status; daily weight; orthostatic blood pressures; heart rate; I&O; serum sodium levels; urine-specific gravity; serum osmolality; periodic hemo-dynamic readings; safety interventions provided; client teaching; response to fluid restriction; response to any teaching; medications administered; IV fluid administered; seizure activity
- Prevention
  - Seek treatment for conditions that cause hyponatremia.
  - Take medications as prescribed and directed.
  - Maintain adequate fluid intake.

- Avoid drinking excessive amounts of tap water.
  - Monitor fluid output.
  - Increase fluid intake with strenuous activity or in hot, humid climates.

APPLICATION AND REVIEW

11. Which assessment data support the conclusion that a client is experiencing hyponatremia, resulting in blood loss? *(Select all that apply.)*
    1. Tachycardia
    2. Orthostatic hypertension
    3. Increased artery wedge pressure
    4. Increased central venous pressure
    5. Decreased pulmonary artery pressure

12. Which interventions should the nurse be prepared to implement when an admitted client is found to have a serum sodium level of 118 mEg/L and signs of fluid volume overload? *(Select all that apply.)*
    1. Monitor IV therapy of 0.9% normal saline.
    2. Monitor the client for signs of respiratory distress.
    3. Transfer the client to the intensive care unit.
    4. Administer furosemide as prescribed.
    5. Administer tolvaptan as prescribed.

13. Which of the following are considered risk factors for the development of hyponatremia? *(Select all that apply.)*
    1. Infancy
    2. Pregnancy
    3. Asian ethnicity
    4. Corticosteroid therapy
    5. History of cigarette smoking

14. How often will the nurse record fluid intake for a client experiencing a sodium imbalance?
    1. Every 2 hours
    2. Every 8 hours
    3. Every 12 hours
    4. Every 24 hours

15. Which fluids will the nurse record as lost fluids when strictly monitoring output? *(Select all that apply.)*
    1. Urine
    2. Emesis
    3. Liquid stool
    4. Nasogastric tube irrigate
    5. Chest tube drainage

See Answers on pages 128–130.

Hypernatremia

- Hypernatremia is less common than hyponatremia.
- Serum sodium levels are greater than 145 mEq/L.
- Serum sodium levels greater than 160 mEq/L are considered a medical emergency.
- Hypernatremia can occur with an excess or a decrease of body water.
- Is most commonly caused by the loss of water
- The risk is higher in older adults and breastfed infants.
- Is most common in older adults
  - May have decreased thirst sensation
  - May be unable to access fluids independently
- Hypernatremia may be sudden or gradual.
  - Sudden onset is associated with a greater risk of death.
- Kidney dysfunction places clients at a greater risk of developing hypernatremia.

- The kidney may be unable to react to ADH in the renal tubule, decreasing the ability of the body to reabsorb water.
- Clients with decreased glomerular filtration rates have low sodium and water reabsorption into the bloodstream, which causes the excretion of aldosterone.
- Aldosterone increases the rate of reabsorption of sodium and water from the tubules of the kidneys, increasing the sodium level.
- Clients with decreased thirst sensation or the ability to drink fluids are at an increased risk of developing hypertension.
- Hypernatremia is associated with an increased risk of death.
- Pathophysiological factors
  - When serum sodium levels increase, fluid begins to move from inside the cells into the vascular space to dilute the rising sodium level.
  - As fluid exits the cells, the cells shrink (Figure 6.3).
  - Cells respond by osmotically moving electrolytes across the cell membrane, changing the rest potentials of electrically charged membranes.
  - Within a very short time of excessive serum sodium levels, the body produces intracellular organic solutes in an attempt to improve cellular fluid volume and to protect the membranes from damage.
  - The dehydration and shrinking of the cell causes the client to develop changes in neurological functioning.
  - Clients may develop fluid volume overload if the amount of fluid shifting to the vascular space is significant.
  - Brain hemorrhage is possible as a result of the stretching and rupturing of connecting veins.
  - Deficient water volume is a cause of hypernatremia.
  - Hypernatremia occurs when the loss of water or the gain of sodium is significant.
  - A combination of water loss and sodium gain can contribute to the development of hypernatremia (Box 6.1)

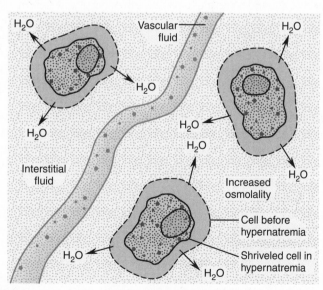

FIGURE 6.3   Cell shriveling in hypernatremia. (From Banasik, J. L., & Copstead, L. E. C. [2019]. *Pathophysiology*, [6th ed.]. St. Louis: Elsevier.)

| **BOX 6.1** | **Causes of Hypernatremia** |

Gain of Relatively More Salt Than Water	**Loss of Relatively More Water Than Salt**
Tube feeding	Diabetes insipidus (deficient antidiuretic hormone)
Intravenous infusion of hypertonic solution	Tube feeding (causes obligate water loss in urine)
Near drowning in salt water	Osmotic diuresis
Overuse of salt tablets	Prolonged emesis, diarrhea, or diaphoresis without
Food intake with reduced fluid intake	water replacement
Difficulty swallowing fluids	
No access to water	
Inability to respond to thirst	

From Banasik, J. L., & Copstead, L. E. C. (2019). *Pathophysiology,* (6th ed.). St. Louis: Elsevier.

- Hypernatremia is a development of a state of hyperosmolality.
- Sodium concentration is regulated by thirst, and urinary concentration is controlled by the pituitary gland and renal effects of the ADH.
- Fever and heat can result in several liters of insensible fluid loss. Types of insensible fluid loss include perspiration and respirations.
- Clients with hyperventilation can lose significant amounts of fluid through respirations.
- Burns can cause excessive fluid and sodium losses.
- Vomiting may result in a significant fluid loss, promoting an increased serum sodium level.
- Diarrhea can cause water loss, which can elevate sodium levels.
- Diuresis can cause large amounts of water to exit the body and affect the sodium level and can be a symptom of an illness or an effect of a drug.
- Excessive intake of sodium can also shift the fluid balance of the vascular space.
- Intake of high amounts of protein by diet or tube feedings can increase sodium levels.
- Diabetes insipidus can cause the loss of fluids in excess of 4 gallons per day. Severe dehydration and hypernatremia can result without adequate replacement.
- Cushing syndrome and excessive adrenocortical secretion are associated with high serum sodium levels.
- Increased sodium in the body from dietary sources, fluid administration, or medications can cause hypernatremia.
- Drugs associated with hypernatremia: cation exchange resins such as sodium polystyrene sulfonate (kayexalate); antacids; osmotic diuretics; antibiotics; IV fluids containing sodium chloride; sodium bicarbonate; salt tablets
- Assessment: heart rate; blood pressure; serum sodium levels; urine-specific gravity; urine osmolality; daily weight; history of fluid imbalances; current medications; signs of fluid volume overload (bounding pulses, weight gain, and bulging neck and hand veins); signs of fluid volume deficit (tachycardia, dry mucous membranes, and orthostatic hypotension)
- Diagnostic factors
  - Serum sodium levels greater than 145 mEq/L
  - Serum osmolality greater than 300 mOsm/kg
  - Urine-specific gravity greater than 1.030; may be decreased with diabetes insipidus
- Signs and symptoms:
  - Symptoms can vary, depending on cause of hypernatremia.
  - General symptoms: flushing; agitation; low-grade temperature; thirst; muscle twitching; weakness; lethargy

- If caused by increased sodium in the vascular space: bounding pulse; shortness of breath; elevated blood pressure; water retention; weight gain; mental changes; pulmonary edema; distended neck and hand veins
- If caused by fluid loss: orthostatic hypotension; thirst; irritability; flushed skin; oliguria (small amounts of concentrated urine); dry mucous membranes

- Goals of care
  - Return serum sodium levels to between 135 and 145 mEq/L.
  - The client will remain free from injury.
  - Fluid volume status will return to normal; no signs and symptoms of fluid volume deficit or fluid volume excess.
  - Prevent mortality. High mortality rates are associated with hypernatremia.
- Treatment
  - Depends on the cause of hypernatremia
  - Correct the underlying cause.
  - Provide oral fluid replacement.
  - Administer diuretic medications.
  - Provide dialysis.
  - Administer oral glucose-electrolyte replacement solutions for infants.
  - Gradually and slowly administer IV fluids.
  - Restrict food and fluids containing sodium.
  - If caused by diabetes insipidus: hypotonic fluid administration; diuretic administration
- Complications: seizures; coma; permanent neurological damage
- Nursing interventions
  - Identify clients at high risk.
    - Infants
    - Young children
    - Adults older than 60 years of age
    - Clients taking medications: antibiotics; IV solutions; diuretics; corticosteroids; over-the-counter medications
  - Decrease oral sodium intake.
    - Processed meats: luncheon meats; smoked fish; bacon; sausage
    - Canned goods: soups; vegetables; meats
    - Processed grains: crackers; cereals
    - Condiments: ketchup; margarine; pickles; salad dressings; soy sauce; Worcestershire sauce
    - Fast food
    - Snack food
    - Soda
  - Ensure adequate water intake. Clients without renal failure or heart failure may require higher than usual fluid intake to dilute sodium levels.
  - Monitor blood pressure.
  - Check pulse regularly.
  - Administer medications as prescribed: loop diuretics (furosemide); thiazide diuretics (hydrochlorothiazide).
  - Initiate IV access.
  - Monitor IV fluids.
    - Hypotonic IV fluids such as 0.225% or 0.45% sodium chloride may be administered if hypernatremia is caused by fluid loss.

- Isotonic fluids such as 0.9% normal saline may be administered if sodium and fluid loss are the issue.
- Be alert to the development of signs of cerebral edema: headache; vision changes; nausea; vomiting; inability to speak; stupor
- Frequently assess neurological status.
  - Monitor level of consciousness.
  - Assess for signs of stupor or coma.
  - Assess pupils for PERRLA.
  - Determine if the client is alert and oriented.
  - Compare alertness and orientation with the baseline.
- Carefully monitor I&O, and measure and record all I&O from all sources.
- Perform daily weights.
  - Weigh at the same time each day.
  - The client should wear the same type and amount of clothing.
- Assess skin for signs of breakdown.
- Evaluate serum sodium levels.
  - Normal serum sodium: between 135 and 145 mEq/L
- Monitor urine-specific gravity.
- Encourage the client to drink fluids to ensure adequate fluid intake.
- Record fluid intake from all sources at least every 8 hours: parenteral medications; IV fluids; oral intake; any IV flushes; flushes for tube feedings
  - Record ice chips as approximately one-half their volume.
- Record the amounts and types of all fluids lost by the client: urine; liquid stool; emesis; tube drainage (chest, wounds, nasogastric tubes); any fluids aspirated out of the body
  - Subtract any fluids used in tube irrigation from the total fluid output.
- Measure output in calibrated containers.
  - Observe the container at eye level.
  - Record the amount using the bottom of the meniscus as a guide.
- I&O collection can be delegated to unlicensed personnel, if properly instructed.
- Provide oral hygiene. Increased sodium levels cause dry mucous membranes.
- Initiate safety measures.
  - Reduce environmental stimuli.
  - Limit visitors.
  - Place the client in a room within view of the nurse.
- Institute fall precautions.
  - Assess the risk for falls.
  - Place the bed in the low position.
  - Lock the wheels of the bed.
  - Clear pathways.
  - Use nightlights.
  - Place assistive devices within reach of the client.
  - Place necessary items such as water, telephone, and remote controls within reach of the client.
  - Have the call light within reach.
  - Instruct the client to call for help with ambulating.
  - Encourage the family to sit with the client, if needed.
- Reorient the client as needed.

- Prepare for seizure activity.
  - Suction should be available at the bedside.
  - Oxygen should be available.
  - Pad the side rails.
  - Prepare for intubation.
  - Prepare for cardiac defibrillation.
- Client and caregiver education
  - Causes of sodium excess
  - Medical diagnoses
  - Interventions
  - Treatment recommendations
  - Instruct the client on how to prevent sodium excess.
    - Instruct the client on how to follow a low sodium diet.
    - Avoid foods high in sodium.
      - Foods low in sodium should contain less than 140 mg per serving.
      - Foods with very low sodium should contain less than 35 mg per serving.
      - Sodium-free foods should contain less than 5 mg per serving.
    - Recommend salt substitutes.
      - Teach the client to consult with the primary care provider for safety of using salt substitutes.
      - Some salt substitutes contain high amounts of potassium, which may be contra-indicated for those with heart failure or renal dysfunction.
    - Recommend seasoning foods with herbs, spices, and juices.
    - Instruct the client on reading food labels.
  - Educate the client and caregiver on common over-the-counter medications that can increase sodium, such as Alka-Seltzer and some antacids.
- Documentation: orthostatic blood pressures; heart rate; temperature; daily weight; I&O; safety measures initiated; client and caregiver education; serum sodium levels; urine-specific gravity; medications administered; response to medications; response to IV fluid administration
- Prevention
  - Educate clients and caregivers about the causes of hypernatremia: medical diagnoses; diets high in salt; dehydration; medications; increased perspiration
  - Include the signs and symptoms of hypernatremia in the teaching plans: thirst; tachycardia; restlessness; muscle spasms and cramps
  - Teach clients to take medications as prescribed.
  - Teach clients to report adverse drug effects.
  - Educate clients on dietary sources of sodium: canned soups; canned vegetables; processed meats; table salt; processed snack foods (chips, crackers); seafood; condiments, (ketchup, soy sauce); cheese; fast food

APPLICATION AND REVIEW

16. At which conclusion should the nurse arrive when a client's serum sodium level is 161 mEq/L?
    1. It is below normal limits and requires attention.
    2. It is within normal limits and does not require attention.
    3. It is above normal limits but not enough to require attention.
    4. It is considered a medical emergency and requires immediate attention.

17. Which assessment detail suggests the client is experiencing fluid volume overload?
    1. Reports of thirst
    2. Orthostatic hypotension
    3. Bilateral bulging hand veins
    4. Moist oral mucous membranes

18. For which client should the nurse consider as having a priority need for an assessment focused on possible hypernatremia?
    1. Client who is reporting to be lethargic.
    2. Client who is developing general weakness.
    3. Client who has developed a low-grade fever.
    4. Client noted to have muscle twitching in the face.

19. What is the primary goal of care for the client diagnosed with a sodium imbalance?
    1. Prevention of injury to the client
    2. Identification of the cause of the imbalance
    3. Education of the client to minimize the risk of a reoccurrence of the imbalance
    4. Selection of the appropriate treatment with input from health care professionals and the client

20. Which intervention included in the plan of care for an older adult client will **best** ensure adequate fluid intake?
    1. Encourage the client to include adequate fluids when selecting meal choices.
    2. Ensure that the client drinks fluids at least every 2 hours while awake.
    3. Place the priority on keeping accurate I&O records.
    4. Ensure that the client's favorite beverages are available.

See Answers on pages 128–130.

ANSWER KEY: REVIEW QUESTIONS

1. **Answer: 1, 3, 5**
   1 Sodium is the most plentiful solute in the ECF. **3** Sodium controls the distribution of water. **5** Sodium contributes to osmotic pressure.
   2 The chemical symbol is Na^+. **4** Normal serum sodium level is between 135 and 145 mEq/L.
   Client Need: Physiological Integrity; **Cognitive Level:** Understanding; **Integrated Process:** Teaching and Learning

2. **4 Dehydration, associated with sweating, can lead to an increase in serum sodium levels attributable to blood concentration.**
   1 Drinking 6 cups of fluid over 5 hours is going to cause an increase of serum sodium levels since it will not affect blood concentration. **2** Eating 1 cup of salty peanuts while watching television is not likely to affect blood concentration significantly. **3** Administering 1000 cc of IV fluid over 2 hours will likely result in a dilution of sodium by expanding vascular fluid levels.
   Client Need: Physiological Integrity; **Cognitive Level:** Analysis; **Nursing Process:** Analysis

3. **3 Cerebral (brain) cells are highly sensitive to changes in the sodium level and fluid volume.**
   1 Although affected, cardiac cells are not as sensitive to the sodium level and volume fluid shifts as are brain (cerebral) cells. **2** Although affected, kidney cells are not as sensitive to the sodium level and volume fluid shifts as are brain (cerebral) cells. **4** Although affected, skin cells are not as sensitive to the sodium level and volume fluid shifts as are brain (cerebral) cells.
   Client Need: Physiological Integrity; **Cognitive Level:** Understanding; **Integrated Process:** Teaching and Learning

4. **2 Although sodium requirements vary according to the age and size of a person, he or she should ingest at least 0.5 to 2.7 grams of sodium per day.**
   1, 3, 4 Although sodium requirements vary according to the age and size of a person, he or she should ingest at least 0.5 to 2.7 grams of sodium per day.
   Client Need: Physiological Integrity; **Cognitive Level:** Understanding; **Integrated Process:** Teaching and Learning

5. **4 Thirst is triggered by the thirst center, which is located in the anterior hypothalamus; damage to that portion of the brain would result in an impaired need to drink fluids.**

   1 Brain cells shrink in response to an increase in blood osmolarity and is not directly related to the anterior hypothalamus. **2** By drinking fluids, the ECF volume is increased, reducing osmolarity. **3** By drinking fluids, the ECF volume is increased, reducing osmolarity.

   Client Need: Physiological Integrity; **Cognitive Level:** Understanding; **Integrated Process:** Teaching and Learning

6. **Answers: 3, 4, 5**

   Aldosterone, from the adrenal gland, and ADH, or vasopressin, from the pituitary gland, adjust the way the kidneys respond with water and sodium to maintain the appropriate total amount of sodium and water in the body.

   1 Water is regulated, rather than serving as an influence. **2** Potassium is not relevant to the kidneys' role in sodium management.

   Client Need: Physiological Integrity; **Cognitive Level:** Understanding; **Integrated Process:** Teaching and Learning

7. **4 Clients with stomach and bowel disorders may have more problems with electrolyte absorption and excretion.**

   1 A bladder infection, although a serious problem, does not affect kidney function and therefore is not relative to sodium excretion. **2** Although sodium is excreted through the skin via perspiration, a rash would not affect that process. **3** A mitral valve issue would not directly affect sodium absorption or excretion.

   Client Need: Physiological Integrity; **Cognitive Level:** Analysis; **Nursing Process:** Analysis

8. **3 Clients experiencing pain and anxiety may have increased respirations, which can result in excess water loss.**

   1 Vasocontraction is not directly affected by anxiety. **2** Kidney function is not directly affected by anxiety. **4** The thirst drive is not directly affected by anxiety.

   Client Need: Physiological Integrity; **Cognitive Level:** Understanding; **Integrated Process:** Teaching and Learning

9. **2 In response to ADH, the kidneys retain water to help dilute the blood volume and restore normal osmolality.**

   1 The thirst response is triggered by several events but not by ADH. **3** Aldosterone is necessary for sodium conservation. **4** As sodium levels decrease, osmolality decreases, thirst and ADH are stopped, and the kidneys begin to excrete more water.

   Client Need: Physiological Integrity; **Cognitive Level:** Understanding; **Integrated Process:** Teaching and Learning

10. **2 To counteract the natural tendency of sodium and potassium movement, the sodium-potassium pump is at work in every cell of the body.**

    1 With diffusion, sodium tends to move inward toward the cells, and potassium tends to move outward toward the ECF. **3** BNP increases the glomerular filtration rate. **4** ANP increases the glomerular filtration rate.

    Client Need: Physiological Integrity; **Cognitive Level:** Understanding; **Integrated Process:** Teaching and Learning

11. **Answers: 1, 2, 5**

    If hyponatremia occurs with hypovolemia, symptoms may include tachycardia, orthostatic hypertension, and decreased pulmonary artery pressure.

    3 Clients with accompanying hypervolemia may experience an increase in artery wedge pressure. **4** Clients with accompanying hypervolemia may experience an increase in central venous pressure.

    Client Need: Physiological Integrity; **Cognitive Level:** Applying; **Nursing Process:** Assessment

12. **Answers: 2, 3, 4, 5**

    2 Fluid overload often results in respiratory distress. **3** A serum sodium level of 118 mEg/L is a medical emergency, and the client should be transferred to an intensive care unit for care. **4** The client's fluid status requires diuretic therapy. **5** Tolvaptan is prescribed for the treatment of hypervolemic hyponatremia with a serum sodium of 125 mEq/L or less.

    1 This client's condition would be treated with a slow infusion of a 3% or 5% saline solution rather than isotonic 0.9% normal saline.

    Client Need: Physiological Integrity; **Cognitive Level:** Analysis; **Nursing Process:** Planning

13. **Answers: 1, 4**

    Both infancy and corticosteroid therapy are considered risk factors for the development of hyponatremia. **2** Pregnancy does not necessarily raise the risk of hyponatremia. **3** Asian ethnicity is not a risk factor for hyponatremia. **5** Although a general health risk, smoking is not associated with an increased risk for hyponatremia.

    Client Need: Physiological Integrity; **Cognitive Level:** Understanding; **Integrated Process:** Teaching and Learning

14. **2 Fluid intake from all sources should be recorded at least every 8 hours.**

    1 Ordinarily, recording fluid intake this frequently is not necessary. **3, 4** Fluid intake from all sources should be recorded at least every 8 hours.

    Client Need: Physiological Integrity; **Cognitive Level:** Applying; **Nursing Process:** Implementation

15. **Answers: 1, 2, 3, 5**

    When monitoring lost fluids, urine, emesis, liquid stool, and chest tube drainage should be documented. **4** The amount of any fluids used in nasogastric tube irrigation should be subtracted from the total fluid output.

    Client Need: Physiological Integrity; **Cognitive Level:** Applying; **Nursing Process:** Implementation

16. **4 A serum sodium level greater than 160 mEq/L is considered a medical emergency.**

    1 Sodium levels below 135 mEq/L are considered low. **2** Normal sodium levels are between 135 and 145 mEq/L. **3** Serum levels above 145 mEq/L are high but not yet considered a medical emergency.

    Client Need: Physiological Integrity; **Cognitive Level:** Applying; **Nursing Process:** Evaluation

17. **3 Signs of fluid volume overload include bulging neck and hand veins.**

    1 Although unreliable, thirst is associated with a fluid volume deficit. **2** Orthostatic hypotension is associated with a fluid volume deficit. **4** Moist oral mucous membranes are associated with adequate hydration and fluid volume.

    Client Need: Physiological Integrity; **Cognitive Level:** Applying; **Nursing Process:** Analysis

18. **4 Of the general signs and symptoms of hypernatremia, muscle twitching is most specific to this sodium imbalance.**

    1 Lethargy is common and can be associated with a wide variety of causes. **2** General weakness is common and can be associated with a wide variety of causes. **3** A low-grade fever is associated with a variety of causes including hypernatremia but also with bacterial infections.

    Client Need: Physiological Integrity; **Cognitive Level:** Analysis; **Nursing Process:** Assessment

19. **1 Prevention of injury and the preservation of client safety is the primary goal of client care.**

    2 Although an appropriate goal, identifying the cause of the imbalance is not the primary concern. **3** Although an appropriate goal, client education is not the primary concern. **4** Although an appropriate goal, collaborative treatment is not the primary concern.

    Client Need: Physiological Integrity; **Cognitive Level:** Analysis; **Nursing Process:** Planning

20. **2 Being aware of the client's fluid intake by physically ensuring the ingestion of fluids is the most effective way to address this client's fluid needs.**

    1 Although appropriate, encouraging, alone, is not the most effective intervention to ensure adequate fluid intake. **3** Although appropriate, monitoring and accurately documenting I&O is not the most effective intervention to ensure adequate fluid intake. **4** Although appropriate, keeping favorite beverages available is not the most effective intervention to ensure adequate fluid intake.

    Client Need: Physiological Integrity; **Cognitive Level:** Analysis; **Nursing Process:** Implementation

CHLORIDE IMBALANCE OVERVIEW

Significance of Chloride

- The major anion in the blood is chloride.
  - Chloride is represented by the chemical symbol Cl^-.
  - Chloride is the first electrolyte to be measured.
  - It is the "queen" of electrolytes.
    - Sodium is the principle electrolyte.
    - Molecular weight of chloride is 35.5.
    - Chloride is the human body's chief anion.
    - Chloride accounts for 70% of the total negative ion content in the human body.
  - Chloride accounts for approximately 33% of plasma tonicity (osmolarity of a solution compared with plasma).
    - Hypertonic
    - Isotonic
    - Hypotonic
  - On average, an adult body is comprised of 115 grams of chloride, which makes up 0.15% of the aggregate body weight.
  - Chloride has many functions.
    - Maintains osmotic pressure
    - Maintains balance between acid and base
    - Produces muscular work and activity
    - Promotes the flow of water among sections at a cellular level

APPLICATION AND REVIEW

1. The nurse is monitoring a client's serum chloride. The laboratory result associated with which chemical symbol is relevant?
   1. Ca
   2. Cl^-
   3. Cr
   4. Ce
2. The nurse is teaching a group of clinical nursing students about the functions of chloride. Which information should the nurse include about the functions of chloride? *(Select all that apply.)*
   1. Maintaining osmotic pressure
   2. Producing muscular work and activity
   3. Maintaining a balance between acid and base
   4. Promoting healthy nerve and muscle function
   5. Promoting the flow of water among sections at the cellular level

See Answers on pages 146–148.

Sources of Chloride

- Dietary sources of chloride are primarily found through the ingestion of sodium (Na^+) and food containing chloride.
  - Sources of chloride in the diet occur with the daily ingestion of sodium chloride (NaCl).
    - The daily oral intake of chloride is approximately 150 mmol/L, which is equal to a liter of 0.9% saline a day.
    - For adult men, this intake is between 7.8 and 11.8 g/day, which is equal to between 133 and 201 mmol/day.
    - For adult women, this intake is between 5.8 and 7.8 g/day, which is equal to between 99 and 133 mmol/day.
  - Chloride must be consumed by a person in his or her diet.
  - The primary source of chloride in the diet is table or sea salt.
    - 0.5 teaspoon equals 750 mg of chloride.
  - Other food sources of chloride include dairy products, meat, and processed foods; any food high in Na^+ is also high in chloride.
  - Percentages of the U.S. diet that can provide sources of NaCl
    - Salt (restaurants, fast food, and home): 29%
    - Breads, grains, and cereals: 19%
    - Poultry, red meats, and eggs: 12%
    - Dairy items: 8%
    - Gravies: 7%
    - Soy and teriyaki sauces: 4%
    - Soups: 3%
    - Pickles and olives: 1.5%
    - Baking powder and baking soda: 1.4%
    - Margarines: 1.3%
  - Chloride has many functions.
    - Maintains osmotic pressure
    - Balances acids and bases
    - Promotes muscular activity
    - Promotes the movement of water between fluid sections

Control of Chloride

- Review of the key principles of acid-base balance
  - Hydrogen (H^+) ions are the smallest ions (atomic weight of 1).
  - H^+ ions comprise the smallest concentration in the body.
    - H^+ ions, although small, are important.
    - H^+ ions are responsible for driving the production of adenosine triphosphate (ATP).
    - From the perspective of providing energy from fuel oxidation, the charge on proton is more important than the concentration.
  - An acid is a mixture that can donate an H^+ ion.
  - A base is a mixture that is able to accept an H^+ ion.
  - H^+ concentration in body fluids is a narrow range that must be maintained for health.
  - If the concentration of H^+ rises, it will bind with other compounds (proteins) and change the shape, charge, and potentially the function with dire outcomes.
  - A concentration high in H^+ stimulates breathing.

- When work is performed by the body, energy is provided when the high-energy ATP phosphate bond is hydrolyzed and results in the production of the antidiuretic hormone (ADH).
- Electrolytes are the primary component of body fluids—extracellular fluid (ECF) and total water content.
- Water is the most plentiful molecule in the body.
  - On average, 60% of the adult body is comprised of water.
  - Over 66% of the water in the human body is found inside cells.
  - The percentage of body weight relative to water is dependent on the amount of muscle and fat in the human body.
  - Skeletal muscle consists of the largest organ in the human body. Therefore one-half of the entire body of water is situated in the ECF or intracellular fluid (ICF) compartments of muscle.
  - Women have a have a greater percentage of body fat than men (60% versus 50%) and therefore have a decreased amount of water.
  - Older adults have a smaller proportion of muscle and therefore have less water per body weight.
  - Newborns are made up of almost 70% of water, which is due to less adipose tissue.
  - Fat stores vary among individuals.
  - Adults who are obese have higher fat stores and therefore have less water as a percentage of body weight.
  - Water crosses the cell membranes until an osmotic equilibrium is achieved.
  - Particles confined to the ECF area are Na^+, attendant anions chloride, and bicarbonate (HCO_3^-).
  - Na^+ that enters the ICF compartment is transferred out of the cell by the Na^+-potassium (K^+)-adenosinetriphosphatase (ATPase) positioned in the cell membranes.
- Chloride assists with stabilizing metabolic acid-base balance.
- Chloride in the body combines with cations (positively charged ions) to form NaCl, potassium chloride (KCl), calcium chloride ($CaCl_2$), and hydrochloric acid (HCl).
- Chloride provides electroneutrality, in particular with Na^+ and K^+.
- Chloride and Na^+ work together to balance osmotic pressure.
- Normal serum chloride values
  - Newborns: between 98 and 104 mEq/L
  - Infants: between 95 and 110 mEq/L
  - Children: between 101 and 105 mEq/L
  - Adult: between 95 and 110 mEq/L
  - Critical level: less than 80 mEq/L and greater than 115 mEq/L
- The ECF contains 80% of the chloride in the body, which is the largest concentration in the lymph and interstitial fluids.
- Cerebrospinal fluid is comprised of NaCl.
- Chloride is found in specialized cells, such as the nerve cells.
- Absorption of chloride primarily occurs in the colon.
  - Absorption rate of chloride exceeds Na^+ in the colon.
  - Chloride is absorbed to a lesser degree in the ileum when exchanged with HCO_3^-.
  - The stomach produces chloride in the form of HCl.
- Chloride is excreted by the renal system.
  - 90% of chloride is excreted in the urine.
  - Remaining 10% is excreted in sweat and feces.

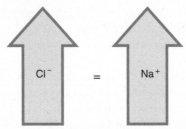

FIGURE 7.1 When body fluids are alkalotic, more chloride and sodium are reabsorbed by the kidneys. (From Chernecky, C., Macklin, D., & Murphy-Ende, K. [2006]. *Saunders nursing survival guide: Fluids and electrolytes*, [2nd ed.]. St. Louis: Saunders.)

- Rate of excretion is dependent on the amount of chloride ingested and adequate hydration and fluid.
- Acid-base balance is accomplished by the renal tubules.
  - Reabsorption of chloride is accomplished in response to the pH level of the ECF.
  - Chloride is vying with HCO_3^- for Na^+.
  - Acidic body fluids result in the excretion of NaCl by the kidneys.
    - HCO_3^- is reabsorbed.
  - Basic body fluids (alkalotic) result in the retention of NaCl by the kidneys (Figure 7.1).
    - There is an inverse relationship with chloride and HCO_3^- levels.
- Cystic fibrosis is an autosomal recessive genetic disease that involves chloride imbalance.
  - Results in an abnormal chloride transport
  - Results in a lack of NaCl in secretions from the endocrine glands: pancreas; intestine; bronchi
  - The bronchi and pancreas are blocked by thick mucus, resulting in malabsorption, steatorrhea, chronic pancreatitis, sweat with high chloride content, and respiratory infections.
- Role of chloride
  - The major roles of NaCl in the body are controlling the osmotic pressure and water balance and maintaining electroneutrality.
  - Chloride is vital for the production of HCl.
  - Chloride is a buffer and enzyme activator for HCl in the stomach.
    - In the stomach, HCl is essential for digestion.
    - Nausea, vomiting, or suctioning of stomach secretions can alter gastric juices and affect chloride levels.
  - Chloride aids in acid-base balance.
    - Chloride shift describes the process of how the pH in the body is maintained.
      - In response to low blood pH
      - The diffusion of HCO_3^- (a weak acid ion) occurs as movement from the red blood cells to the plasma.
      - In exchange of chloride (a strong acid ion) occurs as movement from the plasma to the red blood cells.

APPLICATION AND REVIEW

3. Which client understands the education regarding the necessary daily requirements of chloride?
   1. Man who consumes 6 grams per day
   2. Woman who consumes 7.6 grams per day
   3. Man who consumes 12 grams per day
   4. Woman who consumes 12.8 grams per day

4. A client receiving nutritional information should learn that chloride is best introduced into the diet by consuming what?
   1. Green, leafy vegetables
   2. Animal protein
   3. Dairy products
   4. Table salt

5. Which food choice best demonstrates the client's understanding of food sources that provide NaCl?
   1. Bowl of fortified cereal
   2. Cup of low fat yogurt
   3. Bowl of chicken soup
   4. Hardboiled egg

6. When considering the chemical composition of the human body, which element should the nurse assess when a client demonstrates a rapid respiratory rate?
   1. H^+
   2. Cl^+
   3. Na^+
   4. K^+

7. Which one of these clients has the smallest percentage of body water?
   1. Newborn girl
   2. 70-year-old man
   3. 25-year-old young man
   4. 25-year-old woman

8. The nurse identifies which individual as demonstrating an abnormal serum chloride level?
   1. Male newborn: 100 mEq/L
   2. 10-year-old girl: 104 mEq/L
   3. 35-year-old male adult: 108 mEq/L
   4. 55-year-old female adult: 115 mEq/L

9. The nurse understands that careful monitoring of serum chloride is **most** important in the care of a client with which medical diagnosis?
   1. Stomach cancer
   2. Kidney cancer
   3. Bladder cancer
   4. Colon cancer

10. Which intervention is a **priority** when caring for a client with _____ ____sis?
   1. Falls precautions
   2. Consuming a low-fat diet
   3. _____ ____ng respiratory function
   4. Monitoring for chronic constipation

See Answers on pages 146–148.

Functions of Chloride

- Chloride is one of the most integral extracellular anions.
- Chloride assists with many bodily functions.
  - Balance and maintenance of osmotic pressure
  - Maintenance of acid-base balance
  - Muscular activity
  - Movement of water between fluid compartments
- Descriptions of chloride channels
  - Pore-forming membrane proteins
  - Permitting chloride to be transported through membranes
  - Existing in any cell with a membrane and nucleus (eukaryotic cells)
  - Genetic studies have determined mutations in genes.
    - These changes in the gene encode chloride channels.
    - Mutations lead to a loss of chloride channel activity.
    - Loss of chloride functions can result in the evolution of a variety of diseases.
      - Dystrophia myotonica: decrease in conductance attributable to a loss of activity of the chloride channel (CIC-1)
      - Cystic fibrosis: defective permeability of cell membranes to the Na^+ or chloride ions
      - Chronic pancreatitis: trapped chloride and water in the cell as a result of the cystic fibrosis transmembrane conductance regulator (CFTR) gene and a defect in protein

- Bronchiectasis: surface mucus becomes thick and sticky as a result of the lack of movement of chloride and water in the cells
- Hereditary hyperekplexia: lowering of chloride conductance
- Epilepsy: dysfunction of chloride channels thought to inhibit the electrical activity in the neurons
- Cataracts: decreased movement of chloride channels of the lens through the plasma membrane
- Bartter syndrome: lower Na^+ and chloride reabsorption through a reduction in renal tubular chloride transport

- Chloride and the gastrointestinal (GI) tract
  - Chloride intake is important since it is absorbed by the intestinal track during digestion.
  - Chloride ions are secreted in HCl in gastric juices.
    - HCl promotes the digestion of protein.
    - HCl activates the conversion of pepsinogen to pepsin.
    - Pepsin is responsible for
      - Destroying foodborne pathogens
      - Controlling the overgrowth of fungus and bacteria in the small intestine
      - Promoting the secretion from the pancreas, including bile and other enzymes
      - Promoting the absorption of folic acid, ascorbic acid, betacarotene, nonheme iron, and some forms of calcium (Ca), magnesium, and zinc
    - HCl promotes the release of iron and its transformation to ferrous from the digestion of certain iron-rich foods.
      - Secretes 11 mmol of basal HCl per hour, increasing with meals to between 10 and 63 mmol
      - The HCl suspension has a pH of approximately 0.8 and contains 160 mmol of HCl per liter.
      - With the pH at 0.8, the H^+ concentration in the gastric acid is approximately three million times more than the pH of arterial blood, and this pH level is responsible for the effect of gastric acid.
      - On an average day, 8 liters of gastric fluid are released into the digestive tract and secreted into the intestinal tract.
      - HCl is the catalyst for the movement of fluid across the osmotic gradient into the mucosa and the opening of the intestine.
      - The osmotic gradient is accountable for transporting water into the intestine.
        - Primarily chloride and HCO_3^-
        - Na^+ travels across the paracellular space.
        - Three paths exist in which chloride can travel into the intestine, creating an osmotic gradient for the production of fluid.
          - CFTR
          - Ca-activated chloride channels (CaCCs)
          - Chloride type-2 channels (CICC-2)
- Extracellular space
  - A specific amount of chloride in serum is critical to make a diagnosis and to select the best treatment.
  - Plasma chloride concentrations can vary between assays.
  - Chloride is accountable for 100 out of 300 mOsm/L of ECF and accounts for more than 66% of negative charges in plasma.
  - Excess chloride is excreted in the urine.
  - Na^+ and chloride interact to control balance of serum osmolarity and fluid levels.

- Movements in Na^+ or chloride concentrations are catalysts for changes in fluid volume, obtaining a balance in normal solution, and restoring a balance in water ratios.
- To preserve acid-base balance, chloride and HCO_3^- have an inverse relationship.
  - The buffering system helps maintain a normal pH when the intestines or kidneys lose HCO_3^-.
  - Chloride and HCO_3^- shift in and out of cells, such as erythrocytes and tubules, to preserve acid-base balance.
  - Chloride is an important anion because of its large concentration.
    - Assists in maintaining equilibrium between extracellular cations and anions
    - Ensures the electrical impulses conduct charges
- Intracellular space
  - The presence of chloride is less in the intracellular space.
    - Muscle cells have an estimated resting membrane potential of -68 megavolt (mV) and a chloride level between 2 and 4 mEq/L.
    - Red blood cells (RBCs) have an estimated resting membrane potential of -15 mV and an average chloride concentration of 70 mEq/L.
    - The erythrocytes with higher intracellular chloride promote movement in and out of the RBCs.
  - The electrical charge on either side of the cell membrane determines the movement of chloride.
  - The chloride shift and the movement of chloride from plasma to erythrocytes are unique.
    - Blood flows from the arterial to the venous capillaries.
    - The chloride shift occurs because of bodies attempt to reestablish ratios for chloride and HCO_3^-, and there is a special HCO_3^-–chloride carrier protein in the RBC membrane.
    - Chloride content of the venous RBCs is larger than arterial RBCs.
    - Most of the carbon dioxide transported in the blood is through HCO_3^-.
    - The chloride shift is essential and promotes the capacity of the blood to carry HCO_3^-.
    - The function of the chloride shift is to lessen fluctuations in the pH.
- Kidneys and chloride
  - The regulation of chloride concentration is primarily performed through the GI tract and kidneys.
  - Chloride is primarily excreted through the kidneys.
  - An average of 19,440 mmol/day is filtered through the kidneys.
    - 99.1% of chloride is reabsorbed by the kidneys.
    - Only 180 mmol is excreted per day.
  - Reabsorption of Na^+, chloride, and HCO_3^- occurs in the renal proximal tubule.
  - Volume of chloride excreted in urine is determined by the amount included in the diet, infused, and required by the body.
  - Chloride ingested by diet and/or infusion or the amount required by the body determines how much chloride will be excreted in the urine daily.
  - The Henle loop is responsible for reabsorbing approximately 15% to 25% of filtered NaCl.
  - Aldosterone acts on the distal nephron to increase the reabsorption of Na^+ and chloride and to secrete K^+ and H^+.
    - Aldosterone deficiency, resistance, or inhibition can be exhibited in a variety of conditions— hyperkalemia, hyperchloremic acidosis, hyperkalemia, and renal tubular acidosis (RTA).
      - RTA is a syndrome attributable to a dysfunction in the renal tube and results in continual metabolic acidosis. Hyporeninemic hypoaldosteronism is the most common cause of RTA.
      - Often, older adults with diabetes and mild renal insufficiency have this disorder.

- The excretion of chloride by the kidneys is the mechanism for adapting to metabolic acidosis and chronic respiratory acid-base disturbance.
  - Metabolic acidosis
    - Kidney increases net acid excretion.
      - Ammonium chloride (NH_4Cl) excretion is enhanced.
      - A maximum is reached in 5 days.
      - Chloride ion excretion, without the associated increase in Na^+ ion excretion, is increased, returning HCO_3^- and transitioning the pH level toward normal.

Pathophysiological Conditions of Hypochloremia

- Hypochloremia
  - Serum level of chloride is less than 95 mEq/L.
  - Multiple causes of hypochloremia are based on how chloride is excreted through perspiration, the GI tract, and the kidneys.
  - Water gain in excess of chloride absorption is exhibited in congestive cardiac failure, syndrome of inappropriate antidiuretic hormone (SIADH) secretion, and excessive infusion of hypotonic IV solutions.
  - Chloride is a negative ion (anion).
    - Chloride is usually attached to a positive ion (cation), such as Ca or K^+.
    - A decrease in Na^+ or K^+ will result in a decrease in chloride levels.
  - Chloride also has an inverse relationship with HCO_3^-.
    - When chloride levels are decreased as a result of renal or GI loss, HCO_3^- reabsorption increases.
    - The increase in HCO_3^- can lead to metabolic alkalosis.
    - Frequently, excessive vomiting and nasogastric suctioning are the primary causes of hypochloremia.
  - Diabetic ketoacidosis and Addison disease that alter the acid-base and electrolyte balance can lead to hypochloremia.
  - Emphysema, pneumonia, and pulmonary edema result in hypoventilation and, ultimately, respiratory acidosis, as well as hypochloremia.
  - Increased acid in the body causes the renal tubules to compensate by increasing the excretion of acid in the form by H^+ ions. In addition, this increase in renal excretion occurs with loop, osmotic, and thiazide diuretics.
  - Any medical condition that affects the fluid balance in the body can cause a decrease in chloride levels, including congestive heart failure, cardiac fluid overload, and the removal of large amounts of pleural or ascetic fluid.
  - Large administration of HCO_3^- or HCO_3^- precursors, such as Na^+ lactate or Na^+ citrate, can result in an increase in HCO_3^- levels and a decrease in chloride levels.
  - Metabolic alkalotic state can result in the binding of Ca to protein, therefore resulting in hypocalcemia.
    - A decrease in Ca levels cause changes in the Ca pump needed for muscle relaxation and contraction.
    - The decrease in Ca levels can result in muscle irritability.

Hypochloremia

- Signs and symptoms
  - Hypoventilation
  - Excretion of chloride to compensate for increased serum HCO_3^-

- Muscle cramps
- Symptoms related to metabolic alkalosis: tetany; hyperactive deep-tendon reflexes; burning sensation (paresthesia) of the upper or lower extremities; psychomotor agitation; confusion; convulsions

Nursing Care of the Client With Hypochloremia

- Assessment
  - Client history, including the risk factors for decreased chloride levels: cystic fibrosis; chloride loss attributable to diuretic therapy; excessive gastric drainage; vomiting; diarrhea; excessive fluid loss attributable to perspiration and kidneys; renal disease; history of diabetes or ketoacidosis; Addison disease
  - Symptoms analysis: location; duration; onset; intensity; description and/or character; aggravating and alleviating factors
  - Medical history: general health history; infectious disease(s); allergies; hospitalizations
  - Physical findings
    - Assess the client for the signs and symptoms related to hypochloremia.
    - Observe for neurological and other changes in the client, including
      - Altered level of consciousness
        - Mental status
        - Changes in the level of consciousness
        - Confusion
        - Agitation
      - Cranial nerves: II through XII intact
      - Sensory alterations: light touch (sharp or dull); paresthesia (tingling of extremities)
      - Motor-related changes: range of motion in the extremities (active or passive); deep-tendon reflexes; gait
    - HEENT (head, ears, eyes, nose, and throat)
      - Assess the client for pathophysiological conditions affecting the head, face, ears, and eyes.
      - Assess the client for PERRLA (pupils equal, round, react to light, and accommodation).
    - Cardiovascular system
      - Auscultate heart rate and rhythm
      - Test capillary refill
      - Check pulse rate
      - Observe for pulmonary edema
    - GI system
      - Auscultation
      - Percussion
      - Palpation (all four quadrants)
      - Genitourinary factors: urine color and clarity; output volume
  - Personal history: medical conditions; hospitalizations; obstetric history; immunizations; allergies; current medications; occupation; habits and diet; present living environment; psychosocial factors
  - Family history: metabolic conditions; history of prematurity in infant; diabetes; Addison disease; respiratory diseases (emphysema, pneumonia); pulmonary edema; renal disease
- Diagnostic findings
  - Assess laboratory values of serum: chloride; Na^+; anion gap; Ca; creatinine (renal function); pH; HCO_3^-
  - Analysis of electrolytes in the body fluids: urine; sweat; cerebrospinal fluid; gastric fluids

- Goals of care
  - Restore normal values of serum: chloride; Na^+;pH
- Treatment
  - If the client is able to eat and drink, promote the consumption of
    - Foods and liquids high in salt and chloride: tomatoes; leafy vegetables, such as lettuce and celery; olives; kelp; seaweed; rye; and foods high in Na^+
  - Correct GI losses by treating vomiting and diarrhea with antiemetic medications and acid inhibitors.
  - Consider discontinuing diuretic medications to minimize the excretion of acid.
  - Correct metabolic alkalosis or electrolyte imbalance.
  - Administer NH_4Cl for severe cases of metabolic alkalosis.
  - Assess the client for seizures; implement seizure precautions.
  - For severe cases of metabolic alkalosis, consider the intravenous (IV) administration of NH_4Cl.
- Complications
  - Metabolic alkalosis is classified as either chloride responsive or chloride resistant.
    - Chloride-responsive metabolic acidosis is often due to vomiting, the use of diuretic medications, or long-term hypercapnic acidosis.
      - Normal kidney function excretes high levels of HCO_3^-.
      - Therefore metabolic alkalosis is an impairment of renal HCO_3^- excretion and an increase in alkali.
      - Evaluation of urine chloride concentration will assist in determining whether the classification is chloride-responsive metabolic alkalosis (the majority of cases) or chloride-resistant metabolic alkalosis.
- Nursing interventions
  - Implement supportive interventions for comfort and to minimize nausea, vomiting, and diarrhea.
    - Administer acid inhibitors.
    - Monitor strict intake and output.
- Prevention
  - Address and intervene to minimize gastric loss before the appearance of symptoms of hypochloremia.
  - Monitor laboratory values when a client is taking diuretic medications.
  - Provide client education to identify the potential causes of hypochloremia.

APPLICATION AND REVIEW

11. The effects of decreased chloride on HCO_3^- levels causes which condition?
    1. Metabolic acidosis
    2. Metabolic alkalosis
    3. Respiratory acidosis
    4. Respiratory alkalosis
12. What is the **major** cause of hypochloremia among postoperative clients recovering from neck or facial surgery?
    1. Excessive nasogastric suctioning
    2. Ineffective pain management
    3. Ineffective respirations
    4. Nutritional deficiencies
13. Which chronic conditions could contribute to the development of hypochloremia? (Select all that apply.)
    1. Renal disease
    2. Cystic fibrosis
    3. Diabetes mellitus
    4. Addison disease
    5. Congestive heart failure

14. The consumption of which foods should the nurse encourage when considering the treatment for the client with hypochloremia? *(Select all that apply.)*
    1. Olives
    2. Tomatoes
    3. Animal protein
    4. Various lettuces
    5. Various dairy items
15. Which nursing intervention is the nurse's **priority** when considering the treatment of a client diagnosed with hypochloremia?
    1. Educating the client on the importance of effective diet management
    2. Conducting an effective assessment of past medical conditions
    3. Documenting client allergies
    4. Administering an antiemetic medication as prescribed

See Answers on pages 146–148.

Pathophysiological Considerations of Hyperchloremia

- Hyperchloremia
  - Has a blood serum level of chloride greater than 110 mEq/L
  - Rarely occurs and is often due to dehydration
  - Hyperchloremia is a concern for critical care and perioperative clients in acute care.
    - Reported incidence for acute hyperchloremia
      - 22% for unselected postoperative clients
      - 57% for intensive care postoperative clients
    - Severe hyperchloremia has occurred in 6.2% of clients in intensive care.
  - Hyperchloremia causes renal vasoconstriction, which results in a decreased glomerular filtration rate (GFR).
  - Hyperchloremia can affect splanchnic circulation, which is circulation of the GI tract.
    - Splanchnic circulation could predispose a client to gastric distention and decreased motility.
  - Metabolic acidosis is due to an increase in chloride.
    - Loss of HCO_3^-
      - Causes for the loss of HCO_3^- can be attributable to renal loss or GI losses.
      - HCO_3^- can be lost in the stool through severe diarrhea with, subsequently, an increase in chloride.
        - Decreases in the ECF volume results in a larger concentration of Na^+ and chloride.
  - Hyperchloremia can be caused by an excessive management of NaCl, $CaCl_2$, and NH_4Cl.
  - Medications can also potentiate the development of hyperchloremia.
    - Cortisone preparations result in Na^+ retention and, subsequently, a rise in chloride.
      - Acetazolamide increases the excretion of HCO_3^-.
      - Triamterene lowers the secretion of H^+ ions by the kidney (distal tubes).
  - Metabolic acidosis is due to the anion gap.
    - Increased levels are noted in organic acids: (lactic acid, ketone acids), sulfates, phosphates, and proteins.
    - Decrease in HCO_3^- concentration and an increase in chloride causes normal anion gap acidosis or hyperchloremic metabolic acidosis to occur (See Fig. 7.2).
    - Acidosis results from an abundance of chloride ions in acidifying salts with fewer HCO_3^- ions.
      - High chloride level
      - Low HCO_3^- level

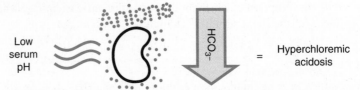

FIGURE 7.2   When retained anions are excreted by the kidneys to compensate for low serum pH, hyperchloremia acidosis occurs. (From Chernecky, C., Macklin, D., & Murphy-Ende, K. [2006]. *Saunders nursing survival guide: Fluids and electrolytes*, [2nd ed.]. St. Louis: Saunders.)

- ▪ Unmeasured anions are unchanged.
- ▪ Laboratory testing includes a calculation of the anion gap, which measures the difference between the anions and the cations.
- ▪ Anion gap: add serum chloride and HCO_3^- and subtract from the Na^+ level.
  - ○ $Na^+ - (Cl^- + HCO_3^-)$
  - ○ The anion gap is the amount of other anions, such as proteins, lactic acid, sulfates, phosphates, and ketone acids, that are stable in metabolic acidosis.
  - ○ The anion gap is a secondary measure of the primary relationship between the anions and the cations.
- ▪ If the anion gap is normal, then the assumption can be made that metabolic acidosis, not hyperchloremia, is the primary cause of the acidotic condition (Box 7.1).

BOX 7.1   Causes of Metabolic Alkalosis

Net Loss of Hydrogen From the Extracellular Fluids

Gastrointestinal Loss (Extracellular Fluid Volume Depletion)
- Vomiting or nasogastric suction*
- Chloride-losing diarrhea

Renal Loss
- Loop or thiazide-type diuretics* (NaCl restriction + ECF depletion)
- Mineralocorticoid excess*
- Hyperaldosteronism
- Cushing syndrome; exogenous corticosteroid therapy
- Excess licorice ingestion
- High-dose carbenicillin or penicillin
- H^+ movement into cells
- Hypokalemia*

Retention of Bicarbonate
Excess administration of $NaHCO_3$
Milk-alkali syndrome (antacids, milk, $NaHCO_3$)

Massive (>8 units) bank blood (citrate)
Posthypercapnia metabolic alkalosis (after correction of chronic respiratory acidosis)
- Mechanical ventilation: rapid decrease in $PaCO_2$ but HCO_3^- remains high until kidneys can excrete excess

Chloride-Responsive Metabolic Alkalosis (Urinary Chloride <10 mEq/L)
Is usually associated with ECF volume contraction
- Vomiting or nasogastric suction
- Diuretics
- Posthypercapnia

Chloride-Resistant Metabolic Alkalosis (Urinary Chloride <20 mEq/L)
Is not usually associated with ECF volume contraction
- Mineralocorticoid excess
- Edematous states (congestive heart failure, cirrhosis, nephrotic syndrome)

ECF, Extracellular fluid; *H⁺*, hydrogen; *HCO₃⁻*, bicarbonate; *NaCl*, sodium chloride; *NaHCO₃*, sodium bicarbonate.

---

*From Price, S. A., & Wilson, L. M. (2012). *Pathophysiology: Clinical concepts of disease processes*, (6th ed.). St. Louis: Mosby–Elsevier.

- Conditions associated with hyperchloremia
  - Administration of chloride-enhanced IV fluids
    - Na^+ 0.9%
      - Serum chloride is usually below 110 mmol/L.
      - 0.9% saline is 154 mmol/L.
      - Human albumin solution is up to 160 mmol/L.
    - Total parenteral nutrition
    - Lysine HCl
    - Arginine HCl
  - IV infusion of chloride
  - Water loss (water loss only or water loss in excess of chloride) through the skin: dehydration; exercise; fever; hypermetabolic conditions
  - Renal losses: osmotic diuresis; central and nephrogenic diabetes insipidus; postobstructive diuresis; intrinsic renal failure; diuretics
  - Extrarenal loss: diarrhea; burns
  - Water loss (water loss only or water loss in excess of chloride)
  - Increase in tubular chloride resorption: renal tubular acidosis; stage 1 renal failure; acetazolamide; posthypocapnia; starvation
  - Diabetic ketoacidosis
  - Metabolic acidosis attributable to ingestion of acid precursors: salicylate; ethylene glycol; methanol
  - Other medications
    - NH_4Cl: used as an expectorant, urinary acidifier, or acidifier for metabolic alkalosis
    - Na^+ polystyrene sulfonate (Kayexalate) K^+-removing resin: causes excretion of K^+ and chloride to be reabsorbed by the colon
  - Miscellaneous
    - Bromide intoxication (increased concentration of chloride in laboratory assays that use an ion electrode)

APPLICATION AND REVIEW

16. What clinical sign observed in a postoperative client is associated with the vasoconstriction caused by hyperchloremia? (*Select all that apply.*)
    1. GFR
    2. Abdomen distention
    3. Constipation
    4. Depression
    5. Anxiety
17. The nurse identifies which client risk that is associated with hyperchloremia? (*Select all that apply.*)
    1. Hypoventilation
    2. Diabetes insipidus
    3. Salicylate poisoning
    4. Early-stage renal failure
    5. Second degree burns over 15% of the body

See Answers on pages 146–148.

Signs and Symptoms of Hyperchloremia

- Tachypnea or hyperventilation
  - Respiratory compensation enables the lungs to blow off carbon dioxide.
  - Carbon dioxide combines with water to form carbonic acid (H_2CO_3).

- Lowered cardiac output
  - Peripheral vasodilation
  - Compensation for decreased fluid balance
  - Headache
  - Lethargy
  - Hypotension
    - Decreased cardiac output
    - Volume depletion and associated headache and lethargy
  - Hyperchloremia is frequently associated with metabolic acidosis, as well as decreased level of consciousness, Kussmaul respirations, and weakness and lethargy.
  - Hypernatremia is often associated with hyperchloremia and the following corresponding symptoms: agitation; tachypnea; tachycardia; hypertension; edema.

APPLICATION AND REVIEW

18. Which situations increase the client's risk for hyperchloremia? *(Select all that apply.)*
    1. Treatment for anaphylactic shock
    2. Current IV replacement therapy
    3. Second trimester of pregnancy
    4. Diagnosis of malnutrition
    5. On a respirator
19. What situation suggests the resolution of hyperchloremia?
    1. Denies headache
    2. Normal deep-tendon reflexes
    3. No seizure activity in 36 hours
    4. Denies burning sensations in any extremity
20. Which diagnostic laboratory report suggests the achievement of a goal for the treatment of hyperchloremia?
    1. Decreased blood pH
    2. Increased serum iron level
    3. Increased HCO_3^- level
    4. Decreased serum albumin level

See Answers on pages 146–148.

Nursing Care of the Client With Hyperchloremia

- Assessment
  - Analyze laboratory values for elevated chloride and Na^+ levels.
  - Analyze laboratory values for lower serum pH and HCO_3^- levels, indicating an acidotic state.
  - Analyze laboratory values for anion gap.
    - Normal anion gap will be reflected with low pH and HCO_3^- levels, which indicates metabolic acidosis.
  - Client history
    - Risk factors for increased chloride levels: recent IV fluid replacement; decreased respiratory effort of ventilation; history of shock or starvation; history of medications
    - Symptom analysis: location; duration; onset; intensity; description and/or character; aggravating and alleviating factors
  - Medical history: general health history; infectious diseases; allergies; hospitalizations
  - Physical findings
    - Assess the client for signs and symptoms related to hyperchloremia.
      - Neurological changes
        - Altered level of consciousness
        - Headache

- Edema in the extremities
- Cardiac-related changes: decreased cardiac output; volume depletion
  - Vascular-related conditions
  - GI-related changes
    - Bowel sounds: present, quality, and activity in all four quadrants
    - Percussion for resonance
    - Palpation for tenderness, guarding, and masses noted in each quadrant
  - Genitourinary-related changes
    - Strict intake and output
    - Weight changes
  - Neuromuscular-related changes
  - Respiratory-related changes: hyperventilation; tachypnea
- Personal history: occupation; habits; present living environment; psychosocial
- Family history: metabolic conditions; renal disease
- Diagnostic factors:
  - Serum blood levels; elevated serum chloride; elevated NaCl; low pH; elevated HCO_3^-
- Goals of care
  - Correct the underlying pathological conditions, and restore hemostasis of chloride to normal levels; restore fluid balance; increase blood pH; increase HCO_3^- levels
  - Nurse should assess laboratory values for elevated chloride level; elevated Na^+ level; low serum pH (acidotic); low HCO_3^- level; anion gap
- Treatment
  - Administer IV hydration (IV fluids).
  - Replace HCO_3^- with sodium bicarbonate ($NaHCO_3$) to increase the pH of the blood.
- Complications
  - Blood pH and the HCO_3^- replacement should not occur rapidly.
    - Rapid replacement may result in paradoxical cerebrospinal fluid acidosis.
  - Hyperchloremia has been associated with an increase in associated conditions: renal dysfunction; splanchnic circulation; sepsis; increase risk of hemorrhage.
    - Hypocoagulable thromboelastography (TEG) measures the hypercoagulable state, which is increased in clients with metabolic acidosis and is attributable to hyperchloremia.
- Nursing interventions
  - Continual monitoring of the client for changes: level of consciousness; respiratory status (rate, rhythm, effectiveness)
  - Physical assessment
    - Neuromuscular-related changes: level of consciousness and other neurological changes; reflexes; muscle tone
    - Cardiac-related changes: murmur; cardiac status (rate and rhythm); electrocardiographic (ECG) readings, if applicable
    - Respiratory-related changes: lung sounds; respiratory status (rate and depth)
    - Integumentary-related changes: edema in the extremities
  - Careful monitoring of IV fluid rates and amounts: IV replacement rates; volume of normal saline infusion; daily weights
  - Additional assessments: other sources of fluid intake and output; volume of normal saline infusion
- Prevention
  - Monitor medications and IV fluids that could result in hyperchloremia.
  - Assess fluid loss in clients, and monitor symptoms and laboratory values for hyperchloremia.

- Provide close assessment and continual monitoring of clients with renal disease, fluid replacement therapy, diarrhea, reduced respiratory effort (encourage deep breathing and coughing).
- Review the client's medications, including oral and IV.

ANSWER KEY: REVIEW QUESTIONS

1. **2 Cl⁻ is the chemical symbol for chloride.**

   1 Ca is the chemical symbol for calcium. **3** Cr is the chemical symbol for chromium. **4** Ce is the chemical symbol for cerium.

   Client Need: Physiological Integrity; **Cognitive Level:** Understanding; **Integrated Process:** Teaching and Learning

2. **Answers: 1, 2, 3, 5**

   Chloride has many functions. It maintains osmotic pressure, produces muscular work and activity, maintains a balance between acid and base, and promotes the flow of water among sections on a cellular level. **4** Na⁺ is responsible for promoting healthy nerve and muscle function.

   Client Need: Physiological Integrity; **Cognitive Level:** Understanding; **Integrated Process:** Teaching and Learning

3. **2 Normal chloride consumption for a woman is between 5.8 and 7.8 grams per day.**

   1, 3 Normal chloride consumption for a man is between 7.8 and 11.8 grams per day. **4** Normal chloride consumption for a woman is between 5.8 and 7.8 grams per day.

   Client Need: Physiological Integrity; **Cognitive Level:** Application; **Nursing Process:** Evaluation

4. **4 The primary source of chloride in the diet is table salt or sea salt.**

   1 Although green, leafy vegetables are considered a healthy food, the primary source of chloride in the diet is table or sea salt. **2, 3** The primary source of chloride in the diet is table salt or sea salt.

   Client Need: Health Promotion and Maintenance; **Cognitive Level:** Application; **Integrated Process:** Teaching and Learning

5. **1 Breads, grains, and cereal provide 19% of the daily-required NaCl for the average adult.**

   2 Dairy products provide 8% of the daily-required NaCl for the average adult. **3** Soups provide 3% of the daily-required NaCl for the average adult. **4** Poultry, red meats, and eggs provide 12% of the daily-required NaCl for the average adult.

   Client Need: Health Promotion and Maintenance; **Cognitive Level:** Application; **Nursing Process:** Evaluation

6. **1 A high H⁺ concentration stimulates breathing.**

   2, 3, 4 A high H⁺ concentration stimulates breathing.

   Client Need: Physiological Integrity; **Cognitive Level:** Application; **Nursing Process:** Assessment

7. **4 Women have a greater percentage of body fat (60% versus 50%) and a smaller proportion of muscle; therefore they have a decreased amount of water than men.**

   1 Newborns have almost 70% of water per body weight due to less adipose tissue. **2** Older adult men have a smaller proportion of muscle and therefore have less water per body weight but not as low as comparable-aged women. **3** Women have a greater percentage of body fat (60% versus 50%) and therefore have a decreased amount of water than men.

   Client Need: Physiological Integrity; **Cognitive Level:** Analysis; **Nursing Process:** Evaluation

8. **4 Normal serum chloride values for adults are between 95 and 110 mEq/L. A value of 115 mEq/L is high and is considered abnormal.**

   1 Normal serum chloride values for newborns are between 98 and 104 mEq/L. **2** Normal serum chloride values for children are between 101 and 105 mEq/L. **3** Normal serum chloride values for adults are between 95 and 110 mEq/L.

   Client Need: Physiological Integrity; **Cognitive Level:** Analysis; **Nursing Process:** Assessment

9. **4 Chloride is primarily absorbed in the colon.**

   1, 2, 3 Chloride is primarily absorbed in the colon and excreted by the kidneys.

   Client Need: Physiological Integrity; **Cognitive Level:** Analysis; **Nursing Process:** Planning

10. **3 Cystic fibrosis causes blockage of the bronchi, which results in respiratory infections.**
    1 Falls are not a primary effect of cystic fibrosis. **2** Cystic fibrosis affects the absorption of nutrients requiring a high-fat, high-calorie diet. **4** Cystic fibrosis results in steatorrhea, which is loose but bulky stools with globs of fat and noticeable oil separation.
    Client Need: Physiological Integrity; **Cognitive Level:** Analysis; **Nursing Process:** Planning

11. **2 When chloride levels are decreased, HCO_3^- reabsorption increases, leading to metabolic alkalosis.**
    1, 3, 4 When chloride levels are decreased, HCO_3^- reabsorption increases, leading to metabolic alkalosis.
    Client Need: Physiological Integrity; **Cognitive Level:** Understanding; **Integrated Process:** Teaching and Learning

12. **1 Frequent and excessive vomiting and nasogastric suctioning are the primary causes of hypochloremia.**
    2, 3, 4 Frequent and excessive vomiting and nasogastric suctioning are the primary causes of hypochloremia.
    Client Need: Physiological Integrity; **Cognitive Level:** Analysis; **Integrated Process:** Teaching and Learning

13. **Answers: 1, 2, 3, 4**
    A decreased chloride level, which is a risk factor for hypochloremia, is increased by renal disease, cystic fibrosis, diabetes, and Addison disease.
    5 Congestive heart failure is not generally considered a risk factor for hypochloremia.
    Client Need: Physiological Integrity; **Cognitive Level:** Understanding; **Integrated Process:** Teaching and Learning

14. **Answers: 1, 2, 4**
    Consumption of foods and liquids high in salt and chloride, such as olives, tomatoes, and lettuces, should be encouraged.
    3 Animal protein is not necessarily considered a good source of Na^+ or chloride. **5** Dairy items are not necessarily considered good sources of Na^+ or chloride.
    Client Need: Physiological Integrity; **Cognitive Level:** Understanding; **Nursing Process:** Planning

15. **4 Correcting the cause of the imbalance has priority. Hypochloremia is commonly caused by excessive vomiting.**
    1 Although appropriate, diet management is not the priority. **2** Although appropriate, an assessment of past medical conditions is not the priority **3** Although appropriate, identifying and documenting allergies is not the priority.
    Client Need: Physiological Integrity; **Cognitive Level:** Analysis; **Integrated Process and Nursing Process:** Implementation

16. **Answers: 1, 2, 3**
    1 Hyperchloremia causes renal vasoconstriction, which results in decreased GFR. **2** Hyperchloremia can affect splanchnic circulation, which is the circulation of the GI tract, causing gastric distention. **3** Hyperchloremia can affect splanchnic circulation, causing decreased gastric motility.
    4 Although psychosocial disorders may be observed in these clients, depression is not a result of vasoconstriction. **5** Although psychosocial disorders may be observed in these clients, anxiety is not a result of vasoconstriction.
    Client Need: Physiological Integrity; **Cognitive Level:** Application; **Nursing Process:** Assessment

17. **Answers: 2, 3, 4, 5**
    2 Central and nephrogenic diabetes insipidus is a risk factor for hyperchloremia. **3** Salicylate poisoning is a risk factor for hyperchloremia. **4** Early-stage renal failure is a risk factor for hyperchloremia. **5** Burns are a risk factor for hyperchloremia.
    1 Hypoventilation increases the risk of hypochloremia.
    Client Need: Physiological Integrity; **Cognitive Level:** Understanding; **Integrated Process:** Teaching and Learning

18. **Answers: 1, 2, 4, 5**
    Risk factors for increased chloride levels include recent IV fluid replacement, decreased respiratory effort of ventilation, and a history of shock or starvation.

3 Second trimester of pregnancy is not generally considered a risk factor for hyperchloremia.

Client Need: Physiological Integrity; **Cognitive Level:** Analysis; **Nursing Process:** Assessment

19. **1 Reports of a headache are associated with hyperchloremia.**

    2 Abnormal deep-tendon reflexes are associated with hypochloremia. **3** Seizures are associated with hypochloremia. **4** Paresthesia is associated with hypochloremia.

    Client Need: Physiological Integrity; **Cognitive Level:** Analysis; **Nursing Process:** Evaluation

20. **3 Goals for restoring hemostasis related to normalizing chloride levels include increasing HCO$_3^-$ levels.**

    1 Goals for restoring hemostasis related to normalizing chloride levels include increasing blood pH.

    2 Goals for restoring hemostasis related to normalizing chloride levels do not include iron levels.

    4. Goals for restoring hemostasis related to normalizing chloride levels do not include albumin levels.

    Client Need: Physiological Integrity; **Cognitive Level:** Analysis; **Nursing Process:** Evaluation

POTASSIUM IMBALANCE OVERVIEW

Significance of Potassium

- Potassium is the most plentiful solute in the intracellular fluid (ICF).
  - Potassium is represented by the chemical symbol K^+.
    - Potassium comprises 98% of the ICF cations.
    - Only 2% of potassium is found in extracellular fluid (ECF).
  - Is a major cation
  - Is measured in serum levels
  - Is necessary for many metabolic cellular functions and for neuromuscular activity
  - Is critical to heart function
    - Low levels in the body lead to irregular heart contractions.
    - Potassium is specifically needed for voltage-gated potassium channels to work in the outer membranes of the cardiac muscle cells.
    - Voltage-gated channels open in response to a change in polarization and are responsible for changing action potentials and contractions while initiating repolarization.
    - Hyperkalemia causes reduced electrical conduction and often leads to palpitations and disrupted heart rhythm.
  - Helps maintain acid-base balance
    - Acidosis causes potassium to move from the cells into the ECF in exchange for hydrogen ions.
    - Alkalosis causes the reverse movement of potassium and hydrogen ions.
  - Normal range of serum potassium: between 3.5 and 5 mEq/L
    - Potassium levels are tightly controlled by body functions.
    - Major alterations can occur with slight changes in potassium levels.
  - Inside the cell, potassium can be as high as 140 mEq/L.
  - The primary source of potassium is dietary intake.
  - The recommended daily allowance for adults is 4700 mg.
  - Adult diets are usually low in potassium as a result of a low consumption of fruits and vegetables.

Sources of Potassium

- Primary dietary sources: oranges; bananas; avocadoes; cantaloupe; apricots; dried fruit; nuts; seeds; chocolate; meats; potatoes; mushrooms; celery; tomatoes; beans
- Approximately 90% of ingested potassium is absorbed in the small intestines.
- Potassium is excreted through the urine after filtering through the kidneys.

Potassium-Containing Foods

- Control of potassium (Box 8.1)
  - Potassium enters the body through dietary intake.
  - The daily adult requirement is approximately 40 mEq or 4700 mg.
  - The average adult consumes between 60 and 100 mEq of potassium daily.

BOX 8.1 Potassium Content of Foods	
Foods High in Potassium Fruits: oranges, avocados, bananas, and cantaloupe Dried fruits: apricots Nuts and seeds Chocolate Meats Yogurt	Vegetables: potatoes, celery, mushrooms, tomatoes, beans (white, soy), beets, and spinach **Foods Low in Potassium** Fruits: apples, cherries, and grapefruit Eggs Vegetables: green beans, peppers, lettuce, and eggplant

- ECF gains potassium when cells are destroyed.
- ECF may also gain potassium with fluid shifts from the intracellular space into the vascular space.
- Kidney function
  - Potassium is excreted in the urine.
    - Each liter of urine contains between 20 and 40 mEq of potassium.
    - Even when there is no potassium intake, between 10 and 15 mEq/day will be excreted through the urine.
  - The body rids itself of excess potassium through the kidneys.
  - As the body detects elevated serum potassium levels, the renal tubules excrete more potassium.
  - In the presence of aldosterone, the kidneys reabsorb more sodium and excrete more potassium.
  - The kidneys do not have a mechanism to prevent the excretion of potassium.
  - Some potassium is excreted with perspiration.
  - The body loses some potassium through the gastrointestinal (GI) tract.
    - Approximately 9 mEq/day is lost through the intestines.
    - Hyperaldosteronism can increase potassium loss through the intestines to approximately 12 mEq/day.
- Sodium-potassium pump (Figure 8.1)
  - The sodium-potassium pump is an active transport mechanism that helps maintain stable sodium and potassium levels in the body.
  - With diffusion, sodium tends to move inward toward the cells and potassium tends to move outward toward the ECF.
  - To counteract this natural tendency, the sodium-potassium pump is at work in every cell of the body.
  - The sodium-potassium pump requires energy in the form of adenosine triphosphate (ATP).
  - ATP consists of phosphorous and magnesium.
  - Phosphorous and magnesium drive sodium out of the cell and potassium inside the cell wall.
  - The sodium-potassium pump works to prevent the swelling of cells.
  - An electrical charge is created by the movement of the sodium-potassium pump, which allows the transmission of neuromuscular impulses.

Functions of Potassium
- Maintains cellular osmolality
- Maintains neutrality of cells
- Affects acid-base balance
- Necessary for skeletal muscle contraction
- Required for cardiac muscles to contract

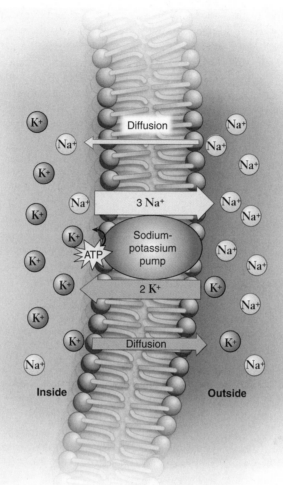

FIGURE 8.1   The sodium-potassium pump in the plasma membrane actively pumps sodium ions out of a cell and potassium ions into a cell to help maintain stable sodium and potassium levels in the body. For every three sodium ions leaving a cell, two potassium ions enter it. (From Patton, K. T., & Thibodeau, G. A. [2019]. *Anatomy & physiology*, [10th ed.]. St. Louis: Mosby.)

- Necessary for electrical conductivity of the heart
- Helps transmit nerve impulses
- Makes normal digestion possible
- Uses amino acids in making protein

APPLICATION AND REVIEW

1. A client's potassium level at 3.3 mEq/L determines the priority of which safety-related nursing intervention?
   1. Monitoring cardiac rhythm
   2. Implementing falls precautions
   3. Monitoring the level of consciousness
   4. Administering a potassium supplement as prescribed

2. Which statement made by a client demonstrates an understanding of correcting a dietary deficiency related to potassium?
   1. "I need to eat dairy items to get more potassium into my diet."
   2. "Increasing my consumption of healthy dietary fat will be appropriate."
   3. "I need to alter my diet to be certain I consume at least 4000 mEq of potassium daily."
   4. "I don't particularly like vegetables, but I need to find several that I can add to my regular diet."
3. Which dietary choices added to a salad best demonstrate the client's understanding of food sources high in potassium? *(Select all that apply.)*
   1. Green peppers
   2. Dried cherries
   3. Spinach
   4. Apples
   5. Beets
4. Which client is at an increased risk for developing acute hypokalemia?
   1. Marathon runner
   2. Tobacco smoker
   3. Vegetarian
   4. Hispanic

See Answers on pages 165–167.

DISORDERS OF POTASSIUM

Hypokalemia

- Serum potassium level: less than 3.5 mEq/L
- Associated with hypertension
- Can cause death as a result of cardiac dysrhythmias
  - Abnormal cardiac rhythm is caused by a disruption in the electrical conduction system of the heart.
- Small changes in potassium levels can produce significant symptoms.
- The body can compensate for gradual changes in potassium levels.
- Symptoms may not appear until the potassium level is significantly low.
- Moderate hypokalemia
  - Serum potassium level: between 2.5 and 3.0 mEq/L
- Severe hypokalemia
  - Serum potassium level: less than 2.5 mEq/L
- Symptoms of hypokalemia can worsen if accompanied by hypocalcemia.
- Metabolic alkalosis can enhance the symptoms of hypokalemia.
- Digoxin therapy can increase the symptoms of hypokalemia.
- Muscle weakness from hypokalemia can progress to involve the respiratory muscles.

Pathophysiological Considerations of Hypokalemia

- Inadequate intake of potassium
- Excessive output of potassium
- Causes of hypokalemia (Box 8.2): gastrointestinal suction; ileostomy; prolonged vomiting; diarrhea; severe diaphoresis; diuresis; high glucose levels; Cushing syndrome; stress; liver disease; alcoholism; heart failure; leukemia; nephritis; anorexia; bulimia
- Drugs that can cause hypokalemia: diuretic medications (thiazides, furosemide); corticosteroidal medications; insulin; cisplatin; antibiotics (gentamicin, amphotericin B, carbenicillin); epinephrine; albuterol; laxatives
- Symptoms that are present are often from the underlying cause of the hypokalemia rather than the low potassium level.

BOX 8.2	Causes of Hypokalemia

Decreased potassium intake
Anorexia
NPO (nothing by mouth [*nil per os*]) orders and
  intravenous solutions without potassium
Fasting
Unbalanced diet
Shift of potassium from extracellular fluid to
  the cells
Alkalosis
Excess insulin (e.g., during total parenteral nutrition)
Excess β-adrenergic stimulation
Hypokalemic familial periodic paralysis
Increased potassium excretion through normal
  routes

Renal Route
Potassium-wasting diuretic medications
Corticosteroid therapy

Cushing disease
Hyperaldosteronism
Excessive ingestion of black licorice (glycyrrhizin)
Hypomagnesemia
Parenteral piperacillin or similar agents
Amphotericin B, cisplatin, cyclosporine, and many
  other medications

Fecal Route
Diarrhea (includes laxative overuse or abuse)

Skin Route
Excessive diaphoresis
Loss of potassium through abnormal routes
Emesis
Gastric suction
Fistula drainage

From Banasik, J L., & Copstead, L. C. (2019). *Pathophysiology*, (6th ed.). St. Louis: Elsevier.

- Symptoms of hypokalemia are nonspecific.
- Symptoms related to muscular or cardiac function: weakness; fatigue; muscle cramps; pain in muscles; polyuria; difficulty controlling diabetes; depression; heart palpitations
- Severe hypokalemia may lead to bradycardia with cardiac arrest.
- Respiratory failure from muscle paralysis can develop in rare cases.

Assessment of Hypokalemia

- Complete a client history.
- Identify the risk factors for potassium imbalance.
- Determine preexisting conditions predisposing a client for potassium imbalance: gastric suctioning; diarrhea; vomiting; kidney injury.
- Assess the client's ability to ingest food and fluids.
- Complete a diet history.
  - Assess the client for the use of salt substitutes; 1 teaspoon of a salt substitute may contain up to 60 mEq of potassium.
- Review medications. The use of diuretics increases the risk of hypokalemia.
- Evaluate the medication list for the use of digoxin.
  - Hypokalemia increases the risk of digoxin toxicity.
  - Symptoms of digoxin toxicity: confusion; irregular pulse; loss of appetite; nausea, vomiting, diarrhea; fast heartbeat; vision changes (blind spots, blurred vision, changes in appearance of colors, seeing spots, seeing halos around objects)
- Obtain vital signs: heart rate; blood pressure; respiratory rate; temperature.
- Collect laboratory data: serum potassium level; pH level; bicarbonate (HCO_3^-) level; magnesium level; serum glucose level.
- Evaluate electrocardiographic (ECG) results, which measures the force and rate of heart contractions.

Diagnostic Factors of Hypokalemia

- Serum potassium level: less than 3.5 mEq/L
- Elevated pH
- May have elevated HCO_3^- levels
- Increased serum glucose levels
- Decreased magnesium levels
- Increased 24-hour urine level
- ECG changes (Figure 8.2): flattened T wave; inverted T wave; U wave; depressed ST segment
- May have an increased digoxin level; normal digoxin level is between 0.5 and 2.0 ng/mL

Signs and Symptoms of Hypokalemia

- Signs and symptoms: skeletal muscle weakness; progressive weakness; anorexia; nausea; vomiting; constipation; decreased bowel sounds; dilute urine; weak, irregular heart rate; orthostatic hypotension; heart palpitations; ECG changes; paresthesia; paralysis of respiratory muscles (rare); rhabdomyolysis

Goals of Care for the Client With Hypokalemia

- The underlying cause of hypokalemia should be resolved.
- Serum potassium level should return to between 3.5 and 5.0 mEq/L.
- Associated laboratory values should return to within normal limits.
- Vital signs should be stable and within normal ranges for the client.
- Cardiac rate and rhythm should return to baseline.

Treatment of Hypokalemia

- Treatment depends on the cause and severity of hypokalemia.
- The underlying cause of hypokalemia must be resolved.
- Encourage a high potassium and low sodium diet.
- Provide oral potassium supplements (potassium chloride).
- Administer intravenous (IV) potassium replacement therapy.
- Treat low magnesium levels. Low magnesium levels prevent the kidneys from adequately conserving potassium.

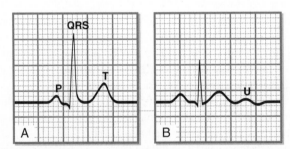

FIGURE 8.2 Electrocardiogram (ECG) shows changes found in a client with hypokalemia. **(A)** Normal ECG. **(B)** ECG with hypokalemia. A positive wave after the T wave is called a U wave, which is a sign of hypokalemia. (From Gaw, A., Murphy, M. J., Srivastava, R., Cowan, R. A., & O'Reilly, D. S. J. [2013]. *Clinical biochemistry: An illustrated colour text*, [5th ed.]. Philadelphia: Churchill Livingstone–Elsevier.)

APPLICATION AND REVIEW

5. The nurse assesses a client with a potassium level of 3.1 mEq/L for which chronic health condition?
   1. Gastroesophageal reflex disease (GERD)
   2. Crohn disease
   3. Hypertension
   4. Asthma
6. The nurse understands which medical diagnoses increase the client's need for education regarding the prevention of hypokalemia? *(Select all that apply.)*
   1. Leukemia
   2. Alcoholism
   3. Anorexia nervosa
   4. Addison disease
   5. Cushing syndrome
7. Which statements by a client suggest the need for an assessment regarding hypokalemia? *(Select all that apply.)*
   1. "I'm always so tired."
   2. "I feel like I'm depressed."
   3. "It's hard to start my urine flow."
   4. "I seem to have a lot of leg cramps."
   5. "Nothing I do seems to manage my diabetes."
8. The nurse should educate a client being treated for hypokalemia the importance of reporting which vision-related events that may indicate digoxin toxicity? *(Select all that apply.)*
   1. Seeing halos around objects
   2. Existence of blind spots
   3. Involuntary blinking
   4. Distortion of colors
   5. Excessive tearing
9. The nurse recognizes which ECG results support a diagnosis of hypokalemia? *(Select all that apply.)*
   1. U wave
   2. Elevated T wave
   3. Flattened T wave
   4. Elevated ST segment
   5. Absence of a U wave

See Answers on pages 165–167.

Complications of Hypokalemia

- Cardiovascular dysrhythmias
- Development of hypertension
- Muscle weakness
- Decreased gut mobility

Nursing Interventions for Hypokalemia

- Identify clients at risk for developing hypokalemia: fluid volume excess; diuretic medications; gastric suctioning; vomiting.
- Monitor serum potassium levels; normal range is between 3.5 and 5.0 mEq/L.
- Monitor laboratory results associated with hypokalemia: blood glucose; serum chloride; serum calcium; urine osmolality.
- Administer oral potassium supplements as ordered.
  - Dilute powdered potassium supplements in liquids as instructed by the manufacturer.
  - Use the correct amount of diluent as indicated on the packaging. Most often, 20 mEq of potassium in 120 mL of water or juice is recommended.

- May mix the diluent in juice to offset the unpleasant taste and consistency of the potassium powder. Do not mix powdered potassium supplements with grapefruit juice.
- Thoroughly stir the product.
- Administer the supplement with food to decrease GI irritation.
- Do not crush the tablets.
- Do not open the capsules. Follow the manufacturer's instructions for sprinkling the capsule contents on soft food.
- Initiate and maintain IV access.
- IV potassium may be administered for potassium levels less than 3.0 mEq/L.
  - Potassium must be diluted before infusing. Dilute no more than the recommended 1 mEq/10 mL.
  - Never administer potassium IV push.
    - Potassium is one of the drugs that is administered in lethal injections to stop the heart.
    - Fluids containing potassium should be clearly labeled.
  - Infuse slowly.
    - Infusing between 5 and 10 mEq/hr is recommended.
    - Do not exceed 20 mEq/hr.
    - Rapid infusion can cause cardiac arrest.
    - Always use an infusion pump to administer potassium.
  - Monitor cardiac functioning when administering potassium.
    - Clients should be on telemetry when receiving IV potassium.
    - Rapid infusion of potassium can cause cardiac arrest.
  - Monitor the IV site for signs and symptoms of infiltration: redness; swelling; leaking at site; irritation; complaints of pain at insertion site.
  - Stop the infusion if infiltration occurs.
  - Notify the primary care provider.
- Do not administer potassium subcutaneously or intramuscularly.
- Observe ECG changes: ST segment depression; low-amplitude T waves; prominent U waves; QRS complexes that become widened with drops in potassium; T waves that flatten and then invert.
- Check pedal pulses.
- Monitor vital signs.
  - Blood pressure may be decreased.
  - May experience orthostatic hypotension.
  - Heart rate may be decreased or irregular.
    - Weak, thready, irregular pulse
    - Bradycardia or tachycardia (dependent on the cause)
  - Respiratory rate may decrease in severe hypokalemia.
- Assess orthostatic blood pressure.
  - Assess blood pressure while the client is in the lying position.
  - Assess blood pressure with the client in the sitting position.
  - Assist the client to a standing position, and assess the blood pressure.
  - Analyze the measurements.
  - A change greater than 10 mm Hg between readings indicates postural hypotension.
  - Use caution as clients may experience dizziness and light-headedness.
  - Document measurements.
- Monitor for changes in cardiovascular function.
  - Ventricular fibrillation: rapid, life-threatening heart rhythm; causes low blood pressure; can lead to loss of consciousness; can cause death

- Ventricular tachycardia: chest pain; fainting; dizziness; shortness of breath
- Premature ventricular contractions (PVCs)
  - Produce a flip-flop type of feeling in the chest
  - May be described as palpitations
  - PVCs lasting longer than 30 seconds can cause life-threatening dysrhythmias.
- Asystole (absence of cardiac electrical activity)
- Assess for symptoms of alkalosis.
  - pH greater than 7.45
  - Partial pressure of carbon dioxide ($PaCO_2$) less than 35 mm Hg
  - HCO_3^- greater than 28 mEq/L
  - Increased heart rate
  - Thready pulse
  - Hypotension
  - Confusion
  - Headache
  - Dizziness
  - Anxiety
  - Tetany
    - Positive Chvostek-Weiss sign
      - To perform this sign, tap on the facial nerve anterior to the ear and below the zygomatic bone.
      - Twitching of the facial muscles is suggestive of neuromuscular excitability.
    - Positive Trousseau sign
      - To perform this sign, a blood pressure cuff is placed around the arm and inflated to a pressure greater than the systolic blood pressure.
      - The pressure is maintained for 3 minutes to occlude the brachial artery.
      - A positive Trousseau sign will result in a spasm of the muscles of the hand and forearm.
  - Hyperreflexia (body overreacts to external stimuli)
  - Numbness of extremities
  - Tingling of extremities
- Assess muscle strength and tone.
  - Monitor the client for changes in the baseline assessment.
  - Assess for signs of weakness.
  - Baseline data might need to be obtained from family members if the client is confused or nonresponsive.
- Check deep-tendon reflexes.
  - The client should be relaxed and in a sitting position or lying supine.
  - Elicit the biceps reflex by tapping the biceps tendon with a reflex hammer at the elbow. There should be a reflex contraction with elbow flexion.
  - Elicit the triceps reflex by flexing the elbow and tapping the triceps tendon just proximal to the elbow with a reflex hammer. There should be a reflex contraction of the triceps muscle that allows elbow extension.
  - Check the knee reflex by slightly lifting up the leg under the knee and using a reflex hammer to tap the patellar tendon. A reflex contraction of the quadriceps muscle with the extension of the knee should occur. This procedure can also be performed with the client dangling the legs off the bed or examination table.
  - The ankle reflex may be assessed by tapping the Achilles tendon with a reflex hammer. Plantar flexion of the foot should occur.

- Deep tendon reflexes should be graded on a scale from 0 to 4.
  - 0 = absent, despite reinforcement
  - 1 = present only with reinforcement
  - 2 = normal
  - 3 = increased but normal
  - 4 = significantly hyperactive, with clonus
- Observe the client for muscle twitching.
- Listen to bowel sounds.
- Record bowel movements.
- Record all intake and output measurements from all sources at least every 8 hours: parenteral medications; IV fluids; oral intake; any IV flushes; flushes for tube feedings.
  - Record ice chips as approximately one-half their volume.
  - Record the amount and type of all fluids lost by the client: urine; liquid stool; emesis; tube drainage (chest, wounds, nasogastric tubes); any fluid aspirated out of the body.
    - Subtract any fluids used in tube irrigation from the total fluid output.
  - Measure the output in calibrated containers.
    - Observe the container at eye level.
    - Record the amount using the bottom of the meniscus as a guide.
  - Intake and output collection can be delegated to unlicensed personnel, if properly instructed.
- Implement fall precautions.
  - Assess the risk for falls.
  - Clients with orthostatic hypotension are at a greater risk for falling.
  - Place the bed in a low position.
  - Lock the wheels of the bed.
  - Clear pathways.
  - Use nightlights.
  - Place assistive devices within reach of the client.
  - Place necessary items such as water, telephone, and remote controls within reach of the client.
  - Have the call light within reach.
  - Instruct the client to call for help with ambulating.
  - Encourage family members to sit with the client, if needed.
- Educate the client and caregiver
  - Causes of hypokalemia: dilution from excess fluid in the extracellular space; diuretic use; gastric suctioning; prolonged vomiting
  - Symptoms of hypokalemia: weak, thready pulse; decreased blood pressure; orthostatic hypotension
  - Notification of the health care provider
    - Reportable signs and symptoms
    - Exacerbation of medical conditions
    - Adverse reactions to medications
  - Prevention of hypokalemia
    - Taking medications as directed
    - Potassium supplementation with potassium-wasting diuretic medications
    - Eating fruits, vegetables, and other foods high in potassium
    - Eating foods containing potassium: bananas; apricots; potatoes; beans (white and soy); dried fruit; yogurt

- Administering oral potassium replacement therapy as directed
  - Follow the manufacturer's instructions.
  - Powders and liquids must be diluted.
  - Use the correct amount of fluid to dilute potassium.
  - Mix thoroughly before drinking.
  - Take potassium supplements with food to avoid GI irritation.
  - May take potassium supplements with juice to make the taste more palatable
  - Avoid taking with grapefruit juice.
  - Do not crush potassium tablets.
  - Avoid opening capsules.
    - Some capsules may be opened and mixed with soft food such as applesauce.
    - Beads inside the capsules should not be crushed.
    - Ensure that the manufacturer's instructions are read and followed.
    - Report nausea, vomiting, diarrhea, and abdominal cramping to the primary care provider; these signs may be adverse effects of potassium supplementation.
- Clients should avoid taking potassium supplements concurrently with potassium-sparing diuretics.
- Teach the client about salt substitutes containing potassium.
- Educate the client to keep regular laboratory appointments.
  - Potassium levels should be checked within 2 weeks of starting the diuretic medications.
- Document serum potassium levels, laboratory values, vital signs, heart rate, heart rhythm, nursing interventions, and response to interventions.

APPLICATION AND REVIEW

10. Which intervention associated with the administration of a powdered form of an oral potassium supplement demonstrates the client's understanding of the appropriate technique?
    1. Diluting the supplement with no more than 100 mL of liquid
    2. Administering the medication at least 1 hour before or 2 hours after eating
    3. Dissolving the supplemental powder in water only to avoid related interactions
    4. Avoiding grapefruit juice as the diluent used to dissolve the powdered potassium
11. Which tetany-related assessment requires access to a blood pressure cuff?
    1. Hyperreflexia
    2. Chvostek-Weiss sign
    3. Trousseau sign
    4. Deep-tendon reflexes

See Answers on pages 165–167.

Prevention of Hypokalemia

- Teach clients who are at high risk and their caregivers the causes of hypokalemia: excessive water intake; alkalosis; vomiting; diarrhea; gastric suctioning; excessive sweating; renal disease; dialysis.
- Teach the client and caregivers the signs and symptoms of hypokalemia: orthostatic hypotension; weak pulse; fatigue; irritability; anxiety; nausea; vomiting; constipation; weakness; muscle aches; muscle twitching.

- Educate the client and caregivers about the drugs that can lead to hypokalemia: insulin; digoxin; corticosteroids.
- Educate the client on the drugs (diuretic medications) that can cause increased excretion of potassium.
- Teach the client about the foods that are high in potassium: bananas; apricots; potatoes; beans (white and soy); dried fruit; yogurt.

Hyperkalemia

- Serum potassium level: greater than 5.0 mEq/L
- May be asymptomatic
- Can cause death
- The body may compensate for gradual increases in potassium levels.
  - The client may not be symptomatic until serum potassium level reaches a critical point; that increase in the potassium level is gradual.
  - Sudden increases in potassium levels can cause rapid development of life-threatening symptoms.
  - Serum potassium levels greater than 7.0 mEq/L have the potential to suppress the electrical conduction system of the heart, causing cardiac arrest.
  - Potassium levels greater than 6.5 mEq/L are a medical emergency.

Pathophysiological Considerations of Hyperkalemia

- Excessive intake of potassium can cause hyperkalemia.
  - Ingestion of excessive mEq of potassium in food and fluid
  - Overuse of salt substitutes that contain potassium
  - Excessive intravenous fluid administration of potassium containing fluids
  - Rapid administration of fluids containing potassium
- Retention of potassium: acute kidney injury; chronic kidney disease; potassium-sparing diuretics; angiotensin-converting enzyme (ACE) inhibitors; Addison disease
  - Occurs when diseased adrenal glands do not produce enough cortisol, estrogen, androgens, and aldosterone
  - Decreased aldosterone levels, resulting in the excretion of sodium and retention of potassium
  - Fluid volume deficit
- Potassium shifts out of the ICF compartment and into the ECF compartment: vomiting; diarrhea; burn injuries; surgical procedures; rhabdomyolysis; metabolic acidosis; cancer

Assessment of Hyperkalemia

- Conduct a client history.
- Identify risk factors for potassium imbalance.
- Determine preexisting conditions predisposing a client for potassium imbalance: gastric suctioning; diarrhea; vomiting; kidney injury
- Assess the client's ability to ingest food and fluids.
- Collect a diet history.
- Assess for use of salt substitutes.
- Review the use of medications: potassium-sparing diuretics; ACE inhibitors
- Obtain vital signs.
- Collect laboratory data.
- Evaluate ECG results.

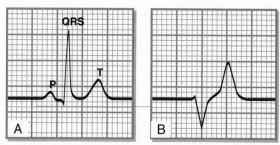

FIGURE 8.3   Electrocardiogram (ECG) shows changes found in a client with hyperkalemia. **(A)** Normal ECG. **(B)** ECG with hyperkalemia. Note the peaked T wave and the widening of the QRS. (From Gaw, A., Murphy, M. J., Srivastava, R., Cowan, R. A., & O'Reilly, D. S. J. [2013]. *Clinical biochemistry: An illustrated colour text*, [5th ed.]. Philadelphia: Churchill Livingstone–Elsevier.)

Diagnostics of Hyperkalemia

- Serum potassium level: greater than 5.0 mEq/L
- pH levels less than 7.35
- ECG changes (Figure 8.3): tall, peaked, tented T waves

Signs and Symptoms of Hyperkalemia

- Serum potassium level: greater than 5.0 mEq/L
- Cardiovascular changes
  - Tall, peaked, tented T waves: first-degree heart block; second-degree heart block; ventricular fibrillation; bradycardia
  - Nausea
  - Diarrhea
  - Hyperactive bowel sounds
  - Fatigue
  - Muscle weakness
  - Cramping
  - Circumoral paresthesia
  - Tingling
  - Can produce respiratory arrest

Goals of Care Hyperkalemia

- Underlying cause of hyperkalemia should be resolved.
- Serum potassium level should return to 3.5 to 5.0 mEq/L.
- Associated laboratory values should return to normal limits.
- Vital signs should be stable and within normal ranges for client.
- Cardiac rate and rhythm should return to baseline.

Treatment of Hyperkalemia

- Treatment depends on the cause.
- To move potassium from ECF to ICF, infuse 50% dextrose, administer 10 units regular insulin, and administer 75 mEq of sodium HCO_3^-.
- Administer a diuretic such as furosemide (Lasix): calcium chloride; calcium gluconate

- Sodium polystyrene sulfonate (Kayexalate) may be administered orally or via an enema to exchange sodium ions for potassium in the intestines.
- Dialysis may be used to reduce potassium levels.

Complications of Hyperkalemia

- Mild ECG changes
- Severe ECG changes (ventricular fibrillation)
- Death

Nursing Interventions of Hyperkalemia

- Stop administering potassium supplements.
- Decrease dietary intake of potassium: fruits; vegetables; meats.
- Discontinue medications that may cause hyperkalemia: potassium-sparing diuretics; ACE inhibitors.
- Monitor vital signs.
  - Blood pressure may be decreased.
  - May develop orthostatic hypotension
  - Blood pressure may elevate depending on its cause.
  - Heart rate may decrease and become irregular.
  - Respiratory rate may decrease with severe hyperkalemia.
- Assess orthostatic blood pressure.
  - Assess blood pressure while the client is in the lying position.
  - Assess blood pressure with the client in the sitting position.
  - Assist the client to a standing position, and assess the blood pressure.
  - A change greater than 10 mm Hg between readings indicates postural hypotension.
  - Use caution as clients may experience dizziness and light-headedness.
  - Document measurements.
- Monitor ECG results.
  - Activate rapid response if T waves become spiked.
    - Monitor heart rate. Rapid response may need to be activated if the heart rate falls below 60 beats per minute.
    - Place the client on telemetry.
    - Evaluate for cardiovascular changes: heart palpitations; slow or absent pulses; hypotension; bradycardia; complete heart block; PVCs; ventricular tachycardia (VT); ventricular fibrillation; asystole.
    - Evaluate for changes in neuromuscular functioning: weakness; cramping; tingling; circumoral paresthesia.
    - Assess for signs of numbness and tingling around the mouth (peripheral numbness).
    - Be alert to the development of respiratory arrest.
    - Assess for signs of metabolic acidosis: pH less than 7.35; $PaCO_2$ normal or less than 35 mm Hg; HCO_3^- less than 21 mEq/L; generalized weakness; tachycardia or severe bradycardia; weak peripheral pulses; hypotension; lethargy; confusion; headache; stupor; Kussmaul respirations; warm, flushed skin; cyanotic mucous membranes; hyporeflexia; hypotonia; muscle twitching.
- Administer IV glucose and insulin as ordered. Increases movement of potassium back into cells
- Administer IV calcium. Acts as an antagonist to treat cardiac and skeletal muscle effects

- Administer IV sodium HCO_3^- as ordered.
  - Increases movement of potassium from the ECF into the ECF
  - Treats acidosis
- Administer cation exchange resins as ordered.
  - Sodium polystyrene sulfonate (Kayexalate) exchanges sodium ions for potassium in the intestine and removes excess potassium from the GI tract.
    - May be administered orally or by enema
    - Is usually followed by sorbitol to ensure that the sodium polystyrene sulfonate clears the intestines if administered orally
    - Removes approximately 40 mEq/day of potassium from the intestines if administered orally
- Administer loop diuretics as ordered to increase potassium excretion through the kidneys: furosemide (Lasix); torsemide (Demadex); bumetanide (Bumex); ethacrynic acid (Edecrin).
- Thiazide diuretics may be administered as ordered: metolazone (Zaroxolyn); hydrochlorothiazide; chlorothiazide (Diuril).
- Observe the client for side effects of the medications: nausea; vomiting; diarrhea; abdominal cramping.
  - Record all intake and output measurements.
  - Record fluid intake from all sources at least every 8 hours: parenteral medications; IV fluids; oral intake; any IV flushes; flushes for tube feedings.
    - Record ice chips as approximately one-half their volume.
  - Record amount and type of all fluids lost by the client: urine; liquid stool; emesis; tube drainage (chest, wounds, nasogastric tubes); any fluid aspirated out of the body.
    - Subtract any fluids used in tube irrigation from total fluid output.
  - Measure output in calibrated containers.
    - Observe the container at eye level.
    - Record the amount using the bottom of the meniscus as a guide.
    - Intake and output collection can be delegated to unlicensed personnel if properly instructed.
- Educate clients and caregivers.
  - Causes of hyperkalemia
  - Signs and symptoms of potassium excess
  - Notify the health care provider concerning symptoms of hyperkalemia.
  - Stress the importance of keeping laboratory appointments.
  - Avoid salt substitutes that contain potassium.
  - Decrease the intake of foods high in potassium: bananas; beets; spinach; apricots; potatoes; beans (white and soy); dried fruit; yogurt.
  - Decrease intake of red meat; 3 ounces of meat contains approximately 375 mg of potassium.
  - Instruct the client on foods with lower potassium content: apples; eggs; cherries; grapefruit; celery; eggplant; lettuce; green beans; peppers.
  - Increase fluid intake if not contraindicated.
    - Increasing fluids can help clear more potassium through the kidneys if the renal system is properly functioning.
  - Read food labels for potassium content.
  - Document potassium levels, laboratory values, vital signs, cardiac rhythm, heart rate, medication administration, nursing interventions, and response to interventions.

Prevention of Hyperkalemia

- Teach clients who are at risk and their caregivers the causes of hyperkalemia: excessive intake of potassium; overuse of salt substitutes; vomiting; diarrhea; severe burns; surgical procedures; Addison disease; fluid volume deficit.
- Teach clients and caregivers the signs and symptoms of hyperkalemia: nausea; diarrhea; muscle weakness; muscle cramps; tingling of extremities; fatigue.
- Educate clients that potassium-sparing diuretics such as furosemide and ACE inhibitors can cause increased retention of potassium.
- Teach the client to decrease the intake of foods high in potassium: bananas; apricots; potatoes; beans (white and soy); dried fruit; yogurt.

APPLICATION AND REVIEW

12. Which outcome represents the achievement of an appropriate clinical goal for the treatment of hyperkalemia?
    1. Achieving a serum potassium level of 4.2 mEq/L
    2. Administering sodium polystyrene sulfonate as prescribed
    3. Providing education regarding related nutritional requirements
    4. Implementing falls precautions related to orthostatic hypotension
13. Which interventions are associated with assessing orthostatic blood pressure? *(Select all that apply.)*
    1. Assessing blood pressure with the client in a supine position
    2. Assessing blood pressure with the client in a prone position
    3. Assessing blood pressure with the client in a sitting position
    4. Assessing blood pressure with the client in a standing position
    5. Reporting a 20 mm Hg difference in blood pressure results
14. Which assessment data would confirm the medical diagnosis of metabolic acidosis of a client being treated for moderate hyperkalemia? *(Select all that apply.)*
    1. pH of 7.25
    2. Hypertension
    3. Kussmaul respirations
    4. HCO_3^- less than 21 mEq/L
    5. $PaCO_2$ greater than 35 mm Hg
15. Which thiazide diuretics would be appropriately prescribed for the treatment of hyperkalemia? *(Select all that apply.)*
    1. Furosemide
    2. Torsemide
    3. Bumetanide
    4. Metolazone
    5. Chlorothiazide
16. The nurse understands that the omission of which food is necessary to manage a client's hyperkalemia?
    1. Chicken
    2. Wheat
    3. Potatoes
    4. Cow's milk
17. A client who is diagnosed with hyperkalemia demonstrates an understanding of the appropriate food selections when adding which items to their lunch salad? *(Select all that apply.)*
    1. Eggs
    2. Celery
    3. Tomatoes
    4. Mushrooms
    5. Red peppers

18. Which statement demonstrates an appropriate understanding concerning fluid intake when attempting to manage the risk of hyperkalemia?
    1. "I need to moderately limit my fluid intake."
    2. "Clear liquids should be my primary source of fluids."
    3. "I make an effort to drink plenty of fluids every day."
    4. "The majority of the fluid I drink each day should be consumed by dinnertime."
19. What assessment question concerning lifestyle choices is appropriate when assessing a client with a slightly elevated serum potassium level?
    1. "Do you drink alcohol daily?"
    2. "Do you use salt substitutes?"
    3. "Do you smoke tobacco products?"
    4. "Do you engage in regular cardiovascular exercise?"
20. What physiological events should be identified for a client as a sign or symptom of hyperkalemia? *(Select all that apply.)*
    1. Diarrhea
    2. Muscles cramps
    3. Tingling of the toes
    4. Ringing in the ears
    5. Red rash on the chest

See Answers on pages 165–167.

ANSWER KEY: REVIEW QUESTIONS

1. **1 Low levels of potassium in the body lead to irregular heart contractions; 3.3 mEq/L of serum potassium indicates hypokalemia.**
   2 Although implementing falls precautions is an appropriate intervention, irregular heart contractions have priority. **3** Although monitoring the level of consciousness is an appropriate intervention, irregular heart contractions have priority. **4** Although supplement administration is an appropriate intervention, irregular heart contractions have priority.
   Client Need: Physiological Integrity; **Cognitive Level:** Analysis; **Nursing Process:** Planning

2. **4 Adult diets are usually low in potassium as a result of the low consumption of fruits and vegetables.**
   1 Dairy items are not a significant source of dietary potassium. **2** Fat is not a significant source of dietary potassium. **3** The recommended daily allowance of potassium for adults is 4700 mg.
   Client Need: Health Promotion and Maintenance; **Cognitive Level:** Analysis; **Nursing Process:** Evaluation

3. **Answers: 3, 5**
   3 Spinach is a high-potassium source. **5** Beets are a high-potassium source.
   1 Green peppers are low in potassium. **2** Dried cherries are low in potassium. **4** Apples are low in potassium.
   Client Need: Health Promotion and Maintenance; **Cognitive Level:** Application; **Nursing Process:** Evaluation

4. **1 Potassium is excreted with perspiration.**
   2 Although a health risk, smoking tobacco is not associated with hypokalemia. **3** An animal protein–free diet is not associated with hypokalemia. **4** Hispanic genetics are not generally associated with hypokalemia.
   Client Need: Physiological Integrity; **Cognitive Level:** Analysis; **Nursing Process:** Assessment

5. **3 Hypokalemia is associated with hypertension.**
   1 Hypokalemia is not generally associated with GERD. **2** Hypokalemia is not generally associated with Crohn disease. **4** Hypokalemia is not generally associated with asthma.
   Client Need: Physiological Integrity; **Cognitive Level:** Application; **Nursing Process:** Assessment

6. **Answers: 1, 2, 3, 5**
   1 Leukemia is associated with hypokalemia. **2** Alcoholism is associated with hypokalemia. **3** Anorexia nervosa is associated with hypokalemia. **5** Cushing syndrome is associated with hypokalemia.
   4 Addison disease is associated with hyperkalemia.
   Client Need: Health Promotion and Maintenance; **Cognitive Level:** Application; **Nursing Process:** Planning

7. **Answers: 1, 2, 4, 5**

    1 Fatigue is a symptom associated with the muscular effects of hypokalemia. **2** Depression is a symptom associated with the effects of hypokalemia. **4** Muscle cramps are a symptom associated with the muscular effects of hypokalemia. **5** Diabetes control is difficult and associated with the effects of hypokalemia. **3** Difficult initiation of urine flow is not a symptom associated with the effects of hypokalemia.
    Client Need: Physiological Integrity; **Cognitive Level:** Analysis; **Nursing Process:** Assessment

8. **Answers: 1, 2, 4**

    1 Seeing haloes around objects is associated with digoxin toxicity. **2** The existence of visual blind spots is associated with digoxin toxicity. **4** Changes in the appearance of colors is associated with digoxin toxicity. **3** Involuntary blinking is not associated with digoxin toxicity. **5** Excessive tearing is not associated with digoxin toxicity.
    Client Need: Physiological Integrity; **Cognitive Level:** Applied; **Integrated Process:** Teaching and Learning

9. **Answers: 1, 3**

    1 Hypokalemia can result in a U wave. **3** Hypokalemia can result in a flattened T wave. **2** Hypokalemia can result in either a flattened or an inverted T wave. **4** Hypokalemia can result in a depressed ST segment. **5** Hypokalemia can result in the presence of a U wave.
    Client Need: Physiological Integrity; **Cognitive Level:** Understanding; **Nursing Process:** Assessment

10. **4 The potassium supplement should not be mixed with grapefruit juice.**

    1 Most often, the potassium supplement is dissolved in 120 mL of water or juice. **2** The potassium supplement should be administered with food to decrease GI irritation. **3** The potassium supplement can be dissolved in certain juices to help manage its unpleasant taste.
    Client Need: Health Promotion and Maintenance; **Cognitive Level:** Application; **Integrated Process:** Teaching and Learning

11. **3 To perform an assessment of the Trousseau sign, a blood pressure cuff is placed around the arm and inflated to a pressure greater than the systolic blood pressure.**

    1 Assessing for hyperreflexia does not require a blood pressure cuff. **2** Assessment of the Chvostek-Weiss sign requires a tap on the facial nerve anterior to the ear and below the zygomatic bone. **4** Assessing deep-tendon reflexes requires a reflex hammer.
    Client Need: Physiological Integrity; **Cognitive Level:** Understanding; **Nursing Process:** Assessment

12. **1 A serum potassium level between 3.5 and 5.0 mEq/L demonstrates resolution of hyperkalemia.**

    2 Administering sodium polystyrene sulfonate is an intervention that should help achieve the goal of resolving the imbalance. **3** Nutritional education is an intervention that should help prevent further potassium imbalance. **4** Implementing falls precautions is an intervention that focuses on client safety.
    Client Need: Physiological Integrity; **Cognitive Level:** Analysis; **Nursing Process:** Evaluation

13. **Answers: 1, 3, 4, 5**

    1 Assessing orthostatic blood pressure requires monitoring the client's blood pressure while he or she is in a supine position. **3** Assessing orthostatic blood pressure requires monitoring the client's blood pressure while he or she is in a sitting position. **4** Assessing orthostatic blood pressure requires monitoring the client's blood pressure while he or she is in a standing position. **5** Reporting a difference in readings greater than 10 mm Hg is required. **2** Assessing orthostatic blood pressure does not require monitoring blood pressure while the client is in a prone position.
    Client Need: Health Promotion and Maintenance; **Cognitive Level:** Application; **Nursing Process:** Application

14. **Answers: 1, 3, 4**

    1 A pH less than 7.35 is associated with metabolic acidosis. **3** Kussmaul respirations are associated with metabolic acidosis. **4** HCO_3^- less than 21 mEq/L is associated with metabolic acidosis. **2** Hypotension is associated with metabolic acidosis. **5** A normal $PaCO_2$ level or a level less than 35 mm Hg is associated with metabolic acidosis.
    Client Need: Physiological Integrity; **Cognitive Level:** Application; **Nursing Process:** Evaluation

15. **Answers: 4, 5**

    4 Metolazone is a thiazide diuretic prescribed for hyperkalemia. **5** Chlorothiazide is a thiazide diuretic prescribed for hyperkalemia.

    1 Furosemide is a loop diuretic. **2** Torsemide is a loop diuretic. **3** Bumetanide is a loop diuretic.

    Client Need: Physiological Integrity; **Cognitive Level:** Understanding; **Integrated Process:** Teaching and Learning

16. **3 Potatoes are high in potassium and should be avoided by clients diagnosed with hyperkalemia.**

    1 Beef does not need to be omitted since it is not high in potassium. **2** Wheat does not need to be omitted since it is not high in potassium. **4** Cow's milk does not need to be omitted since it is not high in potassium.

    Client Need: Health Promotion and Maintenance; **Cognitive Level:** Application; **Integrated Process:** Teaching and Learning

17. **Answers: 1, 2, 5**

    1 Eggs are considered a food low in potassium. **2** Celery is considered a food low in potassium. **5** Red peppers are considered a food low in potassium.

    3 Tomatoes are considered a food high in potassium. **4** Mushrooms are considered a food high in potassium.

    Client Need: Health Promotion and Maintenance; **Cognitive Level:** Application; **Nursing Process:** Evaluation

18. **3 Increasing fluids can help clear more potassium through the kidneys if the renal system is properly functioning.**

    1 Limiting fluid intake is not recommended since increasing fluids can help clear more potassium through the kidneys if the renal system is properly functioning. **2** Increasing fluids of all kinds can help clear more potassium through the kidneys if the renal system is properly functioning. **4** Increasing fluids can help clear more potassium through the kidneys if the renal system is properly functioning; under normal circumstances, it is not necessary to limit fluids after a certain time of day.

    Client Need: Health Promotion and Maintenance; **Cognitive Level:** Analysis; **Nursing Process:** Evaluation

19. **2 Overuse of salt substitutes increases the risk of hyperkalemia.**

    1 Although a health risk, alcohol abuse is a risk factor for hypokalemia. **3** Although a health risk, tobacco use is not directly associated with hyperkalemia. **4** Regular, appropriate cardiovascular exercise is not a risk factor of hyperkalemia; excessive perspiration is a risk factor for hypokalemia.

    Client Need: Physiological Integrity; **Cognitive Level:** Analysis; **Nursing Process:** Assessment

20. **Answers: 1, 2, 3**

    1 Diarrhea can be a sign of hyperkalemia. **2** Muscles cramps can be a sign of hyperkalemia. **3** Tingling of the extremities can be a sign of hyperkalemia.

    4 Ringing in the ears is not associated with hyperkalemia. **5** A red rash is not associated with hyperkalemia.

    Client Need: Health Promotion and Maintenance; **Cognitive Level:** Application; **Integrated Process:** Teaching and Learning

9 Phosphorous Imbalance

PHOSPHORUS IMBALANCE OVERVIEW

Significance of Phosphorus

- Phosphorus is the major anion in intracellular fluid (ICF).
  - Phosphorus is an element represented by the chemical symbol P.
  - Phosphorus has an atomic weight of 15.
  - There is white and red phosphorus.
  - Phosphorus is not found as a free element.
  - Phosphorus is found in nearly all animal- and plant-based foods.
  - Normal serum level of phosphorus is between 2.5 and 4.5 mg/dL (between 1.8 and 2.6 mEq/L).
    - Serum levels of phosphorus are very high in infancy and childhood, especially during bone growth.
    - Phosphorus absorption and reabsorption declines with aging.
  - A normal phosphorus level in the cells is 100 mEq/L.
  - Phosphorus is considered the second most profuse mineral in the human body.
  - It accounts for 1% of the total body weight (TBW).
    - 85% of the body's phosphate is in the bones and teeth.
    - 1% of the phosphate is in the extracellular fluid (ECF).
    - 14% of the phosphate is in other tissues.
  - In the body, phosphorus is contained as phosphate, which is a salt-containing phosphorus.
    - The terms phosphorus and phosphate are considered interchangeable.
    - Phosphorus exists in an approximate 1:2 ratio with calcium.

Sources of Phosphorus

- Dietary sources of phosphorus are primarily through the ingestion of foods containing phosphorus.
  - The dietary daily value (DV) of phosphorus is 1000 mg.
  - Phosphorus is absorbed more easily from meat products.
  - Only approximately 50% of the available phosphorus in plant sources is absorbed.
    - Phosphorus from plants is more readily used by the body than phosphorus from meat sources.
  - The average ingestion of phosphorus is 20 mg/kg/day. Approximately, 16 mg/kg/day is absorbed in the proximal intestine.
    - 3 mg/kg/day is secreted into the intestine as pancreatic enzymes, bile, and other intestinal secretions.
    - Net absorption of the ingested phosphorus is 13 mg/kg/day, and 7 mg/kg/day is excreted in feces.
  - Food sources are considered high in phosphorus.

Food	Amount	Daily Value
Pumpkin and squash seeds	1 oz	35%
Sunflower seeds	1 oz	32%
Parmesan cheese	1 oz	23%
Romano cheese	1 oz	21%
Salmon	3 oz	32%
Whitefish and cod	3 oz	29%
Shrimp	1 oz	26%
Crab	1 oz	24%
Pork	3 oz	26%
Beef	3 oz	24%
Nonfat yogurt	8 oz	36%
Nonfat milk	8 oz	25%
White beans (cooked)	1 cup	36%
Pinto beans (cooked)	1 cup	25%

Control of Phosphorus

- The parathyroid gland is responsible for regulating phosphorus levels by affecting the activity of parathyroid hormone (PTH).
  - PTH keeps the extracellular and intracellular levels of phosphorus in a narrow range (Figure 9.1).
    - Calcium and phosphorus have an inverse relationship.
    - Changes in the serum calcium level affect the release of PTH.
      - PTH leads to an increase in calcium and phosphorus resorption from the bone.
      - PTH leads to a decrease in reabsorption from the proximal renal tubule.
      - Both result in elevated calcium and phosphorus levels.
  - PTH increases phosphorus absorption from the intestines, especially in the presence of vitamin D (calcitriol).
    - PTH is the most important regulator of absorption of phosphate through the intestine.
      - Calcitriol increases the absorption of phosphorus from the gut and bones.
      - Inhibitors of intestinal phosphate absorption include epidermal growth factor (EGF), glucocorticoids, estrogens, and metabolic acidosis.
  - PTH acts on the kidneys to excrete phosphorus.
    - The kidney action on phosphorus is significantly greater that the other aforementioned effects on serum levels.
    - The kidneys excrete approximately 90% of the phosphorus as they try to regulate the levels in the serum.
      - If the intake of phosphorus is increased, the kidneys will excrete the excess.
      - If phosphorus intake is limited, the kidneys will retain phosphorus by increasing reabsorption in the proximal tubule.
      - Reduced PTH allows for increased phosphorus reabsorption and a subsequent rise in the serum phosphorus levels.
- Transcellular shifts
  - Insulin moves phosphorus into the cells.
  - Metabolic acidosis causes the same shift of phosphorus into the cells.

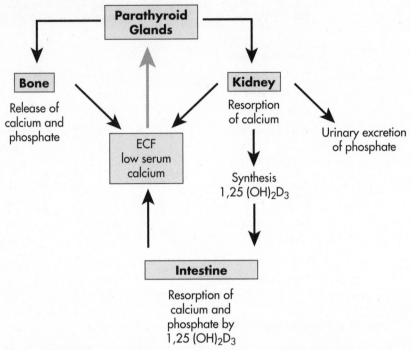

FIGURE 9.1 Mechanisms of action of the parathyroid hormone (PTH). *ECF*, Extracellular fluid; *1,25(OH)₂D₃*, calcitriol. (From Price, S. A., & Wilson, L. M. [2012]. *Pathophysiology: Clinical concepts of disease processes*, [6th ed.]. St. Louis: Mosby.)

- Gastrointestinal-Bone–Renal Axis
  - Phosphate interacts with several minerals.
    - Increased magnesium intake can cause decreased phosphate absorptions.
    - Phosphate needs sodium to ensure its absorption.
- From ingestion to reabsorption
  - Once ingested, phosphorus enters the ECF and moves in and out of bone as needed.
    - Approximately 3 mg/kg/day of phosphorus is absorbed through the intestine.
  - The rate of bone remodeling determines the concentration of plasma phosphorus.
    - Increased bone resorption can cause increased plasma phosphorus levels.
    - Increased bone mineralization can cause decreased plasma phosphorus levels.
  - Plasma phosphorus is completely filtered and enters the renal tubules.
  - The amount of phosphorus excreted in the urine roughly approximates the amount absorbed in the intestine.

APPLICATION AND REVIEW

1. When monitoring a client's phosphorus level, the nurse will refer to the diagnostic results identified with which symbol?
   1. PH
   2. Ph
   3. Pr
   4. P

2. Which client would be expected to have a normally high serum phosphorous level?
    1. 3-year-old girl being treated for asthma
    2. 14-year old boy experiencing a growth spurt
    3. 28-year-old woman during the first trimester of pregnancy
    4. 47-year old man receiving dialysis treatments for acute kidney failure
3. Which information should an older adult client receive concerning the effects of aging on serum phosphorus levels?
    1. Decreased absorption of serum phosphorus causes deficiencies.
    2. Increased reabsorption of serum phosphorus is likely to result in elevated serum levels.
    3. Overuse of supplements containing serum phosphorus can result in acute kidney failure.
    4. Nonfat dairy products are considered poor sources of serum phosphorus because of lactose issues.
4. Which healthy snack is the best source of dietary phosphorus?
    1. White bean hummus
    2. Leafy green salad
    3. Cucumber dill soup
    4. Lemon sherbet
5. Which gland is responsible for the regulation of phosphorus levels?
    1. Pineal
    2. Pituitary
    3. Pancreas
    4. Parathyroid
6. Which vitamin will aid in the absorption of phosphorus for a client who has recently experienced a partial gastrectomy?
    1. A
    2. B_{12}
    3. D
    4. E
7. Which medical diagnosis places a client at increased risk for deficient phosphate levels attributable to an ineffective absorption of phosphorus?
    1. Metabolic acidosis
    2. Metabolic alkalosis
    3. Respiratory acidosis
    4. Respiratory alkalosis

See Answers on pages 178–181.

Functions of Phosphorus

- Provides cell membrane integrity
    - Cell membranes are made of phospholipids, which are similar to fats.
        - The compound made of phosphorus and nitrogen replaces fatty acid molecules.
        - Cell membranes maintain cell growth and repair.
- Phosphorus promotes energy metabolism.
- Regulates subcellular processes
    - Is known as cell signaling through protein phosphorylation of key enzymes
- Promotes metabolism of carbohydrates, fats, and proteins
- Buffers acids and bases
    - Buffers prevent changes in the pH by removing hydrogen ions.
    - Decreases the deleterious effects when changes in the hydrogen ion concentration are abrupt as a result of changing a strong base or acid.
        - Phosphate works as a buffer by regulating the pH of fluids as they pass through the kidneys.
            - Phosphate salts in the renal tubular filtrate as disodium hydrogen phosphate (Na_2HPO_4).
            - Phosphate also acts as a buffer in the ECF.

- Maintains healthy bones and teeth
  - 85% of the body's phosphorus is in the bones and teeth.
  - Skeletal growth
    - Apoptosis of mature chondrocytes in the growth plate begins in puberty as skeletal maturity occurs.
    - Without high levels of phosphorus in early childhood, the chondrocytes will not go through the usual apoptosis, and the formation of new bone will be blocked and bone growth will cease resulting in rickets and/or delayed growth.
- Maintains bone integrity
- Assists in bone remineralization
- Assists the hematological system
  - Helps get oxygen to the red blood cells (RBC) and to the tissues throughout the body
    - 2,3-diphosphoglycerate (2,3-DPG) is inside the RBCs.
      - Phosphorus is the primary ingredient.
  - Assists with white blood cell (WBC) phagocytosis
  - Necessary for normal platelet function

Phosphorus Imbalance

- Hypophosphatemia
  - Pathophysiological factors
    - Common mechanisms that lead to hypophosphatemia
    - Phosphorus is shifted from the ECF to the ICF.
      - Respiratory alkalosis is the most common cause of hypophosphatemia.
        - Is caused by hyperventilation (mechanism unknown) and includes sepsis, alcohol withdrawal, diabetic ketoacidosis, hepatic encephalopathy, acute salicylate poisoning, heatstroke, pain, and anxiety
      - Hyperglycemia
        - Causes the release of insulin, which transports glucose and phosphorus into the cells
      - Severe malnutrition, which is predominantly found in older adults and debilitated individuals, as well as clients who abuse alcohol or have an eating disorder (anorexia nervosa)
      - Refeeding syndrome, which is defined as insufficient phosphorus supplementation in enteral or parenteral feedings that pushes phosphorus into the ICF
      - Hypothermia
        - Decreased absorption of phosphorus from the intestine: malabsorption syndromes; starvation; prolonged use of phosphorus-binding antacids or sucralfate; inadequate vitamin D intake; steatorrhea (fatty stools); decreased dietary intake (rarely a cause of hypophosphatemia since phosphorus is found in most foods)
        - Increased intestinal loss of phosphorus
    - Chronic diarrhea
      - Laxative abuse
    - Increased loss of phosphorus from the kidneys
      - Diuretic use (most common): thiazides; loop diuretics; acetazolamide
      - Diabetic ketoacidosis (second most common)
        - Hyperglycemia causes excessive osmotic diuresis.
        - Phosphorus loss occurs in the urine.

- ▪ Inebriation
  - ○ Affects the phosphorus reabsorption in the kidney, and more phosphorus is excreted
- ▪ Combination of mechanisms
  - ▪ Hyperparathyroidism and hypocalcemia
    - ○ Parathyroid hormone stimulates the kidney to excrete phosphate.
  - ▪ Extensive burns
    - ○ Extensive loss of fluids and salt in the first few days after the burn
    - ○ Respiratory alkalosis
    - ○ Parenteral or enteral carbohydrate administration
- • Assessment
  - ▪ Obtain a thorough client and family medical history.
  - ▪ Obtain a list of client medications including all over-the counter, herbs, and homeopathic preparations.
  - ▪ Monitor for signs of acute or chronic hypophosphatemia.
- • Diagnostic factors
  - ▪ Hypophosphatemia: phosphorus level less than 2.5 mg/dL (1.8 mEq/L)
  - ▪ Severe hypophosphatemia: phosphorus level less than 1 mg/dL
  - ▪ Creatinine kinase is increased in rhabdomyolysis.
  - ▪ X-ray images may show bone softening (osteomalacia) or fractures.
  - ▪ Magnesium levels are decreased.
  - ▪ Calcium levels are decreased.
- • Signs and symptoms
  - ▪ Phosphorus is needed to make ATP for energy; therefore many of the symptoms of hypophosphatemia are related to weakness and low energy.
  - ▪ Acute hypophosphatemia
    - ▪ Generalized muscle weakness (can be subtle or profound): diplopia (double vision); dysarthria (difficulty speaking); dysphagia (difficulty swallowing); weakness in large muscle groups; rhabdomyolysis (skeletal muscle destruction)
  - ▪ Abnormal neurological function
    - ▪ Paresthesia
    - ▪ Diffuse pain and weakness
    - ▪ Cardiac: hypotension; decreased cardiac output; cardiomyopathy
    - ▪ Alterations in mental status: irritability; confusion; altered mental status; coma
  - ▪ Chronic hypophosphatemia
    - ▪ Anorexia (decreased appetite)
    - ▪ Bone weakness: bone pain; fractures; bone loss
    - ▪ Cardiac: hypotension; decreased cardiac output; cardiomyopathy
    - ▪ Hematological symptoms
      - ○ Hemolytic anemia: changes in the structure and function of the RBCs; paleness
      - ○ Increased risk of infection: decreased function of the WBCs
      - ○ Poor platelet function: bruising and bleeding; mild gastrointestinal (GI) bleeding
    - ▪ Loss of appetite
    - ▪ Generalized weakness
- • Goals of care
  - ▪ Ensure client safety.
  - ▪ Monitor for symptoms.
  - ▪ Restore normal serum phosphorus.

- Treatment
  - Increase phosphorus intake by including foods that are high in phosphorus: eggs; nuts; organ meats; milk products; meat; whole grains; fish
  - Avoid drugs that reduce the phosphate level.
  - Drink low-fat or skim milk.
  - Consider a phosphate supplement.
    - Provide an oral phosphorus supplement for moderate hypophosphatemia or if calcium is contraindicated.
    - An oral phosphorus supplement may cause nausea and diarrhea.
    - Administer intravenous (IV) fluid replacement for severe hypophosphatemia.
- Complications
  - Acute hypophosphatemia: dysphagia (difficulty swallowing); profound weakness; rhabdomyolysis (skeletal muscle destruction); cardiomyopathy; alterations in mental status, stupor, coma, or death
  - Chronic hypophosphatemia: fractures; osteopenia; cardiomyopathy; hemolytic anemia; GI bleeding
- Nursing interventions
  - Monitor vital signs (temperature, heart rate, blood pressure).
  - Assess neurological status.
  - Assess muscle strength and tone.
  - Assess pain level, and administer pain medication as needed.
  - Administer oral phosphorus supplements (may cause diarrhea). Mix with juice to improve palatability.
  - Administer parenteral phosphorus as needed.
    - Use an infusion pump.
    - Observe for signs of hypocalcemia.
    - Observe for signs of hyperphosphatemia.
    - IV infiltration of potassium phosphate can cause tissue necrosis and sloughing.
    - Monitor frequent phosphorus levels.
  - Administer vitamin D supplement.
  - Monitor rate and depth of respirations.
  - Avoid hyperventilation.
    - Monitor arterial blood gases (ABGs) for severe hypophosphatemia.
  - Monitor myocardial function (heart failure).
  - Monitor for signs of infection.
  - Order bed rest as needed for safety.
- Prevention
  - Eat a well-balanced diet.
  - Avoid excess sun exposure.
  - Provide a vitamin D supplement.
  - Manage diabetes mellitus.
  - Take medications as prescribed.
  - Drink alcohol in moderation, if at all.
- Hyperphosphatemia
  - Pathophysiological factors
    - Avoid excessive ingestion of vitamin D milk.

- When phosphorus levels rise, phosphorus binds with calcium to create calcium phosphate, which is an insoluble compound that can deposit itself in the lungs, heart, kidneys, and other soft tissues.
  - Called calcification
  - May lead to arrhythmias
  - Decreased urine output
  - May get hazy corneas, conjunctivitis, cataracts, and impaired vision
  - Crystal deposits on the skin that are quite itchy
- Otherwise, hyperphosphatemia is usually related to some underlying condition.
  - Kidney disease
    - Kidney failure is the most common cause of hyperphosphatemia.
    - Glomerular filtration rate (GFR) is less than 30.
      - The kidneys cannot remove the excess phosphorus.
    - Dialysis does does not effectively remove phosphate.
  - PTH-related problems: hypoparathyroidism with a low level of PTH; lack of normal response to normal levels of PTH
  - Shift of phosphorus from ICF to ECF: respiratory acidosis; diabetic ketoacidosis; crush injuries; rhabdomyolysis; chemotherapy
  - Sepsis
  - Heatstroke
  - Cancer: bone tumors; leukemia; lymphoma
  - Burns
  - Prolonged immobilization
  - Ischemic bowel
  - Metabolic or hematological disorders
  - History of neck surgery (manipulated parathyroid gland)
  - Medications: parenteral administration of phosphate; oral phosphate binders; potassium phosphate; antacids; bisphosphonates; laxatives (oral, rectal, enemas that contain phosphate)
- Assessment
  - Obtain a thorough client and family medical history.
  - Obtain a list of client medications, including all over-the counter, herbs, and homeopathic preparations.
  - Monitor for signs of acute or chronic hyperphosphatemia.
- Diagnostic factors
  - Elevated phosphorus: >4.5 mg/dL (>2.6 mEq/L)
  - Severe hyperphosphatemia: phosphorus >6 mg/dL
  - Hypocalcemia: serum calcium <8.5 mg/dL
  - Increased blood urea nitrogen (BUN) and creatinine levels, indicating worsening kidney function
  - Creatinine kinase rhabdomyolysis from tissue destruction and rhabdomyolysis
  - X-ray studies showing skeletal changes attributable to defective bone development in chronic hyperphosphatemia
  - Electrocardiographic changes characteristic of hypocalcemia (prolonged QT syndrome)
- Signs and symptoms
  - Mostly asymptomatic if only hyperphosphatemia

- Crystals (phosphate and calcium) can form on the skin and cause severe itching.
- More severe symptoms, if acute hyperphosphatemia, are associated with hypocalcemia: muscle cramps; paresthesia around the lips and mouth; tetany; neuromuscular hyper-excitability (Chvostek-Weiss sign, Trousseau sign); perioral numbness or tingling; bone or joint pain; osteoporosis; itching; rash; altered mental status (delirium, obtundation, coma, convulsions, seizures).
- Symptoms related to other causes of hyperphosphatemia: uremia causing fatigue; shortness of breath; anorexia; nausea; vomiting; sleeping disturbance
- Goals of care
  - Ensure client safety.
  - Monitor for symptoms.
  - Monitor and treat conditions that might cause hyperphosphatemia.
  - Restore normal levels of serum phosphorus.
- Treatment
  - Recommend a diet low in phosphorus.
  - Administer drugs that bind with phosphate and are taken with meals: sevelamer; lanthanum; calcium compounds.
  - Administer drugs to decrease phosphorus absorption: aluminum; magnesium; calcium gel; phosphate-binding antacids.
  - Treat any other underlying cause of hyperphosphatemia.
    - Diabetic ketoacidosis: administer insulin, which will push the phosphorus back into the cells.
    - Respiratory acidosis
  - Severe hyperphosphatemia
    - Administer parenteral normal saline to promote renal excretion.
    - Administer parenteral diuretic medications.
  - Provide hemodialysis or peritoneal dialysis if hyperphosphatemia is severe and symptoms of hypocalcemia are exhibited.
- Complications
  - Severe hypocalcemia with tetany and seizures
- Nursing interventions
  - Carefully monitor clients with hyperphosphatemia.
  - Avoid additional phosphate infusions, medications, and enemas.
  - Carefully monitor vital signs.
  - Watch for symptoms of hypocalcemia: paresthesia; hyperactive reflexes; tetany.
  - Observe for any signs of calcification: oliguria; visual changes; irritated eyes; palpitations; abnormal electrocardiogram.
  - Carefully monitor intake and output.
    - If urine output falls below 30 mL/hr, immediately notify the health care provider.
  - Monitor electrolytes.
  - Administer medications as ordered.
- Prevention
  - Eat a well-balanced diet.
  - Avoid foods high in phosphorus if there is a preexisting condition that may lead to hyperphosphatemia.
  - Comply with renal failure management.
  - Manage diabetes mellitus.
  - Take medications as prescribed.

APPLICATION AND REVIEW

8. Which medical diagnoses place a client at risk for respiratory alkalosis–induced hypophosphatemia? *(Select all that apply.)*
   1. Client experiencing a hyperglycemic reaction
   2. Teenager diagnosed with chronic constipation
   3. Client on long-term loop diuretic therapy
   4. Severely malnourished older adult
   5. Client in alcohol withdrawal

9. Which interventions should be considered for a client diagnosed with acute hypophosphatemia? *(Select all that apply.)*
   1. Regular pain assessment
   2. Aspiration precautions
   3. Regular blood pressure assessment
   4. Frequent monitoring of level of consciousness
   5. Administering antiemetic medications, as needed

10. Which assessment findings suggests a history of chronic hypophosphatemia? *(Select all that apply.)*
    1. Being treated for hemolytic anemia
    2. Currently being treated for hypertension
    3. Treated for pneumonia twice in the last 2 years
    4. Numerous areas of bruising on the legs and arms
    5. History of two separate bone fractures in the last 3 years

11. Considering the effects of calcium phosphate deposits related to hyperphosphatemia, which body systems would the nurse monitor as a priority? *(Select all that apply.)*
    1. Respiratory
    2. Lymphatic
    3. Nervous
    4. Cardiac
    5. Kidney

12. Which client statement suggests a possible complication of hyperphosphatemia-related calcification?
    1. "My vision, especially in the right eye, seems to be getting more blurry."
    2. "I'm feeling really depressed these past few weeks."
    3. "I'm really craving sugary foods and drinks."
    4. "My fingers are numb and feel cold."

13. Which clients are at risk for developing hyperphosphatemia? *(Select all that apply.)*
    1. 5-year-old child diagnosed with leukemia
    2. 19-year-old athlete who broke an arm skiing
    3. 32-year-old runner who experienced heatstroke
    4. 55-year-old man on long-term antidepressant medication therapy
    5. 75-year-old woman diagnosed with urinary infection–induced sepsis

14. Which client statement suggests an increased risk for hyperphosphatemia?
    1. "I take antacids for indigestion three or four times a week."
    2. "My father abused alcohol as he got older."
    3. "I had my appendix removed last year."
    4. "I work out in the cold quite a bit."

15. Which diagnostic results would suggest hyperphosphatemia? *(Select all that apply.)*
    1. Serum phosphorus level at 5.2 mg/dL
    2. Serum calcium level at 6.8 mg/dL
    3. Serum calcium level at 9.8 mg/dL
    4. Prolonged QT syndrome
    5. T-wave inversion

16. What serum phosphorus level is the baseline used for the diagnosis of severe hyperphosphatemia?
    1. 5 mg/dL
    2. 6 mg/dL
    3. 8 mg/dL
    4. 10 mg/dL

17. Which diagnostic result would the nurse monitor to determine whether the client is experiencing significant muscle injury?
    1. Serum calcium
    2. Serum phosphorus
    3. BUN
    4. Serum chloride

18. A nurse is providing care for a client who has been diagnosed with both uremia and hyperphosphatemia. The nurse demonstrates an understanding of appropriate care planning when implementing which intervention specific for this client?
    1. Monitoring for signs of shortness of breath
    2. Monitoring for signs of muscle tetany
    3. Implementing seizure precautions
    4. Implementing falls precautions

19. Which intervention is a safety priority when caring for a client diagnosed with hyperphosphatemia and a serum calcium level of 7.6 mg/dL?
    1. Monitor appetite
    2. High-calcium diet
    3. Seizure precautions
    4. Low phosphorus diet

20. A client is being treated for hypoparathyroidism. Which instructions should the nurse provide to help the client avoid an associated problem with serum phosphorus?
    1. Eat a well-balanced diet.
    2. Avoid eating organ meat.
    3. Be regularly screened for diabetes mellitus.
    4. Be regularly screened for possible renal failure.

See Answers on pages 178–181.

ANSWER KEY: REVIEW QUESTIONS

1. **4 Phosphorus is an element represented by the chemical symbol P.**

   1, 2, 3 Phosphorus is an element represented by the chemical symbol P.
   Client Need: Physiological Integrity; **Cognitive Level:** Knowledge; **Nursing Process:** Assessment

2. **2 Serum levels of phosphorus are very high in infancy and childhood (during bone growth). Boys tend to show the first physical changes of puberty between the ages of 10 and 16 years. They tend to grow more quickly between the ages 12 and 15 years.**

   1, 3, 4 Physical growth spurts, typically between the ages of 12 and 15 years, are the periods when a child would normally experience high phosphorus levels. Kidney failure is a cause of abnormal hyperphosphorus levels.
   Client Need: Physiological Integrity; **Cognitive Level:** Analysis; **Nursing Process:** Assessment

3. **1 A decline in phosphorus absorption and reabsorption occurs with aging.**

   2 A decline in phosphorus absorption and reabsorption occurs with aging. **3** Overuse of any supplement should be avoided, but it is not necessarily related to the effects of aging. **4** Nonfat dairy products are good sources of phosphorus, but lactose-related issues are not the result of aging.

Client Need: Health Promotion and Maintenance; **Cognitive Level:** Application; **Integrated Process:** Teaching and Learning

4. **1 A hummus spread made with a cup of cooked white beans has approximately 36% of the daily recommended amount of phosphorus.**

   2 Although a healthy snack, a salad of green, leafy vegetables does not have more phosphorus than a serving of white beans. **3** Cucumber dill soup does not have more phosphorus than a serving of white beans. **4** A standard serving of lemon sherbet does not have more phosphorus than a serving of white beans.

   Client Need: Health Promotion and Maintenance; **Cognitive Level:** Analysis; **Integrated Process:** Teaching and Learning

5. **4 The parathyroid gland is responsible for regulating phosphorus levels by affecting the activity of PTH.**

   1 The pineal gland produces melatonin, which helps maintain circadian rhythm and regulate reproductive hormones. **2** The pituitary gland does not regulate the level of serum phosphorus. **3** The pancreas excretes enzymes to break down the proteins, lipids, carbohydrates, and nucleic acids in food.

   Client Need: Health Promotion and Maintenance; **Cognitive Level:** Understanding; **Integrated Process:** Teaching and Learning

6. **3 Vitamin D (calcitriol) increases the absorption of phosphorus from the gut and bones.**

   1 Vitamin A is involved in immune function, vision, reproduction, and cellular communication. **2** Vitamin B_{12} is a nutrient that helps keep the body's nerve and blood cells healthy and helps make deoxyribonucleic acid (DNA), the genetic material in all cells. **4** Vitamin E is a fat-soluble nutrient found in many foods. In the body, it acts as an antioxidant, helping to protect cells from the damage caused by free radical molecules.

   Client Need: Health Promotion and Maintenance; **Cognitive Level:** Applying; **Nursing Process:** Planning

7. **1 Inhibitors of intestinal phosphate absorption include metabolic acidosis.**

   2, 3, 4 Inhibitors of intestinal phosphate absorption include metabolic acidosis.

   Client Need: Physiological Integrity; **Cognitive Level:** Analysis; **Nursing Process:** Assessment

8. **Answers: 1, 3, 4, 5**

   1 Hyperglycemia causes the release of insulin that then transports glucose and phosphorus into the cells. **3** An increase in the loss of phosphorus from the kidneys can occur with loop diuretic therapy. **4** Severe malnutrition, especially in older adults, can result in hypophosphatemia. **5** Respiratory alkalosis, caused by hyperventilation associated with alcohol withdrawal, can result in hypophosphatemia.

   2 Increased intestinal loss of phosphorus occurs with chronic diarrhea.

   Client Need: Physiological Integrity; **Cognitive Level:** Analysis; **Nursing Process:** Assessment

9. **Answers: 1, 2, 3, 4**

   1 Acute hypophosphatemia requires effective assessment for pain. **2** Acute hypophosphatemia requires interventions that focus on possible dysphagia. **3** Acute hypophosphatemia requires frequent assessment for hypotension. **4** Acute hypophosphatemia requires frequent monitoring for levels of consciousness.

   5 Neither nausea nor vomiting are directly associated with acute hypophosphatemia.

   Client Need: Physiological Integrity; **Cognitive Level:** Application; **Nursing Process:** Planning

10. **Answers: 1, 3, 4, 5**

    1 Changes in the structure and function of RBCs are associated with possible chronic hypophosphatemia. **3** A risk for infection is associated with possible chronic hypophosphatemia. **4** Poor platelet function is associated with possible chronic hypophosphatemia. **5** Bone weakness is associated with possible chronic hypophosphatemia.

    2 Hypotension is associated with possible chronic hypophosphatemia.

    Client Need: Physiological Integrity; **Cognitive Level:** Analysis; **Nursing Process:** Evaluation

11. **Answers: 1, 4, 5**

    1 Calcium phosphate is an insoluble compound that can deposit itself in the lungs. **4** Calcium phosphate is an insoluble compound that can deposit itself in the heart. **5** Calcium phosphate is an insoluble compound that can deposit itself in the kidneys.

2 Calcium phosphate is an insoluble compound that is not likely to deposit itself in the lymphatic system. **3** Calcium phosphate is an insoluble compound that is not likely to deposit itself in the nervous system.

Client Need: Physiological Integrity; **Cognitive Level:** Application; **Nursing Process:** Planning

12. **1 Calcification can result in the formation of cataracts.**

2 Depression is not generally associated with calcification problems. **3** Sugar cravings are not generally associated with calcification problems. **4** Paresthesia around the lips, mouth, and eyes is not generally associated with calcification problems. This option suggests a vascular problem.

Client Need: Physiological Integrity; **Cognitive Level:** Analysis; **Nursing Process:** Assessment

13. **Answers: 1, 3, 5**

1 Leukemia increases the risk of developing hyperphosphatemia. **3** A heatstroke increases the risk of developing hyperphosphatemia. **5** Sepsis increases the risk of developing hyperphosphatemia.

2 A bone fracture is not a risk factor for developing hyperphosphatemia. **4** Antidepressant therapy is not a risk factor for developing hyperphosphatemia.

Client Need: Physiological Integrity; **Cognitive Level:** Analysis; **Nursing Process:** Assessment

14. **1 Regular antacid therapy can result in increased serum phosphorus levels.**

2 Although alcohol abuse is a health issue, it is not directly associated with hyperphosphatemia. **3** An appendectomy is not associated with the management of phosphorous. **4** Although a heatstroke can trigger hyperphosphatemia, working out in a cold environment is not associated with this situation.

Client Need: Physiological Integrity; **Cognitive Level:** Analysis; **Nursing Process:** Assessment

15. **Answers: 1, 2, 4**

1 Elevated phosphorus levels are greater than 4.5 mg/dL (2.6 mEq/L). **2** Considering the reciprocal relationship between calcium and phosphorus, hypocalcemia is diagnosed with a serum calcium less than 8.5 mg/dL. **4** Considering the reciprocal relationship between calcium and phosphorus, electrocardiographic changes characteristic of hypocalcemia includes a prolonged QT syndrome.

3 Considering the reciprocal relationship between calcium and phosphorus, hypocalcemia is diagnosed with a serum calcium less than 8.5 mg/dL. **5** T-wave inversion (negative T waves) can be a sign of coronary ischemia.

Client Need: Physiological Integrity; **Cognitive Level:** Analysis; **Nursing Process:** Assessment

16. **2 Severe hyperphosphatemia is diagnosed with a serum phosphorus baseline level at least 6 mg/dL.**

1, 3, 4 Severe hyperphosphatemia is diagnosed with a serum phosphorus baseline level at least 6 mg/dL.

Client Need: Physiological Integrity; **Cognitive Level:** Understanding; **Nursing Process:** Assessment

17. **1 Alterations in calcium levels are associated with muscle injury.**

2 Alterations in serum phosphorus levels are not associated with muscle injury. **3** BUN is associated with renal function. **4** Chloride is not associated with muscle injury.

Client Need: Physiological Integrity; **Cognitive Level:** Application; **Nursing Process:** Planning

18. **1 Uremia is associated with shortness of breath due to cardiovascular complications.**

2 Acute hyperphosphatemia associated with hypocalcemia can trigger muscle tetany. **3** Acute hyperphosphatemia associated with hypocalcemia can trigger seizures. **4** Falls precautions are not specific to a diagnosis of uremia.

Client Need: Physiological Integrity; **Cognitive Level:** Application; **Nursing Process:** Evaluation

19. **3 Hyperphosphatemia coupled with hypocalcemia (serum calcium level <8.5 mg/dL) can trigger seizures. Safety is the priority nursing goal.**

1 The risk of seizures is a safety priority greater than diminished appetite. **2** Although elevating the client's serum calcium is a treatment goal, the safety priority is implementing seizure precautions. **4** Although decreasing the client's serum phosphorus is a treatment goal, the safety priority is implementing seizure precautions.

Client Need: Physiological Integrity; **Cognitive Level:** Analysis; **Nursing Process:** Planning

20. **2 A client diagnosed with an under-functioning parathyroid gland should be encouraged to avoid foods high in phosphorus, such as organ meat, if there is a preexisting condition that may lead to hyperphosphatemia.**

    1 With a preexisting condition that affects the serum phosphorus level, the client needs to manage his or her consumption of that element. **3** Diabetes is a condition that would increase the risk for hyperphosphatemia; identifying the condition would not significantly affect the management of the existing risk. **4** Renal failure is a condition that would increase the risk for hyperphosphatemia; identifying the condition would not significantly affect the management of the existing risk.

    Client Need: Health Promotion and Maintenance; **Cognitive Level:** Analysis; **Integrated:** Teaching and Learning

10 Magnesium Imbalance

MAGNESIUM OVERVIEW

Significance of Magnesium

- Magnesium is the second most available intracellular cation.
  - Magnesium is a cofactor in more than 300 enzymatic reactions involving energy metabolism.
  - Magnesium is involved in protein and nucleic acid synthesis.
- Magnesium has an atomic number of 12.
- Magnesium has a mass of 24.32 daltons.
- The active form of the element is ionized Mg.
- Magnesium is bound to protein and a chelated buffer.
- Magnesium is present in three different states: ionized free, complexed to anions, and bound to protein. Protein bound and complex are both in a form that is not usable for biological activity.
- The half-life of magnesium in the body is between 41 and 181 days.
- Laboratory data concerning serum magnesium may not provide a complete clinical picture. Laboratory values only provide serum values and not the levels of magnesium in the tissues.
- On average for a 70-kg human
  - The human body contains 1 mole of magnesium.
  - One-half of the magnesium is in bone.
  - The other half is in soft tissue (intracellular) and muscle.
  - Less than 1% of the total magnesium is present in the blood. Therefore serum blood levels of magnesium represent a minimal proportion of the total body magnesium level.

Control of Magnesium (Figure 10.1)

- Approximately one-half of magnesium in the body is present in intracellular soft tissue; the other half is present in bone.
- Contrary to other electrolytes, the control of magnesium reabsorption is not dependent on a specific hormone.
- The majority of magnesium is absorbed in the ilium and colon.
- The kidneys maintain control and balance of magnesium.
  - On average, between 70% and 80% of total serum magnesium is filtered by the renal system.
  - Usually, approximately 96% of magnesium is reabsorbed by the kidneys' tubules.
  - Most of the other ions are reabsorbed by the proximal tubule.
    - Only a small amount of magnesium, between 15% and 25%, is absorbed in the proximal tubule.
    - Distal tubules are important in the end urine concentration of magnesium.
    - Factors that affect sodium reabsorption can do the same with magnesium.
    - There is a paracellular reabsorption of magnesium and calcium.
    - Disturbances in calcium (hypercalciuria) will cause a similar rise in magnesium (hypermagnesemia).
  - The volume of magnesium excreted is related to the concentration of magnesium in the plasma.

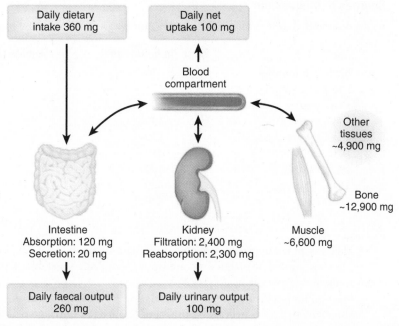

FIGURE 10.1 Normal magnesium balance. (From de Baaij, J. H., Hoenderop, J. G, & Bindels, R. J. [2012]. Regulation of magnesium balance: lessons learned from human genetic disease. *Clinical Kidney Journal*, 5[Suppl 1], i15-i24.)

- Usually only 5% or less of magnesium is excreted in the urine.
- Less than 1% of the total magnesium in the body is present in blood.

APPLICATION AND REVIEW

1. Which statement made by the nurse demonstrates an understanding of the clinical value of the diagnostic laboratory results related to serum magnesium levels?
   1. "Individual responses to abnormal magnesium levels vary greatly, making the results clinically useless."
   2. "Since most magnesium is found in the blood, the results are excellent indicators of client status."
   3. "Serum diagnostic results are seldom reliable and are generally ignored for diagnostic purposes."
   4. "Serum levels are only a part of the client's complete clinical magnesium picture."
2. Which client is at risk for impaired magnesium absorption?
   1. 10-year-old child diagnosed with autism
   2. 20-year-old adult who regularly uses marijuana
   3. 40-year old adult who has had colon resection surgery
   4. 60-year-old man who is being treated for anemia
3. Which chronic condition presents the greatest risk for an increase in serum magnesium levels?
   1. Congestive heart failure (CHF)
   2. Diabetes mellitus (DM) type 2
   3. Crohn disease
   4. Renal failure

See Answers on pages 190–192.

Sources of Magnesium

- Recommended dietary allowances (RDAs) for magnesium are listed in the following table.

Age	Male (in milligrams)	Female (in milligrams)
Birth to 6 months	30	20
7 to 12 months	75	75
1 to 3 years	80	80
4 to 8 years	130	130
9 to 13 years	240	240
14 to 18 years	410	360
19 to 30 years	400	310
31 to 50 years	420	320
51+ years	420	320

- Food
  - Magnesium is extensively available from plants, animal foods, and beverages.
  - The best sources of magnesium are from green, leafy vegetables (spinach), legumes, nuts, seeds, and whole grains.
  - Magnesium is added to breakfast cereals and fortified foods (bread), among others.
  - Some types of food-processing practices remove the nutrient-rich germ and bran, which result in lower levels of magnesium.
  - Tap, mineral, and bottled water can also be sources of magnesium. Amount of magnesium depends on the sources and can range form 1 mg/L to more than 120 mg/L.
  - The amount of dietary magnesium absorbed from the body is approximately 30% to 40% from the food eaten.
  - Foods and the corresponding amounts of magnesium per serving are listed in the following table.

Food	Serving Size	Mg Magnesium	% Daily Value
Almonds, dry roasted	1 ounce	80	20
Spinach, boiled	½ cup	78	20
Cashews, dry roasted	1 ounce	74	19
Peanuts, oil roasted	¼ cup	63	16
Cereal, shredded wheat	Two large biscuits	61	15
Soymilk	1 cup	61	15
Black beans	½ cup cooked	60	15
Edamame (soybeans in pods)	½ cup, shelled, cooked	50	13
Peanut butter, smooth	2 tablespoons	52	12
Bread, whole wheat	Two slices	46	12
Avocado, cubed	1 cup	44	11
Potato, baked	3½ ounces	43	11
Rice, brown, cooked	½ cup	42	11
Yogurt, plain	8 ounces	42	11
Breakfast cereal, fortified	½ cup	40	10
Oatmeal, instant	One pack	36	9
Kidney beans	½ cup	35	9
Banana	One medium size	32	8
Salmon	3 ounces	26	7

- Magnesium consumption is correlated to caloric intake.
- Drinking water is a vital source of magnesium.
  - In the United States, most drinking water contains less than 10 mg/L of magnesium.
  - In some areas in the midwest, the drinking water contains more than 10 mg/L of magnesium.

Functions of Magnesium

- Enhances enzyme reactions within the cells during carbohydrate metabolism
- Promotes neurotransmission and hormone-receptor binding
- Contributes to deoxyribonucleic acid (DNA) and protein synthesis
- Assists with the production and use of adenosine triphosphate (ATP) for energy
- Influences vasodilatation of blood vessels
- Affects irritability and contractility of the cardiac muscles
  - Assists the cardiovascular system to function normally
  - Aids in neurotransmission and hormone-receptor binding
  - Assists in the production of parathyroid hormone (PTH)
  - Facilitates sodium and potassium ions crossing over the cell membrane

Hypomagnesemia

- Pathophysiological factors
  - Hypomagnesemia is found in 12% of hospitalized clients.
  - Incidence in intensive critical care units (ICUs) is approximately 60% of clients.
- Assessment
  - Cardiac assessment includes heart rate, rhythm, and electrocardiographic (ECG) changes.
  - Magnesium regulates multiple cardiac ion channels: calcium channel and outward potassium currents.
  - Decreased myocardial cytosolic magnesium can increase the likelihood of tachyarrhythmias (ventricular); also known as tachycardia: torsades de pointe; monomorphic ventricular tachycardia; ventricular fibrillation
  - Increased risks in clients who are acutely ill: postmyocardial infarction; CHF; ventricular fibrillation
  - Hypomagnesemia has been observed as a comorbidity with insulin resistance, metabolic syndrome, newly onset DM after organ transplantation, migraine headaches, hypertension, and asthma.
  - Clients with unexplained hypocalcemia or hypokalemia should be assessed to evaluate magnesium depletion.
- Diagnostic factors
  - Serum magnesium level is below 1.8 mEq/L.
  - A normal serum magnesium level may occur even when the total body magnesium is exhausted.
  - In clients with hypomagnesemia in ICUs, the risk of morbidity and mortality is significant.
  - There is no consensus on the value of preventing hypomagnesemia and at what level supplementation should begin.
  - Since a small percentage of magnesium is extracellular, decreases in serum magnesium can occur after the total body magnesium is significantly declined.
    - Magnesium retention test
      - Measures the amount of magnesium excreted in the urine in response to a bolus of intravenous (IV) magnesium

- ▪ With hypomagnesemia, the amount of infused magnesium will be absorbed and less will be excreted in the urine.
  - ▪ If less than 50% of the infused magnesium is recovered in the urine, then usually magnesium deficiency is suspected.
  - Differentiate between renal and extrarenal hypomagnesemia. Gastrointestinal causes will result in an extracellular magnesium shift to intracellular.
  - Assess a 24-hour urine collection to calculate the fractional excretion of magnesium. Normal fractional excretion of magnesium is 100 mg/day.
- Signs and symptoms
  - Clients can be asymptomatic or exhibit a wide range of symptoms not specific to hypomagnesemia.
  - Often, no symptoms are exhibited with a mild or gradual development of hypomagnesemia.
  - Severe hypomagnesemia, especially with a rapid onset, can express signs and symptoms related to the cardiovascular, neuromuscular, and central nervous systems.
  - Primary clinical signs and symptoms: apathy; depression; confusion; anorexia
  - Cardiovascular signs and symptoms: cardiac arrhythmias; greater sensitivity to digitalis; ECG changes (prolonged PR and QT intervals, T-wave changes, and widening QRS complex)
  - Neuromuscular signs and symptoms: Chvostek-Weiss or Trousseau sign; muscle cramps; tetany; seizures; muscle weakness; altered level of consciousness (LOC)
  - Associated electrolyte abnormalities: hypokalemia; hypocalcemia
- Goals of care
  - Restore client to normal levels of magnesium.
  - Provide supportive care to manage signs and symptoms.
  - Recommend dietary changes.
- Treatment
  - Reverse the underlying cause of hypomagnesemia.
  - Rate and route of magnesium restoration will be determined by the severity of the clinical symptoms.
  - Plasma magnesium is the major controller of magnesium reabsorption (Henle loop); a major elevation in serum magnesium can result in one half of the amount being excreted in urine.
  - Absorption of magnesium is a slow process.
- Complications
  - Adverse reactions to IV magnesium infusion: facial flushing; loss of deep-tendon reflexes (DTRs); hypotension; atrioventricular block; hypocalcemia
- Nursing interventions
  - Frequently assess vital signs.
  - Monitor respiratory effort. Hypomagnesium can cause laryngeal stridor.
  - Evaluate ECG changes. If the magnesium level is <1 mEq/L, closely monitor for arrhythmias.
  - Neurological considerations: DTR hyperactivity; LOC; Chvostek-Weiss and Trousseau signs (if hypocalcemia is suspected)
  - Muscular considerations: Check for dysphagia before administering fluids or food. Hypomagnesium can interfere with the ability to swallow.
  - Strictly record intake and output measurements.
  - Have calcium gluconate ready if needed for adverse reactions.

- Prevention
  - Prevention begins with the early recognition of clients at risk for developing hypomagnesemia and the clinical setting where it typically develops.
    - Clients in ICUs
      - Poor nutrition
      - Gastrointestinal losses: proton pump inhibitor (PPI) administration; diarrhea; vomiting
      - Renal losses: medications (diuretics, antibiotics); simultaneous electrolyte imbalances
    - Clients with cardiac disease are at a greater risk of sudden death attributable to hypomagnesemia.

APPLICATION AND REVIEW

4. The nurse demonstrates an understanding of the likely comorbid conditions when which assessment questions are asked of a client who has been diagnosed with hypomagnesemia? *(Select all that apply.)*
   1. "Do you have any food-related allergies?"
   2. "Do you experience migraine headaches?"
   3. "Are you currently being treated for hypertension?"
   4. "Do you often have trouble falling or staying asleep?"
   5. "Have you been diagnosed with any form of asthma?"

5. A client diagnosed with hypomagnesemia should be assessed for which other chemical deficiencies? *(Select all that apply.)*
   1. Hypocalcemia
   2. Hypochloremia
   3. Hypokalemia
   4. Hyponatremia
   5. Hypophosphatemia

6. Which clinical information **best** supports the probability that the client is *not* experiencing a magnesium deficiency?
   1. Magnesium retention test results show a 65% recovery.
   2. Patient demonstrates no abnormal cardiac activity.
   3. Patient continues to be awake, alert, and oriented.
   4. Serum magnesium level is 2.0 mEq/L.

7. Which clinical signs and symptoms are associated with hypomagnesemia? *(Select all that apply.)*
   1. Seizures
   2. Depression
   3. Hypercalcemia
   4. Cardiac arrhythmia
   5. Shortness of breath

8. Which client reactions are most possibly the result of an adverse reaction to an IV magnesium infusion? *(Select all that apply.)*
   1. Vomiting
   2. Blurred vision
   3. Facial flushing
   4. Drop in blood pressure
   5. Loss of DTRs

9. What is the focus of the priority nursing assessment for a client with a serum magnesium level of 0.92 mEq/L?
   1. LOC
   2. Cardiac arrhythmias
   3. DTR activity
   4. Dysphagia

10. Which assessment finding is strong supportive evidence of hypocalcemia in a client with a low magnesium level?
    1. DTR hyperactivity
    2. Positive Trousseau sign
    3. Tachycardia
    4. Dysphagia

See Answers on pages 190–192.

Hypermagnesemia

- Pathophysiological considerations
  - Too much magnesium can be as detrimental as having too little in the human body.
  - Hypermagnesium happens when the serum blood level of magnesium is above 2.5 mEq/L.
  - Because the kidneys will often excrete excess amounts of magnesium in the urine, the occurrence of hypermagnesemia is uncommon.
  - Drugs associated with hypermagnesemia: antacids (Maalox, Gaviscon); laxatives (Milk of Magnesia, magnesium citrate); magnesium sulfate (magnesium oxide)
  - Other sources of excessive magnesium intake: magnesium-rich dialysate for hemodialysis; total parenteral nutrition solution with an excess of magnesium; continuous infusion of magnesium sulfate
  - Renal dysfunction is often the reason for hypermagnesemia. Its causes can include advanced age, renal failure, Addison disease, adrenocortical insufficiency, and untreated diabetic ketoacidosis (DKA).
- Assessment
  - Unusually high levels of magnesium can inhibit the neuromuscular system.
  - Hypermagnesemia blocks the neuromuscular transmission, and the nurse may notice lower muscle and nerve activity; decreased DTRs; facial paresthesia (usually with moderately elevated magnesium levels); gastrointestinal disruption (nausea and vomiting); and generalized weakness (weak grasp, inability to reposition oneself in bed). If hypermagnesemia progresses, the weakness can lead to flaccid paralysis.
  - Due to the central nervous system depression, symptoms can include drowsiness, lethargy, and eventually coma.
  - The respiratory system can be impaired as a result of weakened respiratory muscles, exhibiting slow, shallow breathing and the potential for respiratory arrest.
  - Cardiac involvement can occur with hypermagnesemia: weak pulse; bradycardia; heart block; vasodilatation (lower blood pressure); warm, flushed sensation; cardiac arrest
- Diagnostic factors
  - Serum magnesium blood level over 2.5 mEq/L
  - Cardinal ECG changes: prolonged PR interval; widened QRS complex; tall T wave
- Signs and symptoms
  - Magnesium levels between 4 and 6 mEq/L: DTRs disappear; nausea; vomiting; flushing; lethargy; drowsiness
  - Magnesium levels between 6 and 10 mEq/L: respiratory compromise (apnea); mental status changes (sleepiness); hypotension; ECG changes (prolonged PR interval, QRS complex, and QT interval); hypocalcemia
  - Magnesium levels greater than 10 mEq/L: flaccid and paralysis; complete heart block; coma; cardiac arrest
- Goal of care: Correct the underlying cause of the magnesium imbalance.
- Treatment
  - Identify and terminate the source of exogenous magnesium.

- If the client has normal renal function, ending the exogenous source of magnesium may be the only required treatment.
- Life-threatening hypermagnesemia with cardiovascular, neurological, or respiratory complications may require immediate treatment.
  - Administer IV calcium to antagonize the effects of magnesium.
  - Provide supportive care as needed.
  - Volume expansion with IV fluids can enhance the excretion of magnesium through the urine output.
  - Loop diuretics can inhibit the reabsorption of magnesium in the Henle loop.
  - Carefully monitor the calcium levels to maintain hemostasis.
- Complications: paralysis; complete heart block; coma; cardiac arrest
- Nursing interventions for clients with hypermagnesemia
  - Monitor vital signs.
  - Assess the client for hypotension and respiratory depression.
  - Immediately notify the physician of respiratory status decline.
  - Assess the neuromuscular system: DTRs; muscle strength; flushed skin and diaphoresis.
  - Notify the primary health care provider if magnesium levels continue to be elevated. If kidney function is declining, the client may require peritoneal dialysis or hemodialysis using magnesium-free dialysate.
  - Monitor the client for hypocalcemia that can occur with hypermagnesemia. PTH secretion is suppressed by low serum calcium levels.
  - Monitor urine output. Excretion of magnesium occurs in the urine.
  - Evaluate neurological factors: LOC; reorientation, if confused
  - Continually monitor ECG for changes.
  - Make IV access available.
  - Provide oral and IV fluids to flush the kidneys. Strictly monitor and record intake and output.
  - Restrict dietary intake of magnesium.
  - Monitor and restrict client medications with magnesium.
- Prevention: early identification of individuals at high risk for hypermagnesemia
  - Older adults
  - Individuals with renal insufficiency or failure
  - Pregnant women with pregnancy-induced hypertension (PIH) receiving magnesium sulfate therapy
  - Neonates whose mothers received magnesium sulfate during labor
  - Individuals ingesting magnesium sulfate for seizure control
  - Clients ingesting magnesium or products containing magnesium (e.g., laxatives, antacids)
  - Individuals with adrenal insufficiency
  - Individuals with severe DKA
  - Individuals experiencing dehydration
  - Individuals with hypothyroidism (underactive thyroid gland)

APPLICATION AND REVIEW

11. Which client's serum magnesium levels support a diagnosis of hypermagnesemia? *(Select all that apply.)*
    1. 2.0 mEq/L
    2. 2.3 mEq/L
    3. 2.7 mEq/L
    4. 3.5 mEq/L
    5. 5.4 mEq/L

12. What assessment findings support the possibility that a client is experiencing cardinal changes in cardiac function related to an elevated magnesium level? *(Select all that apply.)*
    1. Prolonged PR interval
    2. Widened QRS complex
    3. Tall T wave
    4. Bradycardia
    5. Tachycardia

13. Which nursing interventions should a nurse specifically consider when caring for a client with a magnesium level of 5.2 mEq/L? *(Select all that apply.)*
    1. Regularly monitor the client for nausea.
    2. Assist with daily hygiene as needed.
    3. Regularly monitor the client for hypotension.
    4. Provide dietary snacks high in magnesium.
    5. Assess the client for dehydration related to vomiting.

14. For which specific intervention should a nurse plan when caring for a client with a magnesium level of 10.8 mEq/L?
    1. Supplemental oxygen
    2. Continuous cardiac monitoring
    3. Intermittent blood pressure monitoring
    4. Assessment results to a rapid cardiac response team

15. Which intervention will have the **greatest** effect on preventing an abnormal magnesium level?
    1. Provide adequate hydration for an older adult client after surgery.
    2. Provide effective education to a client scheduled for renal dialysis.
    3. Assess and medicate a woman client in labor for reported pain.
    4. Provide precautions for a client at risk for seizures.

16. For which comorbid chemical deficiency should a client diagnosed with hypermagnesemia be assessed?
    1. Hyponatremia
    2. Hypocalcemia
    3. Hypokalemia
    4. Hypochloremia

17. Which clients have an increased risk for abnormal magnesium levels? *(Select all that apply.)*
    1. 35-year-old woman being treated for PIH
    2. 18-year-old client who is being treated with magnesium sulfate for the control of seizures
    3. 40-year-old individual with a history of long-term antacid therapy
    4. 82-year-old woman receiving dialysis for chronic renal failure
    5. 58-year-old man being treated for hyperthyroidism

See answers on pages 190–192.

See answers on pages 190–192.

ANSWER KEY: REVIEW QUESTIONS

1. **4 Laboratory values provide serum values, not the levels of magnesium in the tissues.**
   1 Although responses to abnormal levels may vary, the clinical knowledge derived from knowing a client's serum magnesium level has value in determining appropriate care. **2** This statement is not accurate; only 1% of the body's magnesium is found in the blood. **3** Serum magnesium values are an important factor in effectively diagnosing and treating clients.
   Client Need: Physiological Integrity; **Cognitive Level:** Analysis; **Nursing Process:** Assessment

2. **3 Since most magnesium is absorbed in the ilium and colon, resection surgery would impair magnesium absorption.**
   1 Autism does not impair the absorption of magnesium. **2** Marijuana does not appear to impair the absorption of magnesium. **4** Anemia does not impair the absorption of magnesium.
   Client Need: Physiological Integrity; **Cognitive Level:** Analysis; **Nursing Process:** Assessment

3. **4 The kidneys maintain control and balance of magnesium with an average of 70% to 80% of total serum magnesium being filtered by the renal system. Renal failure would impair effective filtration.**

    1 No direct relationship exists between CHF and hypermagnesemia. 2 No direct relationship exists between DM type 2 and hypermagnesemia. 3 No direct relationship exists between Crohn disease and hypermagnesemia.

    Client Need: Physiological Integrity; **Cognitive Level:** Analysis; **Nursing Process:** Assessment

4. **Answers: 2, 3, 5**

    2 Hypomagnesemia has been observed as a comorbid condition with migraine headaches. 3 Hypomagnesemia has been observed as a comorbid condition with hypertension. 5 Hypomagnesemia has been observed as a comorbid condition with asthma.

    1 Hypomagnesemia has not been observed as a comorbidity with food allergies. 4 Hypomagnesemia has not been observed as a comorbidity with sleep disorders.

    Client Need: Physiological Integrity; **Cognitive Level:** Analysis; **Nursing Process:** Assessment

5. **Answers: 1, 3**

    1 A client with unexplained hypocalcemia should be evaluated for magnesium depletion. 3 A client with unexplained hypokalemia should be evaluated for magnesium depletion.

    2 Clients diagnosed with hypomagnesemia are not necessarily at risk for hypochloremia. 4 Clients diagnosed with hypomagnesemia are not necessarily at risk for hyponatremia. 5 Clients diagnosed with hypomagnesemia are not necessarily at risk for hypophosphatemia.

    Client Need: Physiological Integrity; **Cognitive Level:** Understanding; **Nursing Process:** Assessment

6. **1 If less than 50% of the infused magnesium is recovered in the urine, then usually a magnesium deficiency can be suspected via a magnesium retention test.**

    2, 3 Often, there are no symptoms with mild or gradual development of magnesium deficiency. 4 A magnesium level of 2.0 mEq/L is within the acceptable normal range.

    Client Need: Physiological Integrity; **Cognitive Level:** Analysis; **Nursing Process:** Assessment

7. **Answers: 1, 2, 4**

    1 The primary clinical signs and symptoms of hypomagnesemia can include seizures. 2 The primary clinical signs and symptoms of hypomagnesemia can include depression. 4 The primary clinical signs and symptoms of hypomagnesemia can include cardiac arrhythmias.

    3 The primary clinical signs and symptoms of hypomagnesemia can include hypocalcemia. 5 Shortness of breath is not a clinical sign directly associated with hypomagnesemia.

    Client Need: Physiological Integrity; **Cognitive Level:** Understanding; **Nursing Process:** Assessment

8. **Answers: 3, 4, 5**

    3 Adverse reactions to an IV magnesium infusion include facial flushing. 4 Adverse reactions to an IV magnesium infusion include hypotension. 5 Adverse reactions to an IV magnesium infusion include loss of DTRs.

    1 Vomiting is not an adverse reaction associated with an IV magnesium infusion. 2 Blurred vision is not an adverse reaction associated with an IV magnesium infusion.

    Client Need: Physiological Integrity; **Cognitive Level:** Understanding; **Nursing Process:** Assessment

9. **2 If the magnesium level is less than 1 mEq/L, the priority nursing assessment is to monitor closely for arrhythmias.**

    1 Although a neurological assessment is appropriate, at this severe level of hypomagnesemia, cardiac function is the priority. 3 Although an assessment of DTR activity is appropriate, at this severe level of hypomagnesemia, cardiac function is the priority. 4 Although muscular assessment is appropriate, at this severe level of hypomagnesemia, cardiac function is the priority.

    Client Need: Physiological Integrity; **Cognitive Level:** Analysis; **Nursing Process:** Planning

10. **2 A positive Trousseau sign is associated with hypocalcemia.**

    1 DTR hyperactivity is associated with hypomagnesemia, not hypocalcemia. 3 Cardiac arrhythmias are associated with hypomagnesemia, not hypocalcemia. 4 Dysphagia is associated with hypomagnesemia, not hypocalcemia.

    Client Need: Physiological Integrity; **Cognitive Level:** Analysis; **Nursing Process:** Evaluation

11. **Answers: 3, 4, 5**

    3, 4, 5 Serum magnesium blood levels over 2.5 mEq/L are generally accepted for a diagnosis of hyperma-gnesemia.

    1 A serum magnesium blood level of 2.0 mEq/L is within the acceptable normal range. **2** A serum mag-nesium blood level 2.3 mEq/L is within the acceptable normal range.

    Client Need: Physiological Integrity; **Cognitive Level:** Understanding; **Nursing Process:** Assessment

12. **Answers: 1, 2, 3**

    1 Cardinal ECG changes associated with hypermagnesemia include a prolonged PR interval. **2** Cardinal ECG changes associated with hypermagnesemia include a widened QRS complex. **3** Cardinal ECG changes associated with hypermagnesemia include a tall T wave.

    4 Cardinal ECG changes associated with hypermagnesemia do not include bradycardia. **5** Cardinal ECG changes associated with hypermagnesemia do not include tachycardia.

    Client Need: Physiological Integrity; **Cognitive Level:** Understanding; **Nursing Process:** Assessment

13. **Answers: 1, 2, 5**

    1 A magnesium level between 4 and 6 mEq/L can trigger nausea. **2** A magnesium level between 4 and 6 mEq/L can trigger lethargy and the need for assistance with daily tasks of living. **5** A magnesium level between 4 and 6 mEq/L can trigger vomiting.

    3 A magnesium level between 6 and 10 mEq/L can trigger hypotension. **4** A magnesium level of 5. 2 mEq/L is elevated and would not indicate a need for additional dietary magnesium.

    Client Need: Physiological Integrity; **Cognitive Level:** Application; **Nursing Process:** Planning

14. **4 A magnesium level above 10 mEq/L places this client at risk for cardiac arrest.**

    1 Magnesium levels between 6 and 10 mEq/L place clients at risk for respiratory compromise. **2** Magne-sium levels between 6 and 10 mEq/L place clients at risk for ECG changes. **3** Magnesium levels between 6 and 10 mEq/L place clients at risk for hypotension.

    Client Need: Physiological Integrity; **Cognitive Level:** Application; **Nursing Process:** Planning

15. **1 Dehydration is a risk factor of abnormal magnesium levels; avoiding dehydration with adequate hydration will prevent the problem.**

    2 Although renal failure is a risk factor for abnormal magnesium levels, education is not as effective as other interventions. **3** Although important, pain is not a common trigger for abnormal magnesium levels. **4** Although an appropriate intervention, seizure precautions will not prevent seizures and there-fore will not affect the magnesium levels.

    Client Need: Physiological Integrity; **Cognitive Level:** Analysis; **Nursing Process:** Implementation

16. **2 Hypocalcemia can occur with hypermagnesemia.**

    1 Hyponatremia is not considered a comorbid condition associated with hypermagnesemia.

    3 Hypokalemia is not considered a comorbid condition associated with hypermagnesemia. **4** Hypochlo-remia is not considered a comorbid condition associated with hypermagnesemia.

    Client Need: Physiological Integrity; **Cognitive Level:** Application; **Nursing Process:** Assessment

17. **Answers: 1, 2, 3, 4**

    1 Individuals at high risk for developing abnormal magnesium levels include the pregnant women with PIH receiving magnesium sulfate therapy. **2** Individuals at high risk for developing abnormal magne-sium levels include those receiving magnesium sulfate for seizure control. **3** Individuals at high risk for developing abnormal magnesium levels include those ingesting antacids that contain magnesium. **4** Individuals at high risk for developing abnormal magnesium levels include older adults and those with renal insufficiency.

    5 Individuals at high risk for developing abnormal magnesium levels include anyone being treated for hypothyroidism, not hyperthyroidism.

    Client Need: Physiological Integrity; **Cognitive Level:** Analysis; **Nursing Process:** Assessment

CALCIUM OVERVIEW

Calcium

- Calcium is found in the intracellular fluid (ICF) and the extracellular fluid (ECF).
- Major electrolytes found in the body: potassium; calcium; sodium; chloride; phosphorus; magnesium
- Electrically charged electrolytes
  - Positive cations: potassium; sodium; magnesium; calcium
  - Negative anions: bicarbonate; chloride; phosphate
- Without electrolytes, the body cannot maintain homeostasis.
- Control of electrolytes
  - Diffusion: movement of molecules from an area of higher concentration to an area of lower concentration; no energy required
  - Active transport: movement of molecules from an area of lower concentration to an area of higher concentration, against a concentration gradient; cellular energy is required
  - Osmosis: movement of water from an area that contains more movement (dilute area) to an area that has less water
- Functions of electrolytes
  - Electrolytes regulate fluid balance.
    - Balance in the body's state is achieved when the required amount of water is present and distributed between the various body fluid compartments (ICF and ECF).
    - Balance is achieved when intake equals output (loss).
  - Electrolytes maintain homeostasis.
  - Electrolytes control acid-base balance.

Significance of Calcium

- Calcium is the most abundant mineral found in the body.
- The body uses this important mineral in many ways.
- Calcium is needed for all cells to function.
- Calcium plays a major role in muscle tone, hormone secretion, transmission of nerve impulses, and contraction of skeletal and heart muscles.

Forms of Calcium

- Two forms of calcium are in the blood.
  - Ionized calcium, also known as free calcium: physiologically active; bound to other minerals (anions); not attached to proteins; associated with the promotion of neuromuscular activity
  - Bound calcium: bound to proteins, particularly albumin; bound to protein cannot pass through the capillary wall

Sources of Calcium

- Dairy products: milk; cheese; yogurt; sour cream; cottage cheese; ice cream
- Canned seafood: salmon; sardines; oysters

- Fruit juices, labeled as fortified
- Dark green, leafy vegetables: spinach; kale; rhubarb; collard greens; broccoli

Control of Calcium

- Calcium is controlled by
  - Parathyroid hormone (PTH)
    - When low levels of serum calcium are present, the parathyroid gland excretes PTH.
    - PTH assists in removing calcium from the bones.
    - PTH increases gastrointestinal (GI) reabsorption of calcium in the ileum and in the renal tubule.
  - Vitamin D
    - Vitamin D is necessary to reabsorb calcium from the GI tract.
  - Calcitonin
    - Calcitonin acts in the opposite manner of the PTH.
    - It prevents absorption of calcium, and promotes excretion through the renal tubules.
- Calcium and phosphate
  - An increase in calcium most often causes a decrease in phosphate (and vice versa) (Figure 11.1).

Functions of Calcium

- Calcium is necessary for the development of strong teeth and bones.
- Assists in maintaining muscle tone.
- Calcium helps maintain cardiac contractility, which contributes to blood pressure (BP) regulation.
- It is the enzyme cofactor in the clotting cascade.
  - Is necessary for the formation of blood clots with the release of thromboplastin from platelets
- Calcium is needed for nerve transmission and contraction of skeletal and cardiac muscles.

Serum Calcium

- An imbalance of serum calcium can present a real medical emergency.
- Serum calcium is the most abundant cation in the body.
  - 99% of serum calcium is found in bones.
  - The remaining 1% is found in the blood plasma or serum.
- Normal range is between 8.5 and 10.6 mg/dL.
- Serum calcium level can be misleading unless it is correlated with the serum albumin level.
- If the total protein in the blood decreases, less serum calcium is bound.

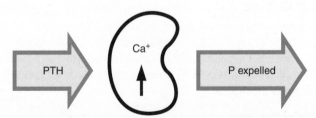

FIGURE 11.1 Parathyroid hormone (PTH) acts on the kidney to reabsorb calcium (Ca) and excrete phosphorus (P). (From Chernecky, C., Macklin, D., & Murphy-Ende, K. [2006]. *Saunders nursing survival guide: Fluids and electrolytes* [2nd ed.]. St. Louis: Saunders–Elsevier.)

APPLICATION AND REVIEW

1. Which menu selection should the nurse make to support sufficient calcium intake?
   1. Spinach and kale salad
   2. Peanut butter sandwich
   3. Chicken salad
   4. Potato soup

2. Which statement made by a nurse demonstrates an understanding of the relationship between calcium and phosphate levels?
   1. An increase in calcium causes an increase in the phosphate level.
   2. A decrease in phosphate results in an increase in the calcium level.
   3. Calcium levels have no affect on phosphate levels.
   4. Phosphate levels are unrelated to calcium levels.

3. Which client assessment notations are related to a calcium imbalance? *(Select all that apply.)*
   1. The client reports, "I'm told that I'm at risk for developing blood clots."
   2. Was recently diagnosed with a seizure disorder.
   3. Demonstrates a negative Trousseau sign.
   4. Muscle tone in the lower extremities is poor.
   5. Has a recent history of renal stones.

4. Which calcium amount demonstrates an acceptable level?
   1. 7.5 mg/dL
   2. 8.6 mg/dL
   3. 10.7 mg/dL
   4. 11.5 mg/dL

5. When analyzing data about a possible calcium abnormality, which hematological result should the nurse also consider?
   1. Serum potassium
   2. Serum phosphate
   3. Serum albumin
   4. Serum sodium

See Answers on pages 202–204.

Hypercalcemia

- Calcium level is higher than 10.6 mg/dL.
  - Because of the increased calcium intake, hypercalcemia rarely occurs.
  - Possible causes (Figure 11.2)
    - Endocrine disorder (hyperparathyroidism); the most common cause
    - Increased intake of vitamin D
    - Prolonged immobilization, attributable to bone loss
    - Malignancies
    - Medications: thiazidine diuretics; lithium
    - Certain forms of cancer of the lungs
    - Paget disease
    - Multiple myeloma
    - Non–weight-bearing activities
    - Elevated levels of calcitriol that can occur with sarcoidosis and tuberculosis
  - Signs and symptoms: thirst; anorexia; renal stones; parenthesis; urinary frequency; bone pain; confusion; abdominal pain; muscular weakness; depression; fatigue; constipation; nausea and vomiting; lethargy; electrocardiographic (ECG) changes (shortened QT interval and ST segment, depressed T wave, bradycardia, heart block); cardiac arrest
  - Goals of treatment: to correct and manage underlying causes and to maintain calcium levels within the normal range

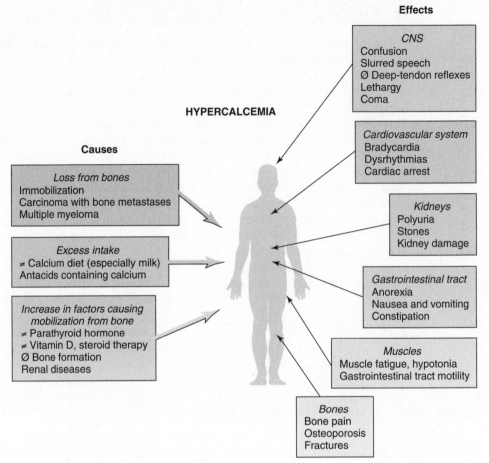

FIGURE 11.2   Causes and effects of hypercalcemia. (From Beare, P. G., & Myers, J. L. [1998]. *Adult health nursing* [3rd ed.]. St. Louis: Mosby.)

- Treatment
  - Administer intravenous (IV) fluid hydration, followed by a loop diuretic agent.
    - Excretion of calcium is followed by excretion of sodium.
  - Administer prednisone, diuretics, and bisphosphonates.
  - Additional pharmacological considerations
    - Pamidronate (Aredia) via IV to assist in reducing bone resorption
    - Calcitonin to promote renal excretion of calcium (via IV infusion)
    - Antiemetic medications to treat nausea
    - Stool softeners to relieve and/or prevent constipation
  - Severe cases may require dialysis.
- Complications
  - Increased pain level; analgesic administration may be helpful
  - Pathogenic bone fractures can occur, secondary to the bone decalcification.

- Hypercalcemia increases clotting times. Leads to increased risk for thrombosis formation with venous stasis
- Nursing assessment
  - Client history and risk factors for increased calcium: hyperparathyroidism; endocrine disorder; increased intake of vitamin D; prolonged immobilization; malignancies; medications
  - Description of symptoms: location; duration; onset; intensity; characteristics; aggravating factors; alleviating factors
- Medical history: general health history; hospitalizations; infectious disease(s); allergies
  - Physical findings
    - Assessment of symptoms related to hypercalcemia
    - Neurological status: altered or changes in the level of consciousness (LOC); mental status; confusion; agitation
      - Cranial nerves: II through XII intact
      - Sensory: touch (light, sharp, dull); paresthesia (tingling in extremities)
      - Motor: range of motion (active, passive); deep tendon reflexes; gait
    - HEENT: head; ears; eyes (PERRLA [pupils equal, round, reactive to light, and accommodation]); nose; throat
    - Cardiovascular system: auscultation of heart rate and rhythm; capillary refill; pulses; assessment of edema
    - GI system: auscultation; percussion; palpation (all four quadrants)
    - Genitourinary (GU) system: urine (color, clarity); output volume
  - Personal history: past medical conditions; hospitalizations; obstetric history; allergies; immunizations; current medications, including any recent medication changes; lifestyle (habits, diet); occupation; living environment; psychosocial considerations
  - Family history of illnesses
- Nursing interventions
  - Magnesium levels are highly associated with calcium levels. Correcting and treating magnesium levels is necessary before calcium levels can be corrected.
  - Keep the client hydrated.
    - Encourage increased fluid intake, between 3 and 4 L/day.
    - An increase in fluid intake will help decrease the chances of renal stone formation.
    - Assess for flank or abdominal pain, and strain the urine to look for stone formation.
  - Initiate safety precautions to compensate for altered gait and muscle weakness.
  - Assess neurological status every 4 hours, including LOC and orientation.
  - Encourage ambulation.
  - Monitor cardiac status.
    - Dysrhythmias: tachycardia (mild hypercalcemia); bradycardia (severe hypercalcemia)
  - Assess IV site for infiltration: erythema; pain.
  - Educate the client on limiting the intake of foods high in calcium and avoiding vitamin preparations that contain vitamin D.
  - Prevention
    - Decrease calcium-rich foods.
    - Assess the intake of calcium-preserving drugs: thiazides; supplements; vitamin D.

APPLICATION AND REVIEW

6. Which clients require focused monitoring for the development of hypercalcemia? *(Select all that apply.)*
   1. Client in skeletal traction for a severely fractured femur
   2. Client being treated for multiple myeloma
   3. Client with a calcium level of 9.8 mg/dL
   4. Client diagnosed with tuberculosis
   5. Client ingesting prescribed lithium
7. Which client assessment findings are indicative of a calcium imbalance? *(Select all that apply.)*
   1. The client reports, "I have to use a lot of pressure to stop bleeding."
   2. Was recently diagnosed with a seizure disorder.
   3. Demonstrates a negative Trousseau sign.
   4. Muscle tone in the lower extremities is poor.
   5. Has a recent history of renal stones.
8. Which client reported symptoms and observed signs support a diagnosis of hypercalcemia? *(Select all that apply.)*
   1. Thirst
   2. Confusion
   3. Bloody stools
   4. Urinary retention
   5. Depressed T wave
9. Which assessment finding in a client diagnosed with hypercalcemia requires the nurse's immediate attention?
   1. Client reports being too tired to ambulate.
   2. Client states, "I'm really feeling depressed."
   3. Client reports consistently eating less than 50% of meals.
   4. Client reports slight swelling in left calf but denies pain.
10. The nurse assesses a client diagnosed with bone pain secondary to hypercalcemia. Which question is most appropriate for the nurse to ask? *(Select all that apply.)*
    1. "When is the pain worse?"
    2. "Where is the pain located?"
    3. "What makes the pain worse?"
    4. "Have you ever experienced cancer pain?"
    5. "How would you rate the pain on a scale of 1 to 10?"
11. Which cardiac-related assessment finding is consistent with a calcium level of 14.4 mg/dL?
    1. Tachycardia
    2. Bradycardia
    3. Spiked T wave
    4. Elongated QT interval

See Answers on pages 202–204.

Hypocalcemia

- Calcium level is lower than 8.5 mg/L
  - Possible causes (Box 11.1): renal disease; malignancies; inadequate dietary calcium; vitamin D deficiency (essential for the absorption of calcium); increased intake of phosphorus (antacids); administration of blood products; low magnesium level; hypoparathyroidism; (with the removal of parathyroid gland); eating disorders; acute pancreatitis
  - Possible medication-related causes: anticonvulsants; alendronate; ibandronate bisphosphonates; rifampin; phenytoin; phenobarbital; corticosteroids; plicamycin

| **BOX 11.1** | Causes of Hypocalcemia |

Decreased Calcium Intake or Absorption
Diet with insufficient calcium and vitamin D
Chronic kidney disease (deficient activated vitamin D)
Excessive dietary phytates and oxalates
Steatorrhea
Pancreatitis
Chronic diarrhea (includes laxative overuse or abuse)
Malabsorption syndromes

Decreased Physiologic Availability of Calcium
Hypoparathyroidism
Excessive phosphate intake
Tumor lysis syndrome (high phosphate)

Hypomagnesemia
Alkalosis
Large transfusion of citrated blood or fresh frozen
  plasma
Rapid infusion of plasma expanders that bind calcium
Elevated plasma-free fatty acids
Chronic kidney disease

**Increased Calcium Excretion Through
Normal Routes**
Steatorrhea
Pancreatitis

From Banasik, J. L., & Copstead, L. C. (2019). *Pathophysiology*, (6th ed.). St. Louis: Elsevier.

- Signs and symptoms: CATS acronym (**C**onvulsions, **A**rrhythmias, **T**etany, **S**pasm and stridor); muscular aches and pains; tingling sensation in the feet, fingers, tongue, and lips; bronchospasm (leading to respiratory problems); seizures; tetany (intermittent muscular spasms); cardiac arrhythmias (can be life threatening); hyperreflexia (repeating, hyperactive reflexes); laryngospasm (vocal cord spasms, making it difficult to speak or breathe); positive Chvostek-Weiss sign (twitching of the cheek in response to tapping the facial nerve); positive Trousseau sign (carpal spasm of the hand when the blood pressure cuff is inflated above the systolic pressure for several minutes)
- Goals of treatment: to correct and manage the underlying causes and to maintain calcium levels between 7 and 9 mg/dL
- Treatment
  - Nonacute hypocalcemia: Administer oral calcium supplements, coupled with vitamin D, and magnesium if the levels are low.
  - Acute hypocalcemia: Administer calcium gluconate or calcium chloride (between 0.5 and 1.0 mL/min) by slow IV push (maximum rate for intermittent infusion is 200 mg/min).
- Complications: life-threatening cardiac arrhythmias
- Nursing assessment
  - Client history
    - Risk factors for decreased calcium: hypoparathyroidism; malnutrition; malabsorption
  - Description of symptoms: location; duration; onset; intensity; characteristics; aggravating factors; alleviating factors
  - Medical history: general health history; hospitalizations; infectious disease(s); allergies
  - Physical findings
    - Assessment of symptoms related to hypocalcemia
    - Neurological status: altered or changes in LOC; mental status; confusion; agitation
      - Cranial nerves: II through XII intact
      - Sensory: touch (light, sharp, dull); paresthesia (tingling in extremities)
      - Motor: range of motion (active, passive); deep tendon reflexes; gait
    - HEENT: head; ears; eyes (PERRLA); nose; throat
    - Cardiovascular system: auscultation of heart rate and rhythm; capillary refill; pulses; assessment for edema

- GI system: auscultation; percussion; palpation (all four quadrants)
- GU system: urine (color, clarity); output volume
  - Personal history: past medical conditions; hospitalizations; obstetric history; allergies; immunizations; current medications, including any recent medication changes; lifestyle (habits, diet); occupation; living environment; psychosocial
  - Family history of illnesses
- Nursing interventions
  - Monitor calcium levels every 4 to 6 hours.
  - Frequently assess IV site for infiltration. Calcium gluconate and calcium chloride can both lead to tissue necrosis.
  - Monitor cardiac rhythm and ECG changes.
  - Monitor vital signs, and assess for low BP.
  - Rapid IV administration could lead to a rapid drop in BP, dysrhythmias, and cardiac arrest. **Avoid rapid administration!**
  - Evaluate client for paresthesias.
    - Pricking sensation of the skin on the hands, arms, legs, and/or feet (may also occur in other areas of the body)
  - Monitor respiratory status.
  - Ensure client safety. Client is at increased risk for bone fractures.
  - Initiate seizure precautions.
  - Administer calcium with vitamin D supplements. When administering calcium orally, do so after meals or at bedtime with a full glass of water.
- Prevention
  - Encourage the intake of foods high in calcium: yogurt; sardines; cheese; spinach; collard greens; tofu; milk; rhubarb.

Ionized Calcium (Free Calcium)

- Normal range
  - Adult: between 4.8 and 5.5 mg/dL
  - Children: between 4.8 and 5.3 mg/dL
- Assess the need for ionized calcium test.
  - The ionized calcium test provides additional information concerning active, ionized calcium.
  - If the balance between bound calcium and free calcium is not normal, ionized free calcium typically makes up 50% to 75% of the calcium.
  - Level needs to be checked if the following are noted:
    - Client has signs of kidney or parathyroid disease. The test can be performed to monitor the progress of treatment of these diseases.
    - Client is receiving a blood transfusion.
    - Client is having major surgery.
    - Client is critically ill and taking IV fluids.
    - Client has abnormal levels of blood proteins.
- Low-ionized calcium levels
  - Abnormal results could mean
    - Malabsorption: alteration in the body's ability to take in nutrients from food
    - Hypoparathyroidism: decreased secretion or activity of PTH
    - Osteomalacia: bone softening caused by vitamin D and/or a calcium deficiency
    - Pancreatitis
    - Renal failure

- Rickets: soft, weakened bones in children caused by an extreme and prolonged vitamin D deficiency
- Vitamin D deficiency
  - Symptoms: variable heart rate; muscle spasms; possible coma; numbness around the mouth, hands, and feet
- High-ionized calcium levels
  - Abnormal results could indicate
    - Decreased levels of calcium in the urine from an unknown cause
    - Hyperparathyroidism: disorder in which the parathyroid glands produce too much PTH
    - Milk-alkali syndrome: caused by ingesting high levels of calcium and absorbable alkali
    - Multiple myeloma: cancer that attacks the plasma cells, a type of white blood cell
    - Paget disease: localized disorder of bone remodeling that begins with excessive bone resorption, followed by increased bone formation
    - Sarcoidosis: inflammatory disease affecting multiple areas of the body, such as the lungs, eyes, skin, and occasionally the heart
    - Thiazides diuretics: used to treat hypertension and to remove excess water from the body
    - Thrombocytosis: disorder of high platelet count
    - Tumors
    - Vitamin A excess
    - Vitamin D excess
  - Symptoms: constipation; dry mouth; continuing headache; irritability; loss of appetite; increased thirst; loss of appetite; metallic taste in mouth; fatigue

APPLICATION AND REVIEW

12. Which dietary deficiency should trigger the nurse's concern about the development of hypocalcemia?
    1. Vitamin D
    2. Vitamin E
    3. Niacin
    4. Iron
13. Which client requires long-term monitoring for the development of hypocalcemia?
    1. Client being treated for psychosis with lithium
    2. Client whose parathyroid was surgically removed
    3. Client with a history of multiple myeloma
    4. Client who recently experienced a severed spinal cord
14. When assessing a client with a low calcium level using the CATS acronym, which finding should cause the nurse the greatest concern regarding hypocalcemia?
    1. Client is currently experiencing constipation.
    2. Client reports that the tinnitus is worsening.
    3. Client reports muscle spasms in the lower extremities.
    4. Client's mobility is affected by arthritic pain.
15. Which client response should indicate a positive Chvostek-Weiss sign?
    1. Involuntary hand spasm triggered by blood pressure cuff–induced pressure to the arm
    2. Voluntary clenching of fists bilaterally after a verbal cue to do so
    3. Voluntary opening of the eyes and mouth simultaneously
    4. Involuntary twitching of the cheek when tapped

16. What is the maximum infusion rate when administering calcium gluconate by IV push?
    1. 50 mg/min
    2. 100 mg/min
    3. 200 mg/min
    4. 300 mg/min

17. Which statement made by the nurse demonstrates a need for further education regarding care of a client being treated for hypocalcemia?
    1. "The client is at risk for bone fractures."
    2. "I need to assess the client for hypotension frequently."
    3. "The infusion of calcium chloride should be rapidly administered."
    4. "Calcium gluconate can kill tissue if an infiltration occurs."

18. When assessing a client for hypocalcemia-related paresthesias, on which parts of the body should the nurse focus the assessment? *(Select all that apply.)*
    1. Legs
    2. Neck
    3. Hands
    4. Genital area
    5. Periorbital areas

19. Which medication instructions should the nurse include when educating a client who has been prescribed an oral calcium supplement? *(Select all that apply.)*
    1. Can be taken at bedtime.
    2. Should be taken on an empty stomach.
    3. Should be taken with a full glass of water.
    4. Should be taken with a vitamin D supplement.
    5. Should not be taken in conjunction with a high-calcium diet.

20. Which food selections indicate the nurse's understanding of high-calcium food sources? *(Select all that apply.)*
    1. Sardines in mustard sauce
    2. Black bean salsa
    3. Cooked rhubarb
    4. Cheese cubes
    5. Fresh pears

See Answers on pages 202–204.

ANSWER KEY: REVIEW QUESTIONS

1. **1 Dark green, leafy vegetables, such as kale and spinach, are foods high in calcium.**
   2, 3, 4 Peanuts, chicken, and potatoes are not good sources of calcium.
   Client Need: Health Promotion and Maintenance; **Cognitive Level:** Evaluation; **Integrated Process:** Teaching and Learning

2. **2 An increase in calcium most often causes a decrease in phosphate (and vice versa).**
   1, 3, 4 An increase in calcium most often causes a decrease in phosphate (and vice versa).
   Client Need: Physiological Integrity; **Cognitive Level:** Understanding; **Integrated Process:** Teaching and Learning

3. **Answers: 1, 2, 4, 5**
   1 Calcium is a cofactor in the clotting cascade; hypercalcemia increases clotting times, which increases the risk for thrombosis formation with venous stasis. **2** Hypocalcemia can trigger seizures. **4** Calcium is a cofactor in maintaining muscle tone; a deficiency in calcium would cause poor muscle tone. **5** Hypercalcemia can trigger renal stones formation.
   3 Hypocalcemia exhibits a positive Trousseau sign.
   Client Need: Physiological Integrity; **Cognitive Level:** Analysis; **Nursing Process:** Assessment

4. **2 A calcium level of 8.6 mg/dL is within the normal range of 8.5 to 10.6 mg/dL.**
   1 A calcium level of 7.5 mg/dL is indicative of hypocalcemia. **3** A calcium level of 10.7 mg/dL is indicative of hypercalcemia. **4** A calcium level of 11.5 mg/dL is indicative of hypercalcemia.
   Client Need: Physiological Integrity; **Cognitive Level:** Understanding; **Nursing Process:** Assessment

5. **3 Serum calcium level can be misleading unless it is correlated with the serum albumin level.**

   1 Serum calcium level can be misleading unless it is correlated with the serum albumin level; serum potassium is unrelated. **2** Serum calcium level can be misleading unless it is correlated with the serum albumin level; serum phosphate is unrelated. **4** Serum calcium level can be misleading unless it is correlated with the serum albumin level; serum sodium is unrelated.

   Client Need: Physiological Integrity; **Cognitive Level:** Understanding; **Nursing Process:** Assessment

6. **Answers: 1, 2, 4, 5**

   1 Possible causes of hypercalcemia are prolonged immobility (skeletal traction is a possible example of such immobility), a diagnosis of multiple myeloma, a diagnosis of tuberculosis, and lithium therapy. **3** A calcium level of 9.8 mg/dL is well within the normal range.

   Client Need: Physiological Integrity; **Cognitive Level:** Analysis; **Nursing Process:** Implementation

7. **Answers: 1, 2, 4, 5**

   1 Calcium is a cofactor in the clotting cascade; a calcium deficiency would cause prolonged clotting time and bleeding. **2** Hypocalcemia can trigger seizures. **4** Calcium is a cofactor in maintaining muscle tone; a calcium deficiency would cause poor muscle tone. **5** Hypercalcemia can trigger renal stones formation. **3** Hypocalcemia exhibits a positive Trousseau sign.

   Client Need: Physiological Integrity; **Cognitive Level:** Analysis; **Nursing Process:** Assessment

8. **Answers: 1, 2, 5**

   Signs and symptoms of hypercalcemia include thirst, confusion, and ECG confirmation of a depressed T wave.

   3 Signs and symptoms of hypercalcemia do not include GI bleeding, resulting in bloody stools. **4** Signs and symptoms of hypercalcemia include urinary frequency.

   Client Need: Physiological Integrity; **Cognitive Level:** Understanding; **Nursing Process:** Assessment

9. **4 Hypercalcemia increases clotting times leading to increased risk for thrombosis formation; calf swelling with or without pain would be a concern.**

   1, 2, 3 Lethargy, depression, and anorexia are symptoms associated with hypercalcemia, but its risk is not as high as possible thrombosis formation.

   Client Need: Physiological Integrity; **Cognitive Level:** Analysis; **Nursing Process:** Planning

10. **Answers: 1, 2, 3, 5**

    Valuable assessment questions related to hypercalcemia and its associated bone pain would include characteristics such as when the pain intensifies, the location of the pain, aggravating factors, and pain intensity. **4** No relationship exists between hypercalcemia-related pain with the pain of cancer; the question would be irrelevant.

    Client Need: Physiological Integrity; **Cognitive Level:** Analysis; **Nursing Process:** Assessment

11. **2 A serum calcium level of 14.4 mg/dL would indicate severe hypercalcemia; bradycardia is consistent with this condition.**

    1 Tachycardia is associated with mild hypercalcemia. **3** A depressed T wave is associated with hypercalcemia. **4** A shortened QT interval is associated with hypercalcemia.

    Client Need: Physiological Integrity; **Cognitive Level:** Assessment; **Nursing Process:** Assessment

12. **1 Vitamin D is essential for the absorption of calcium; a calcium deficiency would likely trigger hypocalcemia.**

    2, 3, 4 Vitamin D is essential for the absorption of calcium; a calcium deficiency would likely trigger hypocalcemia, which is not true of Vitamin E, niacin, or iron.

    Client Need: Physiological Integrity; **Cognitive Level:** Understanding; **Nursing Process:** Assessment

13. **2 Hypoparathyroidism is a cause of hypocalcemia.**

    1 Lithium therapy used in the treatment of psychosis can cause hypocalcemia. **3** Multiple myeloma can cause hypercalcemia. **4** A severed spinal cord triggers some form of immobility, resulting in a risk for hypercalcemia.

    Client Need: Physiological Integrity; **Cognitive Level:** Analysis; **Nursing Process:** Assessment

14. **3 CATS refers to Convulsions, Arrhythmia, Tetany, and Spasm and stridor.**

    1, 2, 4 CATS refers to Convulsions, Arrhythmia, Tetany, and Spasm and stridor, but it does not include constipation, tinnitus, the perception of noise or ringing in the ears, or arthritis.
    Client Need: Physiological Integrity; **Cognitive Level:** Application; **Nursing Process:** Assessment

15. **4 A positive Chvostek-Weiss sign involves the involuntary twitching of the cheek in response to tapping the facial nerve.**

    1, 2, 3 A positive Chvostek-Weiss sign involves the involuntary twitching of the cheek in response to tapping the facial nerve, not involuntary hand spasms, the voluntary bilateral clenching of fists, or the voluntary and simultaneous opening of the eyes and mouth.
    Client Need: Physiological Integrity; **Cognitive Level:** Understanding; **Nursing Process:** Assessment

16. **3 The maximum rate for intermittent infusion of either calcium gluconate or calcium chloride is 200 mg/min.**

    1, 2, 4 The maximum rate for intermittent infusion of either calcium gluconate or calcium chloride is 200 mg/min.
    Client Need: Physiological Integrity; **Cognitive Level:** Understanding; **Integrated Process:** Implementation

17. **3 Rapid IV administration of either calcium gluconate or calcium chloride could lead to a rapid drop in BP, dysrhythmias, and cardiac arrest.** Avoid rapid administration!

    1 A client being treated for hypocalcemia is at risk for bone fracture, resulting from the low levels of calcium and its effect on bones. **2** Hypotension can be an adverse reaction to the medication therapy prescribed. **4** Calcium gluconate and calcium chloride can both lead to tissue necrosis.
    Client Need: Physiological Integrity; **Cognitive Level:** Analysis; **Integrated Process:** Teaching and Learning

18. **Answers: 1, 3**

    1 Although the pricking sensation of the skin may occur in other parts of the body, one of the primary locations is the legs. **3** Although the pricking sensation of the skin may occur in other parts of the body, one of the primary locations is the hands.

    2, 4, 5 Although the pricking sensation of the skin may occur in other parts of the body, the primary locations are the hands, arms, legs, and feet.
    Client Need: Physiological Integrity; **Cognitive Level:** Applying; **Nursing Process:** Planning

19. **Answers: 1, 3, 4**

    1 An oral calcium supplement can be taken at bedtime or after meals. **3** An oral calcium supplement should be taken with a full glass of water. **4** An oral calcium supplement should be taken with a prescribed vitamin D supplement.

    2 An oral calcium supplement should be taken after meals. **5** An oral calcium supplement is prescribed to help increase calcium levels; therefore a high-calcium diet is therapeutic.
    Client Need: Physiological Integrity; **Cognitive Level:** Applying; **Integrated Process:** Teaching and Learning

20. **Answers: 1, 3, 4**

    1 Foods high in calcium include sardines. **3** Foods high in calcium include rhubarb. **4** Foods high in calcium include cheese.

    2 Black beans are not particularly high in calcium. **5** Pears are not particularly high in calcium.
    Client Need: Health Promotion and Maintenance; **Cognitive Level:** Application; **Integrated Process:** Learning and Teaching

Concepts of Minerals and Elements 12

MINERALS AND ELEMENTS OVERVIEW

Concepts of Minerals and Elements

- Minerals found in very small amounts in the body are referred to as trace minerals.
- Trace minerals include fluoride, iodine, iron, selenium, and zinc.
- The trace elements also include copper, nickel, manganese, and molybdenum.
- Although the body only requires limited quantities of these elements and minerals, they are essential for growth and development, as well as for maintaining overall health.
- Excess quantities and deficiencies in trace minerals will result in abnormal health conditions.
- Absorption occurs in the small intestine.
- Clinical conditions affecting the small intestine may alter the absorption of minerals, resulting in an imbalance.

Fluoride

- Fluoride is represented by the chemical symbol F^-.
- Absorption occurs in the gastrointestinal (GI) tract (small intestine).
  - Passive diffusion; as the amount of gastric acid rises, fluoride absorption rises.
  - Bone and teeth deliver and use 50% of the fluoride 24 hours after ingestion.
- Fluoride is largely excreted by the kidneys (20% bowel excretion).
- Fluoride is important for bone strength, teeth strength, and dental cavity prevention.
- Fluoride is not responsible for bone loss. Taking supplements will not improve bone loss.
- Bones and teeth
  - Fluoridated hydroxyapatite: exchanged for fluoride ions; adds stability to structure of enamel; is resilient to acids
- Trace minerals
  - Approximately 2.6 grams of fluoride are present in body tissue. The greatest concentration is found in the bone and teeth enamel.
- Source
  - Small amounts in plants, soil, and fluoridated water
    - Supplemental fluoride is added to the public water source for consumption.
  - Fluoridated consumer dental products: toothpaste; mouthwash (not meant to be ingested)
  - Food sources: seafood (salmon, sardines); tea leaves grown in soil; soup and stew (seafood, bone broth)
  - Recommended daily allowances

Client Age	Daily Allowance of Fluoride (in mg)
Adult	1.5 to 4.0
Children 7 years and older	1.5 to 2.5
Children 4 to 6 years old	1.0 to 2.5
Children 1 to 3 years old	0.5 to 1.5
Infants	0.1 to 1.0

- Function
  - Aids in protection during tooth development
  - Prevents cavities in mature teeth
  - Strengthens bone
  - Strengthens teeth
  - Fluoride found in saliva: prevents the loss of minerals from tooth enamel, protects by replacing fluoride in new cavities
  - Prevents growth of bacteria found in plaque
  - Prevents enzymes produced from bacteria (decreases acid)
  - Increases bone formation: promotes osteoblast activity; increases cells that build bone mass
- Fluorosis (excess fluoride)
  - Fluoride in water >2 ppm; 0.1 mg/kg/day
  - Most commonly caused by ingesting fluoridated toothpaste
  - Fluoride deposited in the tooth enamel during tooth formation, causing discoloration of teeth (brown, gray); white, spotty appearance; and pitting of enamel
  - Chronic excessive ingestion of fluoride
    - Osteosclerosis: crystal formation in bones; risk of fractures; joint pain; joint stiffness
    - Calcification: tendons; ligaments
  - Additional symptoms: nausea; vomiting; diarrhea; itching; chest pain; osteoporosis (loss of bone mass; bones become brittle); loss of muscle mass
  - Treatment: Limit extra fluoride ingestion and the use of supplements; use minimal amounts of toothpaste.
- Conditions caused by a fluoride deficit: tooth formation in children under 14 years of age; cavities (dental caries); osteoporosis as a result of chronic fluoride deficit
- Treatment is focused on preventing a fluoride deficiency.
  - Supplements are recommended.
  - If available, water is fluoridated.

APPLICATION AND REVIEW

1. Which client suggests a high risk for developing a trace mineral imbalance?
   1. A 6-year-old child who is a "picky eater"
   2. An adult's two-pack-a-day smoking habit
   3. An adult's 5-year history of Crohn disease
   4. A teenager diagnosed with exercise-induced asthma
2. Which adult client should be assessed for a fluoride deficiency?
   1. Needs extensive dental reconstruction
   2. Is currently being treated for hypothyroidism
   3. Has had several bone fractures within the last 3 years
   4. Reports a cold intolerance
3. Which result indicates that an adult client has a daily allowance of fluoride that is within normal levels?
   1. 0.5 mg
   2. 1.2 mg
   3. 2.6 mg
   4. 4.5 mg

See Answers on pages 216–218.

Iodine

- Iodine is a trace mineral.
  - Between 20 and 30 mg of total iodine is found in the body.
  - Iodine is stored in the thyroid gland and in the liver.
  - The largest concentration of iodine (75%) in the body is in the thyroid gland.
    - The thyroid gland converts iodine into thyroid hormones: thyroxine (T_4); triiodothyronine (T_3)
  - Thyroid-stimulating hormone (TSH) regulates the production of T_3 and T_4.
  - Tyrosine is attached to serum iodine.
    - Is an amino acid
    - Produces T_3 and T_4
  - Small amounts of the thyroid hormones are found in blood, mucosal lining of the GI tract, mammary glands of lactating women, ovaries, and muscle.
- Laboratory values are obtained from a 24-hour urine collection.
- Sources:
  - Large quantities are found in the ocean.
  - Iodide ions are contained in soil.
    - Exposed to sunlight, causing oxidation and depletion of iodine
    - Plants lacking iodine
  - Fish: saltwater; shellfish
  - Iodized salt
  - Vegetables, if grown in soil containing sufficient iodine
  - Dairy products (iodine content dependent on sufficient iodine ingestion of cattle-producing products)
  - Recommended daily allowances
    - Adults and adolescents: 150 µg
    - Women who are pregnant: 175 µg
    - Women who are lactating: 200 µg
    - Children between ages 7 and 10 years: 120 µg
    - Children between ages 4 and 6 years: 90 µg
    - Children between ages 1 and 3 years: 70 µg
    - Infants up to 1 year: 50 µg
- Function
  - Essential for thyroid gland functioning
  - Essential for the production of the thyroid hormones: T_3 and T_4
  - Regulates bone remodeling, metabolism, and body temperature
  - Enhances growth, development, nerve function, muscle function, use of oxygen within the cells, and collagen production
- Conditions caused by excess iodine
  - Iodism (iodine toxicity)
    - Very rare
    - Not usually caused by regular food intake
    - Caused by chronic ingestion of excess iodine
    - Has 25 times more iodine than the recommended daily allowance
      - Enlarged thyroid gland: goiter; hyperactive; Graves disease (autoimmune disease)
    - Symptoms: anxiety; exophthalmos (bulging eyeballs); hypertension; increased metabolism (weight loss); intolerance to heat; pain in oral mucosa (mouth, gums); tachycardia

- Poisoning from substances other than food
- Acute condition
- Medications
- Chemicals for photography
- Contrast dye for imaging
- Methamphetamine products
  - Symptoms: burning of the GI tract; vomiting; oliguria (decreased urine output); abdominal pain; fever; diarrhea; melena (blood in the stool); metallic taste; delirium; coma
- Treatment
  - Identify the source of the excess iodine.
  - Discontinue the source.
  - Administer radioactive iodine to decrease the production of the thyroid hormones.
  - Administer an antithyroid medication.
  - May include a thyroidectomy (surgical removal of most or all of the thyroid gland)
    - Thyroid hormone replacement will be needed for life.
    - Removing the parathyroid gland is a risk.
    - The parathyroid gland regulates the calcium in the blood.
- Conditions caused by an iodine deficit
  - Iodine deficiency: hypothyroidism; simple goiter
  - Normal function of thyroid hormones initially
    - Iodine stores are depleted.
    - Compensatory release of TSH by pituitary gland occurs in response to the decreased iodine level, which stimulates the thyroid gland to be hyperactive (goiter).
    - T_4 level is low with an elevated TSH level.
  - Symptoms: anemia; bradycardia (slow heart rate); constipation; depression; dry skin; intolerance to cold; menorrhagia (increased menstrual bleeding); decreased reflexes
  - Nonreversible cretinism (iron deficiency in fetal development): severe mental disabilities; major developmental delays; short in stature; gait disturbance (shuffle step); hypothyroidism; deaf; mute; muscle weakness; paralysis
  - Treatment
    - Replacing thyroid hormones
    - Ensuring adequate dietary intake of iodine with 1 teaspoon of iodized salt to meet body requirements
    - Routine monitoring of thyroid function levels
    - May require thyroidectomy (goiter will not diminish in size)

Iron

- Iron is represented by the chemical symbol Fe.
- Iron is a trace mineral.
- The largest concentration of iron (70%) is found in hemoglobin (Hgb).
  - Red blood cells (RBCs)
  - Also found in bone marrow, liver, and spleen
- Absorption
  - Absorption is regulated by the needs of the body.
  - Minor amount of absorption takes place in the stomach.
  - Small intestine is the primary area where iron absorption takes place.
    - Gastric acid is necessary to convert iron into a soluble form.
  - Vitamin C potentiates iron absorption.

- Decreased absorption is caused by decreased gastric acid and increased gastric motility (diarrhea).
- Iron is excreted in feces.
- Serum iron laboratory values for adults: between 50 and 150 µg/dL (increased values in liver disease)
- Sources: iron supplements (difficult to absorb); dietary intake (10% is used); organ meats (liver, heart, kidney); lean meat; poultry; fish; oysters; prune juice; dark green, leafy vegetables; egg yolks; wine; raisins; strawberries; fortified grains; blackberries; nuts; Brussels sprouts; green peas; tomato juice; squash
  - Recommended daily allowance

Client Age	Daily Allowance of Iron (in mg)
Men	10
Women	15
Pregnant women	30
Lactating women	15
Children	10
Infants	6

- Function
  - Carries oxygen to tissues
    - Hemoglobin
    - Millimeters of mercury: protein; oxygen binding site on RBCs; transports carbon dioxide (CO_2) out of cells (CO_2 is exhaled out of lungs)
  - Brain development
  - Brain function
  - Nerve transmission
  - Synthesis of neurotransmitters
  - Immune function
  - Erythropoiesis (RBC production)
- Conditions caused by excess iron
  - Rare; due to dietary intake
  - Absorption regulated by demand
  - Hemochromatosis (abnormally high absorption of iron through the intestinal tract)
    - Genetic disorder: higher incidence in men; iron accumulates in tissues
    - Multiple blood transfusions
      - Liver: hepatomegaly (enlarged liver); cirrhosis
      - Heart: coronary artery disease (CAD); congestive heart failure (CHF); stroke
      - Kidneys: diabetes
      - Joints: arthritis
      - Blood: clots
    - Symptoms: stiffness in joints; dark pigment spots on skin (hyperpigmentation); fatigue; cardiac arrhythmias; CHF (difficulty breathing, swelling of extremities)
    - Treatment: phlebotomy (removal of blood) to maintain Hgb levels within the normal range
      - Women: between 12 and 15 g/dL
      - Men: between 13 and 17 g/dL
- Conditions caused by an iron deficit
  - Iron deficiency
    - Old RBCs are destroyed by the liver and spleen, and iron is recycled. If iron stores are depleted, Hgb production is decreased.

- Intake of food and drink containing iron is inadequate, resulting in the loss of iron.
  - Chronic blood loss: most common cause in older adults
  - Rapid hemorrhage
- Impairment with iron absorption
- Iron-deficiency anemia
  - Decreased RBC production: lack of iron stores; Hgb <7.8 g/dL (may begin to feel symptomatic)
  - Symptoms: altered mental status; pica (eating disorder with persistent eating of nondietary substances such as soil and metal); anemia; cardiac arrhythmias; cold intolerance; fatigue; headache; lethargy; pale skin color; weakness; shortness of breath; cyanosis (bluish discolor of the skin and nail beds); brittle nails
- Treatment
  - Identify the underlying cause: blood loss; issues with the GI tract; malabsorption; inadequate dietary intake.
  - Administer iron supplements: ferrous sulfate (oral, intramuscular [IM] injections [painful and irritating to tissues], intravenous [IV]).
  - Blood transfusions for the treatment of symptomatic anemia (low Hgb levels)
  - Provide education on the foods containing iron and supplements that cause constipation.
    - Increase water consumption.
    - Administer stool softeners.
    - Add dietary fiber.

APPLICATION AND REVIEW

4. Which assessment questions asked of a client diagnosed with an iodine imbalance demonstrate the nurse's understanding of the functions of a trace mineral? *(Select all that apply.)*
   1. "Do you experience bleeding gums?"
   2. "Are you being treated for Graves disease?"
   3. "Is your heart rate considered unusually slow?"
   4. "Would you consider yourself an anxious person?"
   5. "Have you experienced an unexplained weight loss?"
5. The nurse should include information reinforcing which surgical risk that is specifically related to a thyroidectomy?
   1. Postsurgical bleeding
   2. Surgical incision infection
   3. Incision of the parathyroid gland
   4. Postsurgical nausea and vomiting
6. Which dietary information should the nurse include when counseling a client diagnosed with an iron deficiency?
   1. Ingest iron-rich foods during all major meals.
   2. Dietary iron can result in serious diarrhea.
   3. Vitamin C sources should be consumed with iron-rich foods.
   4. The greatest need for iron occurs during the older adult years.
7. Which client's serum iron level is within normal limits?
   1. 11.4 µg/dL
   2. 14.5 µg/dL
   3. 40.2 µg/dL
   4. 75.8 µg/dL
8. Which forms of beef are considered excellent sources of dietary iron? *(Select all that apply.)*
   1. Heart
   2. Tongue
   3. Kidney
   4. Liver
   5. Testes

9. A client has an Hgb level of 7.5 g/dL. Which nursing intervention is the priority for this client?
   1. Provide supplemental oxygen.
   2. Assess for the signs and symptoms of anemia.
   3. Educate the client on the sources of dietary iron.
   4. Suggest the need for a diagnostic assessment of RBCs.
10. Which instructions should the nurse provide to the client who is taking a prescribed iron supplement to help manage a common side effect of the therapy? *(Select all that apply.)*
    1. Increase water consumption.
    2. Use stool softeners as prescribed.
    3. Add dietary fiber to the daily diet.
    4. Consume two servings of seafood weekly.
    5. Avoid caffeine in foods and beverages.

See Answers on pages 216–218.

Selenium

- Selenium is represented by the chemical symbol Se.
- Selenium is a trace mineral.
- Its highest concentration is found in the liver, kidneys, heart, and spleen.
- Small concentrations are found in the glutathione peroxidase enzyme.
- Selenium is absorbed in the small intestine.
  - Its organic forms are more easily absorbed.
  - The inorganic forms are more likely to result in toxic levels.
- Selenium is excreted by the kidneys.
- Function
  - Glutathione peroxidase enzyme component
    - Antioxidant: may contribute to cancer prevention
    - Inflammation response: is a prostaglandin; lipids form at the site of damage or injury
    - RBC protection
    - Cell membrane protection: free radical (an uncharged molecule having an unpaired electron) containing the toxins mercury and cadmium
  - Immunoglobulin production: proteins in the immune system; antibodies
  - Immune system response: macrophage (lymphocyte) is activated; is the first responder to the site of infection
  - Skin protection from ultraviolet rays
  - Eases hot flashes during menopause
- Sources: soil; water; food (Brazil nuts, brown rice, oats and other whole grains, poultry, organ meats, fish)
  - Amounts of selenium found in food are dependent on the concentration found in the soil and water.
  - States with soil containing high concentrations of selenium: Colorado; Montana; New Mexico; South Dakota; Tennessee; Utah; Wyoming
  - Recommended daily allowance
    - Adults: between 40 and 70 µg
    - Children between 7 and 10 years old: 30 µg
    - Children between 1 and 6 years old: 20 µg
    - Infants up to 1 year old: 10 and 15 µg

- Conditions caused by excess selenium
  - Selenosis
  - Rare occurrence
  - Children are more likely to reach toxic levels (tooth decay, tooth loss).
  - Excess selenium is quantified as approximately three times the recommended daily allowance and causes nausea, vomiting, hair loss, problems with skin, damage to nails, fatigue, nerve damage, muscle weakness, edema (in the fingers and toes), and depression.
  - Treatment
    - Limit dietary intake.
    - Medically manage increased excretion with increased fluid intake and diuretic administration.
- Conditions caused by selenium deficiency
  - A selenium deficiency is a rare occurrence.
  - It takes several years for the signs and symptoms to be evident.
  - Causes include decreased ingestion of selenium, total parenteral nutrition (TPN) for an extended period, Down syndrome (more susceptible), and chronic liver disease.
  - Symptoms: cardiac muscle weakness; cardiomyopathy (enlarged heart muscle); jaundice in infants; dermatitis (seborrhea); macular degeneration (macula, the center area of the retina, is responsible for visual acuity); thyroid function impairment
  - Treatment: Increase selenium intake through diet and supplements

APPLICATION AND REVIEW

11. Which classic symptom of menopause is known to improve with selenium therapy?
    1. Insomnia
    2. Depression
    3. Hot flashes
    4. Vaginal dryness
12. Which chronic condition places a client at risk for a selenium deficiency?
    1. Asthma
    2. Diabetes
    3. Down syndrome
    4. Crohn disease

See Answers on pages 216–218.

Zinc

- Zinc is represented by the chemical symbol Zn.
- Zinc is a trace mineral.
- Total body concentration is between 2 and 3 grams.
- Approximately 5 mg of zinc per 1000 calories is ingested daily per individual.
  - Absorption is greatest in the small intestine (stomach, large intestine).
- Excreted in feces and urine
- Found throughout the body
  - Component of proteins and nucleic acid
  - Largest concentrations: liver; pancreas; kidney; muscle; bone
  - Also found in the eyes, prostate gland, skin, hair, nails, and spermatozoa.
- Intracellular zinc concentration: nucleus
- Protein sources high in zinc: oysters (contain the highest concentrations); meat; poultry; fish; shellfish; dairy products; liver; whole grains; legumes; nuts; soy
  - Recommended daily allowance
    - Adults: between 12 and 15 mg/day

- ▪ Children between 1 and 10 years of age: 10/mg/day
  - ▪ Infants: 5 mg/day
- Function
  - Essential in more than 100 varied enzymes
  - Provides ribonucleic acid (RNA) and deoxyribonucleic acid (DNA) structure stability
  - Cell division: RNA functions
  - Maintains cholesterol levels, growth and development, and prostaglandin production (hormonelike substance)
  - Essential for numerous functions throughout the body
  - Immunity support: produces T-lymphocytes (WBCs); increases antibodies; hinders bacterial growth; inhibits viral reproduction
  - Regulates calcitonin secretion from the thyroid gland
  - Helps with wound healing
  - Increases the formation of collagen
- Conditions caused by excess zinc
  - Intake between 100 and 300 mg/day
  - Rare occurrence
  - Impairs the absorption of copper
  - Occurs with kidney dysfunction (hemodialysis)
  - Symptoms: anemia; increased body temperature; central nervous system (CNS) dysfunction
  - Treatment: decrease dietary intake; eliminate supplements
- Conditions caused by a zinc deficiency
  - Immune suppression, resulting in an increased risk of infection and illness
  - Causes: low protein diet; diet high in unrefined grain; diet high in unleavened bread (decreased absorption of zinc); alcoholism; dysfunction with absorption; starvation (anorexia); increased excretion (urinary, pancreatic, exocrine)
  - Symptoms: hypogeusia (lessened sense of taste); delayed growth; delayed sexual development (hypogonadism [decreased production of semen], low sperm count); alopecia (loss of hair); slowed healing of wounds; skin disorders; appetite suppression; decreased immunity; behavioral problems; eye impairments (photophobia [sensitivity to light], night blindness)
    - ▪ Symptoms vary, because zinc has many functions throughout the body.
  - Treatment: identify the underlying cause, increase dietary intake, and add supplements

Copper

- Copper is represented by the chemical symbol Cu.
- Copper is a trace element.
- Normal serum concentration is between 2 and 80 µg/L.
- Copper is considered a heavy metal.
- Absorption occurs in the small intestine and stomach.
- Absorption is higher than the body demands.
- Its highest concentrations are found in the liver.
- Copper is also found in blood.
- It is stored and filtered by the liver and excreted in the biliary tract (bile).
- Sources: eggs; fish; liver; oysters; poultry; legumes; fruit; milk; mushrooms; nuts; peas; whole grains
- Function: energy production; reproductive health; immune support; CNS balance; endocrine system balance; healthy bone and connective tissue

- Conditions caused by excessive copper
  - Excessive copper is harmful in small concentrations.
  - Causes: Wilson disease (genetic component); intrauterine device (IUD) made with copper; exposure to swimming pool and hot tub (cleaning products contain copper); exposure to pesticide (fungicide); ingestion
  - Copper accumulates in the brain, liver, eyes, and other vital organs.
  - Symptoms: nausea; vomiting; headache; diarrhea; abdominal pain; Wilson disease (jaundice, behavioral and memory issues, appendicitis, cirrhosis); scarring of the lung tissue (pulmonary fibrosis); granulomas (fibrous growths)
  - Treatment
    - Dietary management
    - Chelation therapy
      - Treatment is used for heavy metal poisoning.
      - Medication binds to toxins for removal.
- Conditions that cause a deficiency in copper
  - Gastric bypass surgery
    - Malabsorption
  - Disorders that affect intestinal absorption: celiac disease; Crohn disease; inflammatory bowel disease
  - Excess intake of zinc
  - Copper and zinc compete for absorption.
  - Symptoms: fatigue; fragile bones; feeling cold; inflammation (skin, veins); muscles (sore, weak)
  - Treatment: increase dietary intake; administer supplements; may need to decrease zinc intake

Manganese

- Manganese is represented by the chemical symbol Mn.
- Manganese is a trace element.
- Manganese is found in the mitochondria.
- Blood levels are a good indicator of total body levels of manganese.
- Sources: dark, green, leafy vegetables; dried fruit; legumes; nuts; whole grains
- Function
  - Essential cofactor for many enzyme functions
  - Carbohydrate metabolism
  - Production of bone, connective tissue, cholesterol, and fatty acids
- Conditions caused by excess manganese
  - Unknown, due to dietary intake
  - Inhalation: industrial vocations (miners, welders); altered mental status (hallucinations); movement disorders
- Conditions caused by a deficiency of manganese
  - Undetermined
  - Thought to be involved with hypocholesterolemia; weight loss; changes (hair, nails); dermatitis; protein synthesis involving vitamin K

Nickel

- Nickel is represented by the chemical symbol Ni.
- Nickel is a trace element.
- Little is known about nickel and the human body.

- Nickel is rapidly excreted by the kidneys.
- No accumulation is present in the body.
- Sources: soil; water; limited in food sources; foods with high-acid content
- Function: iron metabolism; structural support (nucleic acids, proteins); some enzyme functions cofactor
- Conditions caused by excessive nickel
  - Industrial exposure: metal used for high shine; noncorrosive; nickel carbonyl
  - Toxic exposure assessed by urine
  - Symptoms: dermatitis; GI irritation; respiratory inflammation; cerebral edema
  - Treatment: investigational chelation therapy
- Conditions caused by a deficiency of nickel
  - Extremely rare
  - Limited research
  - Due to very low body requirements

Molybdenum

- Molybdenum is represented by the chemical symbol Mo.
- Molybdenum is a trace element.
- Sources: beans; peas; red meat; whole grains
- Function
  - Enzyme functions: cofactor; xanthine oxidase; sulfite oxidase (binds sulfites)
  - Metabolism functions: fats; carbohydrates
- Molybdenum toxicity is caused by an excess of the element, which can lead to impaired copper metabolism.
- Conditions caused by a deficiency in molybdenum: parenteral nutrition; decreased molybdenum (unable to bind sulfites); uric acid buildup in the body
- Symptoms: painful joints; neurological dysfunctions; death

APPLICATION AND REVIEW

13. Which foods should the nurse suggest to a client who is deficient in dietary copper? (*Select all that apply.*)
    1. Nuts
    2. Fish
    3. Eggs
    4. Organ meat
    5. Whole grains
14. The nurse should monitor a client with skin inflammation consistent with dermatitis for which deficiency? (*Select all that apply.*)
    1. Molybdenum
    2. Copper
    3. Nickel
    4. Manganese
    5. Fluoride
15. The nurse should educate a client diagnosed with a manganese deficiency on the importance of adding which foods to the diet? (*Select all that apply.*)
    1. Peas
    2. Spinach
    3. Peanuts
    4. Cabbage
    5. Avocado
16. Which occupational area poses the greatest risk for exposure to a toxic level of nickel?
    1. Animal husbandry
    2. Industrial exposure
    3. Agriculture and farming
    4. Health care professions

17. Which diagnostic test is used to assess a client for toxic nickel levels?
    1. Urine sample
    2. Blood sample
    3. Bone biopsy
    4. Sputum sample
18. Which body system requires priority assessment by the nurse in a client with an elevated nickel level? *(Select all that apply.)*
    1. Respiratory
    2. Neurological
    3. Cardiovascular
    4. Gastrointestinal
    5. Musculoskeletal
19. The nurse is caring for a client diagnosed with copper toxicity. Which mineral should the nurse monitor in this client?
    1. Molybdenum
    2. Manganese
    3. Nickel
    4. Zinc
20. The nurse is caring for a client deficient in the mineral molybdenum. Which body system should the nurse assess first?
    1. Cardiovascular
    2. Respiratory
    3. Neurological
    4. Gastrointestinal

See Answers on pages 216–218.

ANSWER KEY: REVIEW QUESTIONS

1. **3 Clinical conditions, such as Crohn disease, which affects the small intestine, may alter the absorption of minerals resulting in an imbalance.**
   1 A "picky eater" implies that the child voluntarily eats a limited diet. This habit would not necessarily affect the absorption function of the small intestine. **2** A cigarette habit does not generally affect the absorption function of the small intestine. **4** Asthma does not necessarily affect the absorption function of the small intestine.
   Client Need: Physiological Integrity; **Cognitive Level:** Analysis; **Nursing Process:** Assessment

2. **1 Tooth strength and cavity prevention are associated with fluoride.**
   2 Iodine deficiency is associated with hypothyroidism. **3** Bone fractures are associated with a calcium deficiency. **4** Cold intolerance is associated with an iron deficiency.
   Client Need: Physiological Integrity; **Cognitive Level:** Analysis; **Nursing Process:** Assessment

3. **3 The daily allowance of fluoride for an adult is between 1.5 and 4.0 mg.**
   1, 2, 4 The daily allowance of fluoride for an adult is between 1.5 and 4.0 mg.
   Client Need: Health Promotion and Maintenance; **Cognitive Level:** Understanding; **Nursing Process:** Assessment

4. **Answers: 2, 4, 5**
   2 An overproduction of iodine is associated with hyperthyroidism. Graves disease is an immune system disorder that results in the overproduction of thyroid hormones (hyperthyroidism). **4** Anxiety is a symptom associated with hyperthyroidism. **5** Weight loss is associated with hyperthyroidism.
   1 Oral pain, not bleeding, is associated with an overproduction of iodine. **3** Tachycardia is associated with an overproduction of iodine.
   Client Need: Physiological Integrity; **Cognitive Level:** Evaluation; **Integrated Process/Nursing Process:** Assessment

5. **3 A surgical complication of a thyroidectomy is the removal of part or all of the parathyroid gland.**
   1, 2, 4 Although possible, bleeding, incision infection, and nausea and vomiting are not specific to this type of surgery.
   Client Need: Physiological Integrity; **Cognitive Level:** Application; **Nursing Process:** Planning

6. **3 Vitamin C potentiates iron absorption.**
   1 Although iron ingestion is important, too much can result in an excessive iron level. **2** It is not necessarily true that iron-rich foods can result in serious diarrhea. Iron is associated with constipation, not diarrhea. **4** Iron is most needed by teenage girls who have started menses.

Client Need: Health Promotion and Maintenance; **Cognitive Level:** Application; **Integrated Process:** Teaching and Learning

7. **4 Normal serum iron laboratory values for adults are between 50 and 150 μg/dL.**

   1, 2, 3 Normal serum iron laboratory values for adults are between 50 and 150 μg/dL.

   Client Need: Health Promotion and Maintenance; **Cognitive Level:** Understanding; **Nursing Process:** Assessment

8. **Answers: 1, 3, 4**

   Beef organ meats, such as the heart, are excellent sources of dietary iron.

   2 Tongue is not considered organ meat but is an excellent source of dietary iron. **5** Testes is not considered organ meat but is an excellent source of dietary iron.

   Client Need: Health Promotion and Maintenance; **Cognitive Level:** Understanding; **Integrated Process:** Teaching and Learning

9. **2 An Hgb level less than 7.8 g/dL is often associated with demonstrating symptoms associated with iron-deficiency anemia. The primary intervention would be to effectively assess for the signs and symptoms of anemia.**

   1 An assessment to determine the need for supplemental oxygen should occur before implementing the intervention. **3** An Hgb of 7.5 g/dL is associated with iron-deficiency anemia; dietary counseling would be appropriate, but the priority intervention would be to effectively assess for the signs and symptoms of anemia. **4** The results of a diagnostic assessment to determine the RBC count would be appropriate, but the priority intervention would be to effectively assess for the signs and symptoms of anemia.

   Client Need: Physiological Integrity; **Cognitive Level:** Analysis; **Nursing Process:** Planning

10. **Answers: 1, 2, 3**

    1 Constipation is a common complication of iron supplements. Increasing water intake will help prevent constipation from occurring. **2** Stool softeners will help manage the constipation associated with iron-supplement therapy. **3** Adequate dietary fiber will help manage the constipation associated with iron-supplement therapy.

    4 Seafood is a good source of iodine but not necessarily a good source of iron. **5** Although caffeine consumption should be controlled, avoiding it is not recommended.

    Client Need: Health Promotion and Maintenance; **Cognitive Level:** Application; **Integrated Process:** Teaching and Learning

11. **3 Selenium is sometimes prescribed to ease hot flashes during menopause.**

    1, 2, 4 Selenium is not prescribed to treat insomnia, depression, or vaginal dryness during menopause.

    Client Need: Health Promotion and Maintenance; **Cognitive Level:** Application; **Integrated Process:** Teaching and Learning

12. **3 Clients diagnosed with Down syndrome have an increased risk for selenium deficiency.**

    1, 2, 4 Asthma and diabetes are not known risk factors for the development of a selenium deficiency.

    Client Need: Physiological Integrity; **Cognitive Level:** Understanding; **Nursing Process:** Assessment

13. **Answers: 1, 2, 3, 5**

    1, 2, 3, 5 Nuts **2, 3, 5** Nuts, fish, eggs, and whole grains are good sources of dietary copper.

    4 Organ meat is not considered a good source of dietary copper.

    Client Need: Health Promotion and Maintenance; **Cognitive Level:** Understanding; **Integrated Process:** Teaching and Learning

14. **Answers: 2, 3, 4**

    Skin inflammation, such as dermatitis, is associated with a copper imbalance, and nickel imbalance, and a manganese imbalance.

    1 Molybdenum imbalances are associated with painful joints, neurological dysfunctions, and possible death. **5** Fluoride imbalances are associated with disorders related to the teeth.

    Client Need: Physiological Integrity; **Cognitive Level:** Understanding; **Nursing Process:** Assessment

15. **Answers: 1, 2, 3**

    1, 2, 3 Dietary sources of manganese include legumes (peas, beans), leafy green vegetables, and nuts.

4 Cabbage is not a significant source of manganese. **5** Avocado is not a significant source of manganese.
Client Need: Physiological Integrity; **Cognitive Level:** Understanding; **Integrated Process:** Teaching and Learning

16. **2 Industrial exposure to nickel occurs at levels that can result in nickel toxicity.**

    1 Occupations that involve the raising and care of animals do not generally produce a risk for nickel toxicity. **3** Occupations that involve raising or transporting food stuffs, such as vegetables and fruits, do not generally produce a risk for nickel toxicity. **4** Health care professions do not generally produce a risk for nickel toxicity.
    Client Need: Health Promotion and Maintenance; **Cognitive Level:** Analysis; **Nursing Process:** Evaluation

17. **1 Toxic nickel levels are assessed by an evaluation of the urine.**

    2, 3, 4 Toxic nickel levels are assessed by an evaluation of the urine, not by an evaluation of a blood sample, bone biopsy, or sputum sample.
    Client Need: Physiological Integrity; **Cognitive Level:** Application; **Nursing Process:** Planning

18. **Answers: 1, 2, 4**

    Symptoms associated with an elevated nickel level include respiratory inflammation, cerebral edema, and GI irritation.

    3, 5 An elevated nickel level does not generally cause cardiovascular or musculoskeletal symptoms.
    Client Need: Physiological Integrity; **Cognitive Level:** Analysis; **Nursing Process:** Planning

19. **1 Copper toxicity may be a result of impaired copper metabolism resulting from excessive molybdenum.**
    2, 3, 4 Manganese, nickel, and zinc are not associated with copper toxicity.
    Client Need: Physiological Integrity; **Cognitive Level:** Application; **Nursing Process:** Implementation

20. **3 Symptoms of deficient molybdenum include neurological dysfunctions, which makes a neurological assessment the priority.**

    1, 2, 4 Cardiovascular, respiratory, and gastrointestinal symptoms are not generally associated with a molybdenum deficiency.
    Client Need: Physiological Integrity; **Cognitive Level:** Analysis; **Nursing Process:** Planning

Fluid and Electrolyte Balance in Neonates, Infants, and Children

13

FLUID AND ELECTROLYTE BALANCE OVERVIEW

Fluid and Electrolyte Balance in Neonates

- Body water content and distribution
  - Total body water has two major sections
    - Intracellular water (ICW)
    - Extracellular water (ECW)
      - Interstitial water
      - Plasma volume (intravascular part of ECW)
  - In early fetal development, the body primarily consists of water.
  - The total body water declines as gestation advances, from 94% of the body weight at 3 months to 75% at term (40 weeks' gestation).
    - ECW is 45% of body weight at term.
    - ICW is 34% of body weight at term.
    - Small for gestational age (SGA) infants have a larger total body weight (TBW) per kilogram than term infants with weights within the expected range.
  - After the birth, the infant's TBW per kilogram continues to decline.
    - Is attributable to the reduction in ECW
    - Is attributable to improved renal function after birth
    - For the first several weeks, the ICW is stable but increases in proportion to the body weight.
    - By 3 months, the ICW increases faster than the body weight and exceeds ECW.
      - Is attributable to changes in the body water
      - Partitioning between ECW and ICW is affected by the intake of electrolytes and water.
- Distribution of solute in body fluids
  - Sodium is the major cation in the blood plasma.
  - Remaining elements that constitute the other cations are potassium, calcium, and magnesium.
  - The primary anion is chloride.
  - Remaining elements that constitute the other anions are protein and bicarbonate.
  - Fluid and electrolyte balance in the fetus is dependent on the maternal homeostasis and placental exchange.
    - Likewise, at birth, the infant's fluid and electrolyte balance is affected by the maternal balances in labor.
- Insensible water loss (IWL)
  - IWL is water loss due to evaporation from the respiratory tract or skin.
    - 70% of IWL happens through the skin.
    - 30% of IWL happens through the respiratory tract.
  - Factors that influence IWL
    - Level of maturity
      - Inversely proportional to birth weight and gestational age
      - Premature and smaller infants have a greater IWL per kilogram.
    - Respiratory distress (hyperpnea) that increases with the dry air that is breathed

- Environmental temperature above a neutral thermal zone
- Increased body temperature
- Skin injury
- Congenital skin defects: gastroschisis; neural tube defects; omphalocele
- Radiant warmer
- Phototherapy
- Motor activity and crying
- High inspired humidity
- Plastic heat shield
- Plastic blanket
- Topical agents
  - IWL risk factors are likely to affect the premature infant or the infant who is critically ill.

Neuroendocrine Regulation of Fluid and Electrolyte Balance

- Major organs produce hormones that help maintain water and electrolyte balance in the body.
  - Pituitary gland
    - Intact posterior pituitary gland functioning in newborns
    - Arginine vasopressin (AVP)
    - Antidiuretic hormone (ADH)
  - Adrenal cortex
    - Aldosterone is the most powerful mineralocorticoid.
    - Synthesis is regulated by the renin-angiotensin system, adrenocorticotropic hormone, and concentration of sodium in plasma.
  - Parathyroid glands
    - Regulate calcium concentration in the blood
    - Balance parathyroid hormone (PTH) and calcitonin (produced in the thyroid)
    - PTH is low at birth but steadily rises in term newborns and premature infants.
  - Heart
    - Atrial natriuretic factor (ANF) is present in the fetal heart.
    - ANF levels rise after birth and then return to lower levels than those present at birth.
    - ANF stimulates diuresis and natriuresis.
    - Regulates extracellular fluid (ECF) volume

APPLICATION AND REVIEW

1. At which stage of development is the human body primarily comprised of water?
   1. Fetal (before birth)
   2. At infancy
   3. During the teenage years
   4. An older adult
2. Which newborn has the greatest total body water?
   1. Infant born 10 days prematurely
   2. Infant born 1 week past the due date
   3. Infant diagnosed as SGA
   4. Infant diagnosed as large for gestational age (LGA)
3. Which newborn is at the highest risk for IWL?
   1. Newborn whose rectal temperature is 2° above normal
   2. Newborn diagnosed as SGA
   3. Newborn being treated for respiratory distress
   4. Newborn born 2 weeks prematurely

4. The nurse is caring for a newborn experiencing IWL. Which intervention should the nurse implement?
   1. Apply an extra blanket on the newborn.
   2. Increase the humidity in the newborn's environment.
   3. Swaddle the newborn to reduce crying and motor activity.
   4. Warm the newborn's immediate environment with a radiant warmer.

See Answers on pages 238–240.

Renal Function in Neonates

- Most parts of renal function are not completely developed at birth.
- Glomerular and tubular functions are greater with a higher gestational age and a higher postnatal age.
- Maximum urine concentration on average
  - 600 mOsm/L for premature infants
  - 800 mOsm/L for term newborns
  - 1200 mOsm/L for adults
  - Although newborns can produce diluted urine, they cannot excrete water as rapidly as adults.

Fluid and Electrolyte Therapy in Neonates

- The management of fluid and electrolyte disorders in infants includes three aspects of care.
  - Approximate all fluid and electrolyte deficits.
  - Compute the volume of fluid and electrolytes that are needed for replacing the deficits, maintaining fluid and electrolytes, and replacing continuous abnormal deficiencies.
  - Monitor the infant's response to treatment.

Dehydration and Fluid Deficit

- Assessment
  - Degree of dehydration can help approximate the body water deficit.
  - Acute weight loss can be a measure of the body water deficit.
  - Weight loss of up to 15% can occur during the first week of life.
    - Extracellular water and tissue breakdown
    - Premature infants lose an average of 10% of body weight, despite intravenous (IV) infusion.
    - Smaller infants lose a large percentage of weight after birth.
    - In premature infants, 2% to 3% weight loss per day is typical during the first week of life.
    - Beyond the first week of life, acute weight loss should be indicative of nonphysiological dehydration; water deficit needs to be replaced.
  - If body weight information is not available, other signs of dehydration are urine volume, urine concentration, and physical signs.
- Signs and symptoms
  - Serum sodium levels are indicators of dehydration.
  - Infants with serum sodium concentrations of 130 to 150 mEq/L (isotonic dehydration of 5%): dry mucous membranes; slightly sunken anterior fontanel; decreased tear production; oliguria
  - Infants with isotonic dehydration of 10%: dry mucous membranes; absent tears; sunken eyes and fontanel; cool extremities; poor skin turgor; oliguria
  - Infants with isotonic dehydration of 15%: dry mucous membranes; absent tears; sunken eyes and fontanel; cool extremities; poor skin turgor; oliguria; hypotension; tachycardia; weak pulses; mottled skin; altered sensorium

- Serum sodium concentration above 150 mEq/L
  - Symptoms are less severe than in infants with isotonic dehydration (same percentage of body water).
  - Intravascular volume is better maintained in infants with hypernatremia than with isotonic dehydration.
  - Infants with hypotonic dehydration (i.e., serum sodium below 130 mEq/L) have acute symptoms with the same level of dehydration.
- Signs of dehydration are hard to evaluate in small, premature infants.
  - Skin and mucous membranes are dry (thermal and mechanical injury), especially in infants under radiant warmers.
  - Skin turgor is more difficult to assess as a result of a lack of subcutaneous fat.

APPLICATION AND REVIEW

5. The nurse teaches new parents about the initial change in a newborn's weight. Which information should the nurse provide the parents concerning the infant's first week after discharge?
   1. "It's likely that your baby will start to gain weight starting today."
   2. "We expect that your baby will lose approximately 15% of her birth weight over the next week."
   3. "It is important, in the first week, that your baby not drop below her birth weight."
   4. "There is not steadfast expectation about weight gain until 1 month after the baby's birth."
6. The nurse is caring for a newborn diagnosed with dehydration. Which assessment finding should the nurse document?
   1. Amount of fluid the newborn consumes
   2. Number of wet diapers the newborn produces
   3. Amount of awake time the newborn experiences
   4. Degree of in which physical activity the newborn engages
7. The nurse is caring for a 2-day-old newborn diagnosed with 5% isotonic dehydration. Which assessment finding should the nurse expect?
   1. Dry mucous membranes   3. Cool extremities
   2. Poor skin turgor   4. Absence of tears
8. The nurse is teaching the parents of a premature newborn measures to prevent dehydration. Which statement should the nurse make to the parents?
   1. "Preemies generally have some degree of oliguria."
   2. "Tachycardia is fairly common among premature newborns."
   3. "Skin turgor is an unreliable indicator of dehydration among preemies."
   4. "A common characteristic of premature newborns is a slightly sunken anterior fontanel."

See Answers on pages 238–240.

Electrolyte Deficits

- The extent and cause of electrolyte disturbances can be identified by history and a physical examination and serum electrolyte concentrations.
- Sodium concentrations are divided into three categories.
  - Isotonic (10%): serum sodium concentration at 140 mEq/L
  - Hypertonic: serum sodium concentration at 153 mEq/L
  - Hypotonic: serum sodium concentration at 127 mEq/L

- The type of electrolyte disorder is based on the fluid and electrolyte abnormality.
  - Severe acute diarrhea can lead to isotonic dehydration.
    - High IWL (premature infant under radiant warmer)
    - Hypernatremic dehydration
    - If sodium loss from diarrhea is not replaced, then hypotonic dehydration can occur.
- Goals of care
  - Replace fluid and electrolyte deficits.
  - Fluid deficit is computed from the approximate degree of dehydration.
    - Dehydration is measured by body weight loss and/or clinical examination.
    - Dehydration of acute onset (minimal duration) will require fast resolution.
      - An exception is the case of hypertonic dehydration; rapid increase in body water could result in cerebral swelling and convulsions.
    - Electrolyte deficit is computed as the variance between the total body solute that is anticipated before and during the dehydrated state.
    - Typically, one-half of the deficit in water is replaced in 8 hours and the next one-half is replaced in 16 hours.
    - Sodium deficit is restored over a 24-hour period; rapid replacement may risk overcompensation.
    - Potassium deficit is substantial, and it needs to be restored over a longer period (48 to 72 hours).
      - Allow for sufficient renal function to prevent potential cardiac problems associated with accelerated potassium infusion.
      - Postpone potassium replacement until urine flow is adequate.

Maintenance of Fluid and Electrolytes

- Approximate daily maintenance of water requirements should consider three components.
  - IWL
  - Loss through urine
  - Loss through feces
    - Loss is estimated at 5 to 10 mL/kg/day.
    - In the first week of life, loss through feces is low, and no water is transferred to new tissues because growth has not started.
    - Approximately 10 mL/kg/day of water is retained in tissues during growth.
      - Assumes 10 to 20 g/kg/day weight gain
      - Percentage of weight gain due to water: 60% to 70%
    - Once growth begins, the restoration of water may be 20 g/kg/day.
      - Small amount, when contrasted with IWL and urine water loss, both are primary sources that must be considered when computing water intake to maintain fluid balance.
- Nursing interventions and prevention of fluid and electrolyte imbalance
  - Daily caloric intake is approximately 100 kcal/kg/day.
    - Preterm infants, versus term infants, may have decreased metabolic rates.
    - SGA infants have greater metabolic rates versus preterm infants of comparable weights, due to greater brain-to-body mass ratio; SGA and preterm infants require frequent dietary assessment.
  - Assessment
    - Hourly urine output for infants who are critically ill
      - Every 4 to 6 hours of output are needed for infants who require less stimulation.
      - Smallest infants need careful monitoring of fluid balance.

- Infants who are critically ill may develop hyponatremia if fluid replacement is too aggressive when identification of imbalance is delayed.
- Maintenance of fluids
  - Infant stays in zero balance state.
    - Normal loss (water and electrolytes through urine, stool, and IWL—lung and skin)
    - Abnormal or above-average losses include gastrointestinal and diarrhea–related losses, ostomy, and chest tube drainage.
- Prediaper and postdiaper weights
  - Reweigh diaper after urine and/or stool and subtract the prediaper weight.
  - All losses are calculated to the closest milliliter.
- Deficit is calculated before incurred losses.
  - Is uncommon in the newborn (unless unrecognized third-space losses, such as necrotizing enterocolitis [NEC])
  - Deficits in older neonates occur with physiological disorders, such as renal tubular dysfunction and nonviral congenital adrenal hyperplasia.
  - Deficits are estimated by the percent of body weight comparisons.
    - Weight loss greater than 10% to 15% in 1 week is excessive.
    - Keeping weight loss less than 15% in very low–birth-weight (VLBW) infants is difficult.
    - SGA infants have less weight loss than appropriate for gestational age (AGA) infants.
- Replacement
  - All sick infants require IV access for fluid administration.
  - Selection of parenteral solution is based on
    - Weight and postnatal age
    - Incubator or heated humidified environment or radiant warmer
    - Uncovered VLBW infants under radiant warmers
      - Avoid the use of radiant warmers for infants with an average IWL of up to 170 mL/kg/day.
    - Water and glucose maintenance for large infants during the first day of life
      - 10% glucose is infused at 60 to 80 mL/kg/day (4.2 to 5.5 mg/kg/min).
      - Infusion rate can be steadily advanced over 4 to 5 days to 120 to 140- mL/kg/day.

Electrolytes for Neonates

- Sodium and potassium are not administered during the first and second days of life.
- Later, sodium (1 to 4 mEq/kg/day) is added as the salt of acetate, chloride, or phosphate.
- Potassium is never administered via IV fluid until the assessment of renal function and urine output is determined.
- Initially, calcium administration is 1 mEq/kg/day (20 mg/kg/day).
  - Maintenance of 3.0 to 3.5 mEq/kg/day (approximately 60 to 80 mg/kg/day) and preferably elemental calcium
    - Calcium gluconate (600 to 800 mg/kg/day)
    - Vital for VLBW infants or for those who are critically ill
  - Carefully observe the IV site because of tissue necrosis associated with infiltrated IV fluids with calcium.
- Factors that influence IWL should be recognized early and regulated; maintenance needs to prevent water and electrolyte imbalances.
  - Humidified incubators lower IWL of ELBW infants, and they will require less fluid intake and have decreased percent of weight loss, compared with nonhumidified incubator infants.

- Managing VLBW infants includes complex problems that have to be addressed.
  - Total fluid requirements are between 100 and 120 mL/kg/day at birth.
    - Restriction of fluids (excluding dehydration) reduces the risk of patent ductus arteriosus (PDA) and NEC.
  - By day 3 to 5 of life, cumulative weight loss stabilizes at 10% to 15% of birth weight.
  - Sodium requirements are 2 to 3 mEq/kg/day after 24 to 48 hours.
  - The target glucose level is 45 mg/dL or higher before each feeding in VLBW infants.
  - Higher glucose levels of 8 to 9 mg/kg/min for preterm infants versus 6 mg/kg/min for term infants

Common Problems: Calcium, Potassium, Sodium, Magnesium, Phosphorous, and Chloride

- Hypocalcemia
  - Infants with hypocalcemia have a total serum calcium concentration of less than 7 mg/dL.
    - Measurement includes serum and ionized calcium, phosphate, and alkaline phosphatase.
  - Symptoms are asymptomatic or nonspecific: poor feeding; emesis; lethargy; irritability; polyuria; constipation
  - Causes
    - Excessive vitamin D or calcium supplementation
    - Inadequate phosphorus supplementation with parenteral nutrition supplementation
    - Secondary conditions, such as Williams syndrome and hypophosphatasia-associated hyperkalemia, attributable to maternal hypoparathyroidism
    - Drug-induced hypercalcemia, due to thiazide diuretics
  - Treatment: initially adjusting the calcium-phosphorus ratio in supplementation; administering furosemide in critical cases to encourage calcium excretion in the urine
  - Nursing considerations: monitoring electrolytes for the infant's volume status and signs of dehydration; strictly managing intake and output (I&O); frequently screening intravenous (IV) site for irritation
- Hypercalcemia
  - Infants with hypercalcemia have a total serum calcium concentration in excess of 11 mg/dL.
    - Measurement includes both serum and ionized calcium, as well as phosphate and alkaline phosphatase.
  - Nonspecific symptoms: emesis; poor feeding; irritability; lethargy; polyuria; constipation
  - Causes: secondary conditions attributable to maternal hypoparathyroidism and vitamin D intake; neonatal diseases, such as hyperparathyroidism, hyperthyroidism, Williams syndrome, and hypophosphatasia
  - Treatment: adjusting the calcium-phosphorus ratio in parenteral nutrition solutions; providing adequate phosphorus supplementation instead of decreasing the calcium
  - Nursing considerations: carefully monitoring electrolytes; monitoring infant volume status to avoid dehydration
- Hypernatremia
  - Infants with hypernatremia have a total serum sodium concentration greater than 150 mEq/L.
  - Symptoms: rare; seizures can occur later
  - Causes: dehydration; administration of sodium-containing solutions (bolus or other medication); congenital or acquired lowering of ADH, resulting in electrolyte-free water loss, such as in diabetes insipidus; intracranial bleeding

- Treatment: slowly reducing the serum sodium levels to prevent seizures
- Nursing considerations: assessing for potential seizure activity; initiating safety and seizure precautions; monitoring for dehydration (appears better hydrated due to fluid shifts to intravascular spaces); strictly managing I&O
- Hyponatremia
  - Infants with hyponatremia have a total serum sodium concentration less than 140 mEq/L.
  - Symptoms can develop chronically versus acutely with seizures as a late clinical sign.
  - Causes
    - Excess hydration (electrolyte-free solutions)
    - Renal sodium loss due to diuretics
    - Syndrome of inappropriate antidiuretic hormone (SIADH) secretion
      - Lower serum sodium levels and lower urine output
      - Associated with pathological conditions related to the central nervous system (CNS) and respiratory system
  - Treatment: restricting fluid volume until diuresis occurs; resolving the underlying condition
  - Nursing considerations: monitoring electrolytes; strictly managing I&O and daily weights
- Hyperkalemia
  - Infants with hyperkalemia have a serum potassium concentration in excess of 7 mEq/L.
  - Symptoms: muscular weakness; cardiac dysrhythmias; ileus
  - Electrocardiographic (ECG) changes
    - Short QT interval
    - Widening QRS complex
    - Sine wave QRS/T pattern
  - Causes: acidosis; renal failure; adrenal insufficiency (rare); iatrogenic, secondary to potassium administration
  - Treatment
    - Resolve the underlying causes.
    - Treatment depends on severity.
      - Stop potassium administration.
      - Evaluate total and ionized calcium.
    - If hypocalcemia is present, infuse calcium gluconate (100 to 200 mg/kg).
    - Infuse sodium bicarbonate 1 to 2 mEq/kg slowly over 30 minutes or longer.
      - Treat hyperkalemia with acute renal failure with caution; a large volume of fluid may become an issue.
      - Peritoneal dialysis may be necessary.
  - Nursing considerations: careful monitoring of electrolytes; observing for NEC or other bowel injury with peritoneal dialysis
- Hypokalemia
  - Infants with hypokalemia have a serum potassium concentration less than 3.5 mEq/L.
  - Symptoms: muscular weakness; cardiac dysrhythmias; ileus; ECG changes of decreased T waves and ST segment depression
  - Causes: significant intracellular depletion; low body potassium with normal serum levels (most potassium is intracellular); diuretic-induced hypokalemia
  - Treatment: administering supplemental potassium chloride
  - Nursing considerations: careful monitoring of electrolytes; strict management of I&O; recording daily weights; monitoring for ECG changes

APPLICATION AND REVIEW

9. Which total serum calcium level is suggestive of hypocalcemia in an infant?
   1. 5.8 mg/dL
   2. 7.6 mg/dL
   3. 8.4 mg/dL
   4. 9.2 mg/dL

10. The nurse is caring for a postpartum woman diagnosed with hypoparathyroidism. For which electrolyte imbalance should the nurse monitor the newborn?
    1. Hypocalcemia
    2. Hypernatremia
    3. Hyperkalemia
    4. Hypomagnesemia

11. Which total serum calcium level is suggestive of hypercalcemia in an infant?
    1. 9.3 mg/dL
    2. 10.8 mg/dL
    3. 11.0 mg/dL
    4. 11.6 mg/dL

12. Which newborn assessment finding is suggestive of hypercalcemia?
    1. Hyperactivity
    2. Vomiting
    3. Diarrhea
    4. Oliguria

13. Which serum sodium level is associated with a sodium imbalance?
    1. 132.8 mEq/L
    2. 142 mEq/L
    3. 144.4 mEq/L
    4. 150.0 mEq/L

14. An infant is diagnosed as being hypernatremic. Which body system should the nurse assess *first*?
    1. Neurological
    2. Respiratory
    3. Cardiovascular
    4. Gastrointestinal

15. The nurse is caring for an infant with a serum sodium level of 158 mEq/L. Which intervention should the nurse implement?
    1. Seizure precautions
    2. Aspiration precautions
    3. Supplemental oxygen, as needed
    4. Monitoring skin for diarrhea-related trauma

See Answers on pages 238–240.

Fluid and Electrolyte Balance in Infants and Children

- Body water content and distribution (approximate) (Figure 13.1)
  - Premature infant
    - Water content: 90%
    - Blood volume: 85 to 90 mL/kg
  - Newborn infant
    - Water content: 70% to 80%
    - Blood volume: 80 to 90 mL/kg
  - Toddler 12 to 24 months of age
    - Water content: 64%
    - Blood volume: 75 to 80 mL/kg
  - Adult
    - Water content: 50% to 60%
    - Blood volume: 65 to 70 mL/kg
- Fluid requirements
  - Preterm infants
    - Daily: 200 mL/kg/day
    - Hourly: 1 to 10 mL/kg/hr

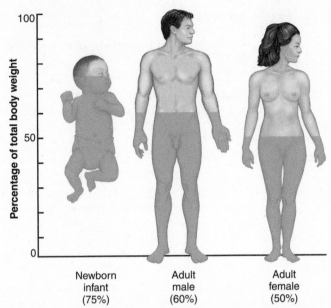

FIGURE 13.1 Proportion of body water varies by age and gender. (From Patton, K. T., & Thibodeau, G. A. [2018]. *The human body in health & disease*, [7th ed.]. St. Louis: Elsevier.)

- Term infants
  - Daily: 150 mL/kg/day
  - Hourly: 11 to 20 kg: 2 mL/kg/hr
- Children and adolescents
  - Daily: 2 to 3 liters
  - Hourly: (weight more than 20 kg) 1 mL/kg/hr
- Factors that increase the risk for fluid loss
  - TBW differs and is due to gender, weight, and age.
  - Infants and young children have higher water concentrations than adults.
  - Infants have a greater water turnover than adults as a result of a higher metabolic rate, larger surface area (relative to body mass), and an infant's inability to concentrate urine because of immature kidneys.
- Normal regulation of water balance
  - Water enters the body through oral intake of fluid and foods.
  - Water from fluids and solids are absorbed in the gastrointestinal tract.
  - Minimal amount of water is generated from body's metabolic processes.
    - At any age, a healthy individual requires
      - 100 mL of water per 100 calories metabolized is needed for dissolving and eliminating metabolic wastes.
      - Metabolism increases with fever or with the need to repair injured tissue.
  - Water loss is primarily through the kidneys, but also through the skin, lungs, and gastrointestinal tract.
  - Two primary mechanisms regulate body water.
    - Thirst and the desire for fluids is controlled by the hypothalamus (thirst center).

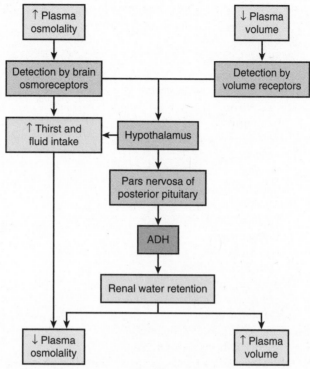

FIGURE 13.2   The antidiuretic hormone (ADH) system. (From Huether, S. E., McCance, K. L., Brashers, V. L., & Rote, S. R. [2017]. *Understanding pathophysiology*, [6th ed.]. St. Louis: Elsevier.)

- Thirst center is stimulated by cellular dehydration caused by extracellular osmosis (detected by osmoreceptors) and a decrease in blood volume.
  - Stretch receptors or baroreceptors in the carotid sinus and aorta are sensitive to arterial blood pressure fluctuations.
  - Low-pressure baroreceptors are located in the left atrium and major thoracic veins.
  - Angiotensin II is secreted in response to low blood pressure or volume.
- ADH (or vasopressin) is responsible for the reabsorption of water by the kidneys (Figure 13.2).
  - Lower ADH production reduces the kidneys' ability to reabsorb water.
  - Levels of circulatory ADH are controlled by ECF volume and osmolality.
- In children and infants who are critically ill, greater production of ADH and aldosterone results in fluid retention.
- Factors that cause fluid retention: hypotension; pain; stress; positive pressure ventilation; severe pulmonary hypertension
  - Cascade effect
    - Increased ADH, resulting in increased intravascular volume
    - Increased secretion of aldosterone, resulting in the retention of sodium and water

Dehydration in Infants and Children

- Causes
  - Types of organisms for common pediatric gastroenteritis

- Dehydration in infants and children, often the result of an infectious process
  - Viral organisms (common)
    - Rotavirus
    - Norwalk
    - Enteric adenovirus
  - Viral organisms (uncommon)
    - Calicivirus
    - Astrovirus
  - Bacterial organisms (common)
    - *Salmonella*
    - *Shigella*
    - *Campylobacter jejuni*
  - Bacterial organisms (uncommon)
    - *Yersinia enterocolitica*
    - *Vibrio cholerae*
    - *Escherichia coli*
    - *Clostridium difficile*
  - Parasitic organisms
    - *Entamoeba histolytica*
    - *Cryptosporidium*
- Nondiarrheal causes of dehydration
  - Water deficit from diabetes insipidus
  - High IWLs after a tracheostomy or with tachypnea
  - Inadequate intake of water from ineffective breastfeeding or child abuse
  - Sodium and water deficits from burns or large amounts of sweating
  - Renal losses resulting from diuretics, diabetes mellitus, and chronic renal disease
  - Other causes include surgical drains and third-spacing
- Pathophysiologic characteristics of dehydration
  - Dehydration can occur at any age.
    - Sick and younger children are at greatest risk.
    - Very young children have greater surface area–to-volume ratios than adults and a high rate of IWLs.
  - Young children cannot actively communicate to let their needs for fluid be known to replace losses.
  - Because of their physiological functioning, infants under the age 2 months are at the greatest risk for dehydration.
  - Regardless of the cause of diarrhea, fluid loss results when intestinal fluid secretion is greater than the rate of absorption.
  - Substantial loss of fluid from the intestine lowers intravascular volume.
    - End-organ hypoperfusion
    - Poor nutrient and oxygen delivery
    - Last, tissue acidosis
    - High aldosterone levels from hypovolemia, resulting in renal potassium loss
    - Last, circulatory collapse and shock, resulting in irreversible organ damage and death
- Assessment
  - Five-point assessment
    - How large is the volume deficit? History and physical examination
    - Is osmolar imbalance present? Serum sodium and serum osmolality measurements

- Is acid-base disturbance present? Serum pH and serum bicarbonate measurements and partial pressure of carbon dioxide ($PaCO_2$)
- Is potassium metabolism present? Serum potassium level
- Is renal function impaired? Blood urea nitrogen (BUN), creatinine, and urine-specific gravity
- Nursing assessment of a child's fluid balance
  - Hourly I&O
  - Continual clinical assessment of body systems: vital signs; pulse volume; blood pressure
  - Physical appearance: skin texture and turgor; moistness of mouth and mucous membranes; tension of the fontanels (when present)
  - Central venous pressure (CVP): measurement of the pressure in the right atrium of the heart, indicating the homeostasis of the body
- Diagnosis
  - Can result from inadequate fluid intake or extensive fluid loss
  - Is associated with abnormal electrolytes
  - Diarrhea is classified on the basis of its severity level and serum (osmolality) levels.
    - Isotonic: equal loss of water and sodium; normal serum sodium; equal distribution of fluid loss between the interstitial and intravascular spaces
    - Hypotonic: proportion of sodium loss is larger than water; serum sodium level decreases; fluid shifts from intravascular space into interstitial and cellular spaces
    - Hypertonic: larger proportion of water loss than sodium; serum sodium rises; fluid shifts from cellular and interstitial spaces into intravascular space
      - Until fluid loss is excessive, the maintained intravascular volume may mask the signs of dehydration.
- Signs and symptoms of dehydration
  - When assessing infants and children for dehydration, a complete history is taken; the infant and child's age is considered.
  - Three classifications of dehydration
    - Mild dehydration
      - Body weight loss: infant 5% (50 mL/kg); child 3% (30 mL/kg)
      - Heart rate (pulse): mild tachycardia
      - Blood pressure: normal
      - Skin color and turgor: pale color, normal-to-warm skin, texture dry, and lightly reduced skin fold return
      - Mucous membranes: slightly dry
      - Eyes: normal
      - Urine output: normal to mildly reduced
      - Neurological factors: normal or irritable
    - Moderate dehydration
      - Body weight loss: infant 10% (60 mL/kg); child 6% (100 mL/kg)
      - Heart rate (pulse): rapid and weak
      - Blood pressure: low orthostatic blood pressure
      - Skin color and turgor: gray, decreased skin turgor
      - Mucous membranes: dry
      - Eyes: decreased tears
      - Urine output: significantly reduced
      - Neurological factors: irritable

- Severe dehydration
  - Body weight loss: infant 15% (150 mL/kg); child >9% (>90 mL/kg)
  - Heart rate (pulse): significant tachycardia and weakness
  - Blood pressure: shock
  - Skin color and turgor: gray, decreased skin turgor
  - Mucous membranes: dry, parched, collapse of sublingual veins
  - Eyes: sunken and absence of tears
  - Urine output: anuria
  - Neurological factors: lethargic, grunting, coma
- Goals of care
  - Replace fluid and electrolyte deficits.
  - Correct the underlying cause.
- Treatment
  - In children, fluid therapy to address dehydration is twofold:
    - Replacement therapy to correct deficit
    - Maintenance therapy to replace ongoing losses and IWLs
  - Goal is to restore and maintain intravascular volume, systemic perfusion, and electrolyte balance
  - Mild dehydration is based on the cause of the dehydration and the age of the child; oral rehydration is administered.
    - A fluid that is designed to promote water and electrolyte absorption is referred to as an oral rehydration solution (ORS).
      - An ORS contains between 70 and 90 mEq/L sodium and not more than 25 g/L of glucose (Pedialyte, Ricelyte, World Health Organization [WHO] and United Nations Children's Fund [UNICEF] oral replacement solutions).
      - Most soft drinks, juices, and punches contain high levels of sugar and minimal to no sodium, therefore these are inappropriate for ORSs.
      - Higher sugar concentrations in fluids can worsen diarrhea by causing a large osmotic load in the intestinal lumen.
      - An ORS can restore both fluid and electrolyte balance.
    - At the end of the rehydration period, sodium and potassium levels are back to within a normal range.
  - The infant or child will become sicker or need parenteral IV fluid therapy.
    - Assess the dehydrated child or infant for signs of shock.
    - Rapidly administer a crystalloid fluid (20 mL/kg), and repeat as needed.
  - Goal of the rehydration phase is to replace the entire fluid deficit in the first 4 to 6 hours.
    - Initially, administer 1 teaspoon (5 mL) per minute for infants, 2 teaspoons (10 mL) per minute for toddlers, and 3 teaspoons (15 mL) per minute for older children.
    - Generally, 300 to 900 mL/hr will replace the fluid deficit in 4 to 6 hours.
    - Continue to administer an ORS even with vomiting, because the entire stomach contents are not expelled. In addition, as dehydration and tissue acidosis recede, the frequency of vomiting declines.
- Complications
  - Moderate and severe dehydration, if left untreated, can lead to a critical decrease in cardiac output and systemic perfusion.
  - If dehydration continues, the body uses compensatory mechanisms to maintain essential organ perfusion, which can lead to metabolic acidosis, multisystem failure, and eventually death.

- Although overhydration can result in transient periorbital puffiness and a 2% to 3% weight gain that is self limiting, overhydrating is preferable than being too cautious with rehydration.
- Nursing interventions
  - Monitor the infant or child for fluid overload.
    - Fluid overload is more circulatory volume than the heart can accommodate and can result in heart failure and pulmonary edema.
    - Manage hourly I&O.
    - Administer fluids (oral and parenteral) as ordered and in response to the needs of the child.
    - Assess for signs of dehydration, and report, if present.
    - Monitor laboratory values for abnormal findings, and report as needed.
- Prevention
  - Parenteral education for the early signs of dehydration
    - Monitor and report to the health care provider the amount of diarrhea and vomiting in a child, especially an infant.
    - Have a hydration solution (Pedialyte) on hand for the early stages of gastrointestinal disturbances.
    - Provide client and child education regarding hand hygiene.

Electrolytes and Children

- Normal values of electrolytes
  - Primary electrolytes: sodium; potassium; calcium; magnesium; chloride; phosphate
- Primary electrolyte values in children

Electrolyte	Premature Infant	Term Infant	Child
Potassium	4.5–7.2 mmol/L	3.6–6.4 mmol/L	3.5–5.0 mmol/L
Sodium	135–145 mmol/L	135–145 mmol/L	135–145 mmol/L
Calcium	2.1–2.7 mmol/L	2.1–2.7 mmol/L	2.1–2.7 mmol/L
Magnesium	0.6–1.0 mmol/L	0.6–1.0 mmol/L	0.6–1.0 mmol/L
Phosphate	1–2.6 mmol/L	1–1.8 mmol/L	1–1.8 mmol/L

- Primary intracellular electrolyte is potassium.
- Primary extracellular electrolyte is sodium.

Sodium

- Sodium is the primary electrolyte in the ECF compartment and has a greater effect on osmosis and osmolality.
- Hyponatremia is defined as a serum sodium level less than 135 mmol/L.
  - Lower sodium levels can alter the cells ability to depolarize and repolarize in a normal pattern.
  - If hyponatremia leads to a loss of ECF, signs of hypovolemia—tachycardia, hypotension, and diminished urine output—may be present.
  - Hyponatremia, attributable to water retention, may result in edema and weight gain.
  - Treatment
    - Depends upon the cause, biochemical laboratory results, and the clinical presentation of hyponatremia.
    - Sodium levels gradually fall, and correction should mirror this gradual reduction.
    - Naturally correct the condition with fluid restrictions.

- Nursing care
  - Educate the parents and client regarding the condition.
  - Weigh the client daily.
  - Manage I&O daily.
  - Monitor laboratory results, and report to the provider.
  - Complete a focused assessment and physical examination of the client.
- Hypernatremia is defined as a serum sodium level greater than 145 mmol/L.
  - Causes excessive water loss; lower water intake; large sodium intake
  - Signs and symptoms: thirst; oliguria or anuria; high specific gravity of urine; increased serum osmolality; lower intravascular volume (tachycardia, hypotension, peripheral shutdown)
    - Neurological symptoms (water moves out of brain cells): headaches; seizures; coma
  - Treatment: identifying the cause of hypernatremia through client history, physical assessment, and monitoring laboratory changes; completing the rehydration phase of treatment
  - Nursing care: educating parents and client regarding the condition; weighing the client daily; managing I&O daily; monitoring laboratory results and reporting them to the provider; completing a focused assessment and physical examination of the client

Potassium

- Potassium (K^+) is the most common intracellular ion (between 140 and 150 mmol/L).
  - Extracellular levels of K^+ are lower.
  - K^+ is regulated through two mechanisms.
    - Kidneys: either conserve or eliminate K^+.
    - Transcellular shifts occur between the ICF and ECF compartments.
      - K^+ enters the cells when plasma levels are high.
      - K^+ leave the cells when plasma levels are low.
  - Deviations from the normal range for K^+ levels can result in life-threatening cardiac dysrhythmias.
    - K^+ is vital for many body functions.
      - Growth
      - Conduction of nerve impulses
      - Acid-base balance
      - Use of carbohydrates for energy
- Hypokalemia is defined as a serum K^+ level less than 3.5 mmol/L.
  - Causes: inadequate intake; unusual losses through the gastrointestinal route and through the skin and kidneys; transcellular shifts between the ICF and ECF compartments
  - Signs and symptoms: polyuria; vomiting; muscle cramps; confusion; metabolic alkalosis; cardiac arrhythmias
  - Treatment: identifying and treating the underlying cause of the K^+ loss; administering oral or IV K^+ supplements
  - Nursing management
    - K^+ is a powerful electrolyte.
    - Children with abnormal K^+ levels need ECG monitoring for arrhythmias and ECG changes.
    - K^+ should be slowly administered and monitored for response (ECG).
- Hyperkalemia is defined as a serum K^+ level greater than 5 mEq/L.
  - Hyperkalemia is an unusual occurrence in a healthy child.
  - Causes of hyperkalemia: rapid administration of K^+; lower renal excretion due to acute renal failure; transcellular shifts of K^+ between the ICF and ECF compartments

- Signs and symptoms: nausea; diarrhea; dizziness; muscle cramps; cardiac dysrhythmias, leading to cardiac arrest
- Treatment: reducing or stopping the intake of K^+; improving renal excretion and cellular uptake
- Nursing management: monitoring vital signs and ECG changes

Calcium

- Hypocalcemia (acute or chronic)
  - Calcium is measured as total or ionized (different ranges).
    - Total calcium: 2 to 27 mmol/L
    - Ionized calcium: 1.2 to 1.3 mmol/L
    - Severe hypocalcemia: plasma levels <1.75 mmol/L
  - Causes of hypocalcemia
    - Children who are critically ill have an increased risk of an impaired ability to use calcium from bone stores.
    - Calcium loss from the kidneys occurs.
    - Calcium can bind with protein, thus making it unavailable in the blood.
    - Maternal hypoparathyroidism
  - Mild signs and symptoms: muscle cramps (legs and back)
  - Acute signs and symptoms: jitteriness; convulsions; ECG abnormalities; encelopathy; arrhythmias; heart failure; papilloedema or cataracts (prolonged hypocalcemia)
  - Treatment: identifying and treating the underlying cause; administering calcium via IV infusion
  - Nursing management: ensuring client safety; initiating seizure precautions; monitoring for ECG changes; monitoring for changes in the physical assessment; providing supportive care
- Hypercalcemia (rare)
  - Causes, due to excessive bone reabsorption
    - Bone metastases
    - Leukemia
    - Lymphoma
    - Multiple myeloma
    - Extensive immobility attributable to a neurological injury (paraplegics or quadriplegics)
    - Endocrine disease
    - Recovery from acute renal failure
    - William syndrome
  - Signs and symptoms: seizures; muscle flaccidity; tachyarrhythmias
  - Treatment (clients are often volume depleted): administering oral and IV fluid replacement supplements, followed by diuretic therapy; addressing the underlying cause of the condition
  - Nursing management: monitor vital signs, symptoms of seizure, and ECG changes.

Phosphate

- Phosphate is critical for several body functions.
  - Assistance with bone formation
  - Formation of adenosine triphosphate (ATP) and enzymes that aid in metabolism
  - Acid-base buffer in ECF and renal excretion of hydrogen ions

- Hypophosphatemia
  - Causes of hypophosphatemia: lower intestinal absorption (severe prolonged diarrhea); lack of vitamin D; renal losses; malnutrition; hypomagnesemia or hypokalemia; severe burns; diabetic ketoacidosis; kidney disease; hyperparathyroidism; hypothyroidism; Cushing syndrome; hemodialysis; prolonged diuretic therapy
  - Signs and symptoms: muscle weakness; respiratory failure; heart failure; seizures; coma; weight loss; osteomalacia
  - Treatment: administering replacement threapy; indentifying and treating the underlying cause
  - Nursing management: monitoring for changes in the physical assessment; monitoring for changes in laboratory values
- Hyperphosphatemia
  - Due to phosphate retention and its accumulation in the bloodstream
  - Will occur with hypocalcemia
  - Causes of hyperphosphatemia: skeletal fractures or disease; hemodialysis; diabetic ketoacidosis; acromegaly; systemic infection; intestinal obstruction
  - Signs and symptoms
    - Mild cases of hyperphosphatemia are asymptomatic.
    - Symptoms of severe hyperphosphatemia: paresthesia; tingling in hands and fingers; muscle spasms and cramps; convulsions; cardiac arrest
  - Treatment: administering replacement therapy; identifying and treating the underlying cause
  - Nursing management: monitoring for changes in laboratory values; monitoring for changes in the client's condition and physical assessment

Magnesium

- Is an important electrolyte
  - Responsible for all reactions that need ATP
  - Replication and transcription of deoxyribonucleic acid (DNA)
  - Cellular energy metabolism
- Hypomagnesemia
  - Causes: impaired intake or absorption; starvation of malabsorption; diuretic therapy; diabetic ketoacidosis
  - Signs and symptoms: tetany; cardiac arrhythmias; nystagmus
  - Treatment: administering IV magnesium replacement
  - Nursing management: monitoring laboratory values; monitoring for changes in the client's condition and physical assessment
- Hypermagnesemia
  - Rare occurrence
  - Primarily caused by renal failure
  - Signs and symptoms: lethargy; confusion; hypotension; cardiac arrhythmias
  - Treatment: discontinuing any administration of magnesium and calcium (antagonist of magnesium)
  - Nursing management: monitoring laboratory values; monitoring for changes in the client's condition and physical assessment

Chloride

- Hyperchloremia
  - Is normal and transient in newborns

- Causes of hyperchloremia: prematurity; gastrointestinal (vomiting, diarrhea); fever; dehydration; high levels of sodium; diabetes; starvation; Addison disease
- Signs and symptoms: gastrointestinal disorder (vomiting and diarrhea)
- Treatment: addressing the underlying cause; administering hydration therapy; changing medications that may be causing the condition; recommending a balanced diet
- Nursing management: providing supportive care to the client
- Hypochloremia
  - Causes of hypochloremia: impaired renal function; prolonged diarrhea or vomiting; metabolic alkalosis
  - Signs and symptoms
    - Is asymptomatic but will notice symptoms of other associated electrolyte imbalances
      - Fluid loss
      - Dehydration
      - Weakness
      - Diarrhea or vomiting
      - Dyspnea
    - Is often associated with hyponatremia
  - Treatment: identifying and treating the underlying cause; making the necessary changes, if the condition is due to medication; administering restorative fluids orally or intravenously
  - Nursing management: providing supportive care to the client

APPLICATION AND REVIEW

17. Which is the nurse's *priority* intervention for a child diagnosed with hyperkalemia?
    1. To manage vomiting
    2. To manage constipation
    3. To monitor for dysrhythmias
    4. To monitor for respiratory distress
18. The nurse is caring for a client diagnosed with leukemia. For which electrolyte imbalance should the nurse monitor?
    1. Hypophosphatemia
    2. Hypomagnesemia
    3. Hypercalcemia
    4. Hyperkalemia
19. The nurse is caring for an infant diagnosed with hyperphosphatemia. For which risk factor should the nurse monitor?
    1. Acromegaly
    2. Hypomagnesemia
    3. Cushing syndrome
    4. Vitamin D deficiency
20. The nurse is caring for an infant diagnosed with hypermagnesemia. For which condition should the nurse monitor?
    1. Renal failure
    2. Premature birth
    3. Respiratory distress
    4. Genetic cardiac anomaly
21. The nurse is caring for several newborns. Which newborns are at risk for developing hyperchloremia? *(Select all that apply.)*
    1. Premature newborn
    2. Newborn experiencing diarrhea
    3. Newborn with an elevated temperature
    4. Newborn diagnosed with hyponatremia
    5. LGA newborn

See Answers on pages 238–240.

ANSWER KEY: REVIEW QUESTIONS

1. **1 In early fetal development, the body is mostly comprised of water.**

   2, 3, 4 The percentage of total body water declines throughout the subsequent stages of development and growth.

   Client Need: Health Promotion and Maintenance; **Cognitive Level:** Understanding; **Integrated Process:** Teaching and Learning

2. **3 SGA infants have a larger TBW per kilogram than term infants weighing within the expected range.**

   1, 2 TBW declines as gestation advances, from 94% of the body weight at 3 months to 78% at term (40 weeks' gestation). **4** SGA infants have a larger TBW per kilogram than term infants weighing within the expected range.

   Client Need: Health Promotion and Maintenance; **Cognitive Level:** Analysis; **Integrated Process:** Teaching and Learning

3. **1 70% of IWL happens through skin; fever would increase this evaporation.**

   2 IWL is water loss attributable to evaporation from the respiratory tract or the skin. **3** 70% of IWL happens through skin, whereas 30% is loss through respirations. **4** IWL is water loss attributable to evaporation from the respiratory tract or the skin.

   Client Need: Health Promotion and Maintenance; **Cognitive Level:** Analysis; **Integrated Process:** Teaching and Learning

4. **3 Motor activity and crying tend to increase IWL. Wrapping a newborn snuggly (swaddling) tends to comfort the infant, thus reducing crying and excessive motor activity.**

   1 Adding an extra blanket will tend to increase the newborn's temperature, which will increase IWL. **2** Increasing the environmental humidity will increase IWL. **4** Raising the temperature of the environment will increase IWL.

   Client Need: Health Promotion and Maintenance; **Cognitive Level:** Analysis; **Nursing Process:** Application

5. **2 Weight loss of up to 15% can occur during the first week of life for a variety of reasons.**

   1, 3, 4 Weight loss of up to 15% can occur during the first week of life for a variety of reasons.

   Client Need: Health Promotion and Maintenance; **Cognitive Level:** Applying; **Integrated Process:** Teaching and Learning

6. **2 Monitoring urine volume is the focus of newborn assessment when considering possible newborn dehydration; a diaper count serves to confirm urine output.**

   1 Although fluid consumption is a focus of newborn assessment, it is not a factor to be considered when monitoring for newborn dehydration. **3** Although awake time is a focus of newborn assessment, it is not a factor to be considered when monitoring for newborn dehydration. **4** Although physical activity is a focus of newborn assessment, it is not a factor to be considered when monitoring for newborn dehydration.

   Client Need: Physiological Integrity; **Cognitive Level:** Analysis; **Nursing Process:** Planning

7. **1 Infants with 5% isotonic dehydration exhibit dry mucous membranes, lightly sunken anterior fontanel, decreased tear production, and oliguria.**

   2, 3, 4 Infants with isotonic dehydration between 10% and 15% exhibit poor skin turgor, an absence of tears, oliguria, and cool extremities, in addition to dry mucous membranes.

   Client Need: Physiological Integrity; **Cognitive Level:** Applying; **Nursing Process:** Assessment

8. **3 Skin turgor is more difficult to assess in premature newborns because of the lack of subcutaneous fat.**

   1 Although oliguria is a characteristic of dehydration, it is not a common characteristic of premature newborns. **2** Although tachycardia is a characteristic of dehydration, it is not a common characteristic of premature newborns. **4** Although a sunken anterior fontanel is a characteristic of dehydration, it is not a common characteristic of premature newborns.

   Client Need: Physiological Integrity; **Cognitive Level:** Analysis; **Nursing Process:** Evaluation

9. **1 Infants with a total serum calcium level less than 7 mg/dL are considered hypocalcemic.**
   2 Infants with a total serum calcium level of 7.6 mg/dL are within the normal range. **3** Infants with a total serum calcium level of 8.4 mg/dL are within the normal range. **4** Infants with a total serum calcium level of 9.2 mg/dL are within the normal range.
   Client Need: Physiological Integrity; **Cognitive Level:** Applying; **Nursing Process:** Assessment

10. **1 This newborn should be monitored for symptoms related to hypocalcemia, secondary to maternal hypoparathyroidism.**
    2 This newborn should be monitored for symptoms related to hypocalcemia, secondary to maternal hypoparathyroidism; hypernatremia is not associated with parathyroid dysfunction. **3** This newborn should be monitored for symptoms related to hypocalcemia, secondary to maternal hypoparathyroidism; hyperkalemia is not associated with parathyroid dysfunction. **4** This newborn should be monitored for symptoms related to hypocalcemia, secondary to maternal hypoparathyroidism; hypomagnesemia is not associated with parathyroid dysfunction.
    Client Need: Physiological Integrity; **Cognitive Level:** Applying; **Nursing Process:** Assessment

11. **4 An infant with a serum calcium level in excess of 11 mg/dL is hypercalcemic.**
    1, 2, 3 Infants with serum calcium levels between 9 mg/dL and 11 mg/dL are within the normal range.
    Client Need: Physiological Integrity; **Cognitive Level:** Understanding; **Nursing Process:** Assessment

12. **2 Nonspecific symptoms that are reflective of hypercalcemia in a newborn include vomiting, irritability, lethargy, polyuria, and constipation.**
    1 Hyperactivity is not a nonspecific symptom reflective of hypercalcemia in a newborn. **3** Diarrhea is not a nonspecific symptom reflective of hypercalcemia in a newborn. **4** Oliguria is not a nonspecific symptom reflective of hypercalcemia in a newborn.
    Client Need: Physiological Integrity; **Cognitive Level:** Analysis; **Nursing Process:** Assessment

13. **1 Infants with serum sodium levels less than 140 mEq/L are diagnosed with hyponatremia.**
    2, 3, 4 Normal serum sodium levels fall between 140 and 150 mEq/L.
    Client Need: Health Promotion and Maintenance; **Cognitive Level:** Understanding; **Nursing Process:** Assessment

14. **1 Hypernatremia in infants is often related to intracranial bleeding, making a neurological assessment a priority.**
    2, 3, 4 Hypernatremia in infants is often related to intracranial bleeding; consequently, an assessment of the respiratory, cardiovascular, or gastrointestinal system would not be a priority.
    Client Need: Physiological Integrity; **Cognitive Level:** Applying; **Nursing Process:** Planning

15. **1 A serum sodium level greater than 150 mEq/L is associated with hypernatremia; seizures can be triggered by elevated sodium levels.**
    2 Hypercalcemia, not hypernatremia, can trigger vomiting. **3** Respiratory distress is not generally associated with hypernatremia. **4** Hypernatremia does not trigger diarrhea.
    Client Need: Health Promotion and Maintenance; **Cognitive Level:** Analysis; **Integrated Process/Nursing Process:** Evaluation

16. **3 Hyperkalemia increases the risk of life-threatening cardiac dysrhythmias; monitoring for dysrhythmias is a primary intervention.**
    1 Hyperkalemia increases the risk of life-threatening cardiac dysrhythmias; monitoring for dysrhythmias is a primary intervention. **2** Diarrhea, not constipation, is associated with hyperkalemia; hyperkalemia increases the risk of life-threatening cardiac dysrhythmias; monitoring for dysrhythmias is a primary intervention. **4** Respiratory distress is not associated with hyperkalemia; hyperkalemia increases the risk of life-threatening cardiac dysrhythmias; monitoring for dysrhythmias is a primary intervention.
    Client Need: Physiological Integrity; **Cognitive Level:** Application; **Nursing Process:** Planning

17. **3 Hypercalcemia is a result of excessive bone reabsorption attributable to leukemia.**
    1 Hypophosphatemia is not associated with excessive bone reabsorption attributable to leukemia. **2** Hypercalcemia is not associated with excessive bone reabsorption attributable to leukemia. **4** Hypercalcemia is not associated with excessive bone reabsorption attributable to leukemia.
    Client Need: Physiological Integrity; **Cognitive Level:** Applying; **Nursing Process:** Planning

18. **1 Causes of hyperphosphatemia include acromegaly.**

    2 Causes of hypophosphatemia include hypomagnesemia. **3** Causes of hypophosphatemia include Cushing syndrome. **4** Causes of hypophosphatemia include vitamin D deficiency.

    Client Need: Physiological Integrity; **Cognitive Level:** Application; **Nursing Process:** Assessment

19. **1 Hypermagnesemia is primarily attributable to renal failure.**

    2 Hypermagnesemia is primarily attributable to renal failure, not premature birth. **3** Hypermagnesemia is primarily attributable to renal failure, not respiratory distress. **4** Hypermagnesemia is primarily attributable to renal failure, not a genetic cardiac anomaly.

    Client Need: Physiological Integrity; **Cognitive Level:** Analysis; **Nursing Process:** Assessment

20. **Answers: 1, 2, 3**

    1 Prematurity is a risk factor for developing hyperchloremia. **2** Diarrhea is a risk factor for developing hyperchloremia. **3** Fever is a risk factor for developing hyperchloremia.

    4 Hyponatremia is not a risk factor for developing hyperchloremia. **5** LGA is not a risk factor for developing hyperchloremia.

    Client Need: Physiological Integrity; **Cognitive Level:** Analysis; **Nursing Process:** Assessment

Fluid and Electrolyte Balance in Special Populations

SPECIAL POPULATIONS OVERVIEW

Older Adults

- Hydration management
  - Older adults require adequate fluid balance, which prevents complications resulting from abnormal fluid levels.
  - A significant number of older adults (up to 85% who are older than 85 years of age) drink less than 1 liter of fluid per day.
  - Recommended fluid intake for this age group is 1500 mL (1.5 liters) per day, with the exception of those requiring fluid restrictions.
- Maintenance of fluid balance is essential to health.
  - Balance is defined as fluid intake equals fluid output.
- Fulfillment of the older person's nutritional needs is affected by numerous factors: changes associated with aging; life-long eating habits; chronic disease; medication regimens; ethnicity and culture; socialization; socioeconomic deprivation; transportation; housing; food knowledge.
- Changes in the older individual: body composition; decreased thirst; decreased renal function; hormonal changes; cardiopulmonary changes
- Body water content and distribution
  - In the older person, body water content decreases; therefore the risk for dehydration increases (Figure 14.1).
  - Water comprises approximately 55% of body weight in the older adult.
- Factors that increase the risk for fluid loss
  - Thirst sensation diminishes.
    - Thirst in older adults is not proportional to his or her metabolic needs, resulting in dehydration.
  - Creatinine clearance declines with age.
    - Kidneys are less able to concentrate urine, which is more pronounced in older individuals with illnesses affecting kidney function.
  - Medications that affect renal function and fluid balance: diuretics; laxatives; angiotensin-converting enzyme (ACE) inhibitors
    - Psychotropic medications with anticholinergic effects result in dry mouth, urinary retention, and/or constipation.
    - The use of four or more medications is also a risk factor.
- Dehydration
  - This complex condition results in a reduction of total body water.
  - Dehydration is a prevalent problem among older adults in all settings.
  - In older people, dehydration most often develops as a result of diseases, such as diabetes, respiratory illness, and heart failure, as well as age-related changes and the side effects of medication(s).
  - Dehydration presents a significant risk factor for delirium, thromboembolic complications, infections, kidney stones, constipation, obstipation (severe form of constipation),

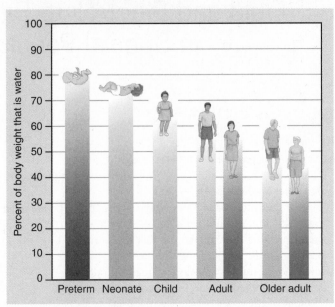

FIGURE 14.1 Percent of body weight that is water over the lifespan. (From Lewis, S. L., Bucher, L., Heitkemper, M. M., Harding, M. M., Kwong, J., & Roberts, D. [2017]. *Medical-surgical nursing: Assessment and management of clinical problems*, [10th ed.]. St. Louis: Elsevier.)

falls, medication toxicity, renal failure, seizures, electrolyte imbalances, hyperthermia, and delayed wound healing.

- Assessment
  - Assessment is complex in older people. Clinical signs may not show up until dehydration is advanced.
  - Diet history
    - A 24-hour diet recall can provide an estimate of nutritional adequacy.
    - If the older person is able, a 3-day dietary record, which includes fluids, foods, and amounts ingested, might be helpful.
  - Physical examination
    - Clinically observable existence
    - Accurate height and weight (always measured, not estimated)
    - Vital signs
    - General condition of the tongue, lips, gums, skin turgor, skin texture, skin color, functional ability, and overall general appearance
    - Simple acronym for dehydration
      Drugs (diuretics)
      End of life
      High fever
      Yellow urine turns dark
      Dizziness (orthostasis)
      Reduced oral intake
      Axilla dry

> _T_achycardia
>
> _I_ncontinence (or fear of)
>
> _O_ral problems
>
> _N_eurological impairment (sunken eyes)

- Diagnostics
  - Diagnosis of dehydration is biochemical.
  - Biochemical examination: blood urea nitrogen (BUN); complete blood count (CBC); total lymphatic count; thyroid level; comprehensive metabolic panel; liver function test; urinalysis; stool sample (fecal occult blood)
- Signs and symptoms: dry mucous membranes (mouth and nose); longitudinal furrows on the tongue; orthostasis (form of low blood pressure which happens when standing up from a sitting or lying position); speech incoherence; extremity weakness; dry axilla; sunken eyes
  - Typical signs and symptoms may not always be present in older people.
  - The large variability in the way different organs are affected by dehydration will cause symptoms to remain atypical in some older adults.
  - Skin turgor is assessed at the sternum.
    - Due to the loss of subcutaneous tissue that comes with aging, skin turgor is an unreliable assessment tool in older adults.
- Goals of care: prevention; education; treating underlying cause(s)
- Treatment: identification of the underlying cause; individualizing the interventions to ensure adequate nutritional intake for older people; hydration management
- Nursing interventions: Use techniques to increase fluid and food intake, and enhance and manage the environment to promote increased fluid and food intake.
- Prevention of dehydration is essential.
  - Education should be provided to older adults: nutritional requirements for health; special dietary modifications; chronic illness management; effects of age-associated changes; medication effects on nutrition; community resources.
- Nursing management of oral intake
  - Calculate a daily fluid goal.
    - Older adults should have an individualized fluid goal determined by a documented standard for daily fluid intake.
    - At least 1500 mL of fluid per day should be provided.
  - Compare the client's current intake with the fluid goal to evaluate hydration status.
  - Consistently provide fluids throughout the day.
    - Deliver between 75% and 80% of fluids at meals, and offer fluids during nonmeal times such as when medications are administered.
    - Offer a variety of fluids and the fluids that the person prefers.
    - Standardize the amount of fluid—at least 6 ounces—that is offered with administered medications.
  - Plan for individuals who are at risk for dehydration.
    - Schedule midmorning and midafternoon fluid rounds.
    - Provide two 8-ounce glasses of fluid in the morning and evening.
    - Provide additional fluids during "happy hour" or "tea time" when clients are able to gather for socialization.
    - Modify the fluid containers, based on the client's ability: lighter cups and glasses; weighted cups and glasses; plastic water bottles with straws; fluid containers that attach to wheelchairs; fluid containers that are delivered with meals.

- Make fluids accessible at all times, and ensure that the client can access them: filled water pitchers; fluid stations; beverage carts in congregate areas.
- Allow adequate time and staff for eating and feeding. Meals can provide two-thirds of the daily fluids.
- Encourage family members to participate in feeding and offering fluids.
  - Perform fluid regulation and documentation.
    - Teach individuals, if able, how to monitor hydration status, such as with a urine chart.
    - Document complete intake including hydration habits.
    - Know the volumes of fluid containers to calculate fluid consumptions accurately.
    - Frequency of documentation of fluid intake will vary among settings and is dependent on the individual's condition.
      - At least one accurate intake and output recording should be documented daily, including the amount of fluid consumed, difficulties with consumption, and urine-specific gravity and color.
      - For incontinent individuals, teach caregivers to observe incontinent pads or briefs for amount and frequency of urine, color changes, and odor, and report all variations from the individual's normal pattern.
- Electrolyte ranges for the older individual
  - Sodium
    - Hypernatremia and hyponatremia are the most common electrolyte abnormalities found in older adults. Both are associated with a high mortality rate.
    - Normal range for older adults: between 135 and 145 mEq/L
    - Hypernatremia: sodium level higher than 145 mEq/L
    - Hyponatremia: sodium level lower than 135 mEq/L
  - Potassium
    - Normal range for older adults: between 3.7 and 5.2 mEq/L
    - Hyperkalemia: potassium level higher than 5.2 mEq/L
    - Hypokalemia: potassium level lower than 3.7 mEq/L
  - Calcium
    - Normal range for older adults: between 8.5 and 10.6 mg/dL
    - Hypercalcemia: calcium level higher than 10.6 mg/dL
    - Hypocalcemia: calcium level lower than 8.5 mg/dL
  - Magnesium
    - Normal range for older adults: between 1.7 and 2.2 mg/dL
    - Hypermagnesemia: magnesium level higher than 2.2 mg/dL
    - Hypomagnesemia: magnesium level lower than 1.7 mg/dL
  - Phosphate
    - Normal range for older adults: between 0.81 and 1.45 molecules per liter
    - Hyperphosphatemia: phosphate level higher than 1.45 molecules per liter
    - Hypophosphatemia: phosphate level lower than 0.81 molecules per liter
  - Chloride
    - Normal range for older adults: between 97 and 107 mEq/L
    - Hyperchloremia: chloride level higher than 107 mEq/L
    - Hypochloremia: chloride level lower than 97 mEq/L

APPLICATION AND REVIEW

1. An 85-year-old client consumes 1.5 liters of fluid daily. Which assumption should the nurse make regarding this client's hydration status?
   1. The client is likely overhydrated and at risk for cardiac complications.
   2. The client requires education regarding the need to hydrate effectively.
   3. The client requires further assessment for physical signs of dehydration.
   4. The client is consuming the recommended fluid intake for this population.

2. Which assessment data are relevant to an older adult's risk for ineffective fluid balance? *(Select all that apply.)*
   1. Female
   2. History of diabetes type 1
   3. Delivered three full-term infants
   4. Adopted a vegan diet 15 years ago
   5. Has lived alone for the past 10 years

3. Which client statements alert the nurse to a client's possible risk for fluid loss? *(Select all that apply.)*
   1. "I'm told that I have age-related renal failure."
   2. "My medications seem to cause me to be constipated."
   3. "My heart condition is being managed with a diuretic."
   4. "I'm not good at managing my preference for salty and spicy foods."
   5. "I control my weight by eating and drinking only when I'm hungry or thirsty."

4. The nurse is caring for an older adult diagnosed with dehydration. Which actions should the nurse take? *(Select all that apply.)*
   1. Encourage the client by stating, "Use your call bell to get help ambulating."
   2. Ask the client, "When did you have your last bowel movement?"
   3. Keep the client's room quiet and dimly lit.
   4. Take the client's temperature every 4 hours.
   5. Complete a detailed medication history.

5. The nurse is caring for a client diagnosed with dehydration. Which client body system should be the nurse's primary focus?
   1. Cardiac
   2. Respiratory
   3. Integumentary
   4. Gastrointestinal

6. Which characteristic is suggestive of dehydration in an 85-year-old client diagnosed with dementia?
   1. Sunken eyeballs
   2. Ruddy complexion
   3. White patches on the tongue
   4. Deep furrows at the corners of the mouth

7. Which interventions should the nurse implement to prevent dehydration in an older adult client? *(Select all that apply.)*
   1. Encourage the client to drink an 8-ounce glass of fluid just before the morning hygiene.
   2. Provide at least 6 ounces of fluids when providing prescribed medications.
   3. Ask the client, "What are your favorite beverages?"
   4. Determine whether the client has a decreased thirst drive.
   5. Ensure that the client has easy access to fresh water.

8. Which serum sodium level suggests hyponatremia?
   1. 129 mEq/L
   2. 138 mEq/L
   3. 145 mEq/L
   4. 151 mEq/L
9. Which is the normal serum potassium range for an older adult?
   1. 1.7 to 2.2 mg/dL
   2. 3.7 to 5.2 mEq/L
   3. 8.5 to 10.6 mg/dL
   4. 97 to 107 mEq/L

See Answers on pages 256–259.

Pregnant Clients

- The body exhibits dynamic changes in composition during pregnancy to support a growing fetus.
- Hormonal changes of pregnancy may result in changes of electrolyte balance.
- Body water changes during pregnancy.
  - During pregnancy, the blood volume increases as much as 40% to 50% above the prepregnancy level.
    - Normally, approximately 5 and 6 liters of water are in the body. During pregnancy, this amount can increase to as high as 9 liters.
- Three conditions can cause dehydration and electrolyte disturbances during pregnancy.
  - Morning sickness
    - Affects approximately 50% to 80% of women
    - Symptoms typically begin at 4 to 6 weeks and peak at 9 to 13 weeks of pregnancy.
    - Symptoms: vomiting; nausea; increased sweating; frequent urination
    - Vomiting, increased sweating, and more frequent urination all speed up the loss of water and electrolytes.
    - Nausea may discourage the individual from voluntarily drinking fluids, making it more difficult to replace lost nutrients.
  - Hyperemesis (severe morning sickness)
    - Is a rare condition, affecting approximately 2% of pregnant women
    - Lasts throughout pregnancy
    - Symptoms: vomiting; extreme nausea; inability to keep down nutrients
    - Symptoms cause a rapid loss of fluids and electrolytes.
    - Fever may be associated with the nausea and vomiting, which can increase sweating and amplify the fluid loss.
  - Diarrhea
    - Can be caused by hormonal changes, dietary changes, or sensitivity to certain foods
    - Is more common during the third trimester
    - Results in severe loss of water and electrolytes
    - Is one of the leading causes of dehydration
- Normal electrolyte ranges for the pregnant woman
  - Sodium
    - First trimester: 133 to 148 mEq/L
    - Second trimester: 129 to 148 mEq/L
    - Third trimester: 130 to 148 mEq/L
  - Potassium
    - First trimester: 3.6 to 5 mEq/L
    - Second trimester: 3.3 to 5 mEq/L
    - Third trimester: 3.3 to 5.1 mEq/L

- Calcium
  - First trimester: 8.8 to 10.6 mg/dL
  - Second trimester: 8.2 to 9.0 mg/dL
  - Third trimester: 8.2 to 9.7 mg/dL
- Magnesium
  - First trimester: 1.6 to 2.2 mg/dL
  - Second trimester: 1.5 to 2.2 mg/dL
  - Third trimester: 1.1 to 2.2 mg/dL
- Phosphate
  - First trimester: 3.1 to 4.6 mg/dL
  - Second trimester: 2.5 to 4.6 mg/dL
  - Third trimester: 2.8 to 4.6 mg/dL
- Chloride
  - First trimester: 101 to 105 mEq/L
  - Second trimester: 97 to 109 mEq/L
  - Third trimester: 97 to 109 mEq/L

APPLICATION AND REVIEW

10. Which is the normal serum magnesium range for a pregnant woman during the third trimester?
    1. 2.8 to 4.6 mg/dL
    2. 130 to 148 mEq/L
    3. 3.3 to 5.1 mEq/L
    4. 8.2 to 9.7 mg/dL

See Answer on pages 256–259.

CLIENTS WITH CANCER

- Electrolyte disorders in clients with cancer are common and may be secondary to the cancer or to its therapy.
- Imbalances may become life threatening when they become extreme or rapidly occur.
- Conditions leading to electrolyte imbalance in cancer clients
  - Loss of body fluids: vomiting; diarrhea; sweating; fever
  - Side effects of certain cancer treatments
    - Chemotherapy (cisplatin, carboplatin); can cause sodium and potassium abnormalities
    - Bone protecting drugs (denosumab, brand name Xgeva); can affect calcium and phosphorus levels
- Hyponatremia
  - Hyponatremia is the most common electrolyte disorder seen in clients with cancer; its prevalence ranges from approximately 4% to as high as 47%.
    - Nearly one-half of these patients represent hospital-acquired hyponatremia, which suggests that the management of these clients significantly contributes to the development of this imbalance.
  - Antineoplastic drugs are well known to cause hyponatremia.
    - The mechanism of action for many of these agents may involve the syndrome of inappropriate antidiuretic hormone (SIADH) secretion.
    - Drugs most commonly associated with SIADH secretion: cyclophosphamide (aggressive hydration protocols, associated with cyclophosphamide, are used to prevent hemorrhagic

cystitis, making cyclophosphamide an important contributor to the development of severe hyponatremia); vinblastine; vincristine; cisplatin (can cause SIADH secretion and lead to salt-losing nephropathy, which can exasperate the development of hyponatremia)

- Causes of hyponatremia in clients with cancer
  - SIADH secretion
  - Gastrointestinal (GI) fluid losses attributable to vomiting, diarrhea, enteric fistula, and nasogastric suctioning
  - Third-spacing: the sequestration of fluid from the intravascular space, resulting in ascites and/or anasarca
  - Kidney failure
  - Drugs: diuretics; cisplatin; carboplatin; selective serotonin reuptake inhibitors; nonsteroidal antiinflammatory agents; steroid withdrawal; cyclophosphamide; vinca alkaloids; narcotics; haloperidol; carbamazepine
  - Adrenal insufficiency
  - Liver failure
  - Heart failure (malignant pericardial disease)
  - Central nervous system (CNS) disorders (primary or metastatic disease)
  - Hypothyroidism
  - Primary polydipsia
  - Cerebral salt-wasting syndrome
  - Natriuretic-peptide–induced kidney salt-wasting syndrome
  - Pain and emotional stress
  - Nausea and vomiting
  - Inappropriate intravenous (IV) fluids
- Treatment of hyponatremia in the client with cancer
  - Therapeutic treatment options are the same as for other causes of hyponatremia and rely on the presence of related symptoms, duration, and volume status of the client.
  - Fluid restriction
    - Is approximately 500 mL less than the daily urine output
    - May present a challenge for clients receiving chemotherapy treatment, during which the regimens require hydration protocols; this restriction of fluids may compromise nutrition and quality of life
- SIADH secretion
  - Essential diagnostic criteria for SIADH secretion
    - Decreased serum osmolality: <275 mOsm/kg
    - Urine osmolality: >100 mOsm/kg
    - Clinically euvolemic hyponatremia
    - Urine sodium: >30 mEq/L on a normal daily sodium intake
    - Normal thyroid and adrenal function
    - No recent use of diuretics
  - Supplemental diagnostic criteria for SIADH secretion
    - Plasma uric acid: <4 mg/dL
    - BUN: <10 mg/dL
    - Failure to correct hyponatremia (or worsening hyponatremia) after 1 to 2 L of 0.9% saline
- Hypercalcemia is also a serious electrolyte disorder in clients with cancer.
  - Hypercalcemia is particularly common in conjunction with breast cancer, lung cancer, or multiple myeloma, which often results from the destruction of bone attributable to bone metastasis.

- Signs and symptoms of hypercalcemia: nausea; vomiting; stomach pain; constipation; anorexia; excessive thirst; dry mouth and/or throat; frequent urination; fatigue; lethargy; moodiness; irritability; confusion; extreme muscle weakness; irregular heart beat; coma
- Hypokalemia associated with cancer
  - Is the second most common electrolyte disorder in clients with cancer
  - Is generally multifactorial
  - Medications that cause tubular damage: cisplatin; ifosfamide; amphotericin B; aminoglycoside antibiotics
  - GI and kidney losses of potassium
  - Causes of hypokalemia in the client with cancer
    - Inadequate potassium intake: poor nutrition; anorexia
    - Excessive GI losses: chemotherapy-induced vomiting; diarrhea (chemotherapy-induced, tumor associated, postsurgical resection); kidney losses; diuretics; hypercalcemia; hypomagnesemia; postobstructive diuresis; drugs (amphotericin B, aminoglycosides, cisplatin, ifosfamide, glucocorticoids); intracellular shifts; use of growth factors and vitamin B_{12} therapy

Tumor Lysis Syndrome

- Tumor lysis syndrome (TLS) is defined as the collection of metabolic disturbances that occurs when large numbers of neoplastic cells are rapidly killed during the treatment of cancer.
- TLS leads to the release of intracellular ions and metabolic by-products into the systemic circulation.
- TLS is characterized by the rapid development of hyperkalemia, hyperphosphatemia, hypocalcemia, hyperuricemia, elevated BUN level, and azotemia (and other nitrogen-containing compounds).
- Most commonly arises after the start of initial chemotherapy treatment
- Clients with acute leukemias and high-grade non-Hodgkin lymphomas may experience TLS.
- Cancer cells are killed by therapy, and the contents are then spilled into the body, accumulating more quickly than they can be eliminated and causing metabolic and electrolyte disturbances.
- Signs and symptoms: shortness of breath; nausea; vomiting; lethargy; joint pain and discomfort; irregular heart beat; cloudy urine
- Diagnostic laboratory results indicative of TLS
  - High levels of potassium, uric acid, and phosphorus
  - Low levels of calcium
- Treatment goal is prevention. Minor imbalances can be corrected by changes in diet.
  - Low potassium level: Eat potassium-rich foods.
  - Low sodium level: Restrict water intake.

Electrolyte Imbalance

- Sodium
  - Plays a primary role in the body's fluid balance and also on the functioning of the body muscles and the CNS
  - Normal range: between 135 and 145 mEq/L
  - Hypernatremia: sodium level higher than 145 mEq/L
    - Possible causes: diabetes insipidus; dehydration (fever, vomiting, diarrhea, Cushing syndrome, extensive and/or excessive exercise, prolonged exposure to environmental heat, diaphoresis)

- Signs and symptoms: agitation; restlessness; thirst; edema; dry mucous membranes; confusion; seizure and coma (severe cases)
- Goal of treatment: to correct and manage the underlying causes and dietary sodium restrictions
- Treatment: Provide oral rehydration therapy and IV fluid replacement.
- Complications: Rapid reduction may lead to a rapid flow of water, which can result in cerebral edema, permanent brain damage (central pontine myolysis), and possible death.
- Nursing interventions
  - Restrict sodium intake.
    - Know foods that are high in salt: butter; bacon; canned food; cheese; hot dogs; processed foods; lunch meat; table salt.
  - Maintain client safety. The individual may be confused and/or agitated.
  - Slowly administer hypotonic fluids.
    - Increased risk to brain tissue is due to the shifting fluids back into the cells.
    - Cells are dehydrated with hypernatremia.
  - Prevention: Encourage a low-sodium diet.
- Hyponatremia: sodium level lower than 135 mEq/L
  - Possible causes: SIADH secretion; medications (diuretics, antidepressants); water intoxication; results of disease; thyroid gland disorder; cirrhosis; heart failure; pneumonia; renal failure; cerebral disorders; cancer; severe diarrhea and/or vomiting; diabetes insipidus; Addison disease; hypothyroidism; primary polydipsia
  - Signs and symptoms: confusion; nausea and/or vomiting; muscle weakness; seizures; headaches; low energy level and/or fatigue; restlessness; irritability
  - Goal of treatment: to correct and manage the underlying causes
  - Treatment: Administer diuretic medications and IV sodium Restrict fluids. Hormone replacement therapy may be necessary to treat Addison disease.
  - Complications: If sodium levels drop too rapidly, the individual is at risk of cerebral edema.
  - Nursing interventions: Monitor cardiac, respiratory, neuromuscular, renal, and GI status.
  - Prevention: Treat conditions that may contribute to hyponatremia (adrenal gland insufficiency).
- Potassium
  - Potassium is an abundant intracellular electrolyte.
  - Potassium promotes and facilitates electrical impulses that are responsible for normal functioning of the brain and also for muscular contractions.
  - Normal range: between 3.7 and 5.2 mEq/L
  - Hyperkalemia: potassium level higher than 5.2 mEq/L
    - Possible causes: renal disease; some medications
    - Signs and symptoms: nausea; muscular weakness; fatigue; paralysis; cardiac dysrhythmias (life-threatening)
    - Goal of treatment: to correct and manage the underlying causes
    - Treatment: Provide renal dialysis; initiate dietary restrictions of potassium-containing foods; and administer potassium-lowering medications (kayexalate) to promote GI sodium absorption, which causes potassium secretion.
    - Complications: can be life threatening
    - Nursing interventions:
      - Monitor cardiac, respiratory, neuromuscular, renal, and GI status.
      - Hold or stop any IV or oral potassium supplements.

- Initiate a potassium-restricted diet; foods high in potassium: potatoes; pork; tomatoes; avocados; strawberries; spinach; fish; mushrooms; cantaloupe; carrots; raisins; bananas
  - Prevention: Adjust diet to decrease potassium dietary load, and manage medications that exacerbate hyperkalemia.
- Hypokalemia: potassium level lower than 3.7 mEq/L
  - Possible causes: commonly the result of bodily fluid loss from diarrhea, vomiting, and diaphoresis; medications (diuretics, laxatives); ketoacidosis
  - Signs and symptoms
    - Mild: asymptomatic
    - Moderate or severe: muscular weakness; tingling and/or numbness; muscle spasms; fatigue; dizziness and/or light-headedness; palpitations; constipation; bradycardia; cardiac arrest (severe cases)
  - Goal of treatment: to correct and manage the underlying causes
  - Treatment: Provide supplemental potassium.
  - Complications: cardiac arrest (severe cases)
  - Nursing interventions: Monitor cardiac, respiratory, neuromuscular, renal, and GI status; and check serial potassium levels.
  - Prevention: Promote a diet rich in potassium.
- Calcium
  - Calcium is essential for bone health and other functions.
  - Normal range: between 8.5 and 10.6 mg/dL
  - Hypercalcemia: calcium level higher than 10.6 mg/dL
    - Possible causes: hyperparathyroidism (endocrine disorder); medications (thiazidine diuretics, lithium); certain forms of cancer of the lungs; Paget disease; multiple myeloma; non–weight-bearing activities; elevated levels of calcitriol (can occur with sarcoidosis and tuberculosis)
    - Signs and symptoms: thirst; anorexia; renal stones; parenthesis; urinary frequency; bone pain; confusion; abdominal pain; muscular weakness; depression; fatigue; constipation; nausea and/or vomiting; lethargy
    - Goal of treatment: to correct and manage the underlying causes
    - Treatment: Provide IV fluid hydration, and administer medications (prednisone, diuretics, bisphosphonates). May require dialysis (severe cases).
    - Complications: increased pain level (analgesia administration may be helpful); pathogenic bone fractures (can occur secondary to the bone decalcification)
    - Nursing interventions
      - Magnesium levels are highly associated with calcium levels. It is necessary to correct and treat magnesium levels before calcium levels can be corrected.
      - Keep the client hydrated, which will assist in decreasing the changes of renal stone formation.
      - Assess for flank or abdominal pain and strain to look for stone formation.
      - Monitor cardiac, neuromuscular, renal, and GI status.
    - Prevention: Decrease calcium-rich foods, and assess the intake of calcium-preserving drugs (thiazides, supplements, vitamin D).
  - Hypocalcemia: calcium level lower than 8.5 mg/dL
    - Possible causes: renal disease; inadequate dietary calcium; vitamin D deficiency (essential for the absorption of calcium); low magnesium level; hypoparathyroidism; eating disorders; pancreatitis; medications (anticonvulsants, alendronate, ibandronate bisphosphonates, rifampin, phenytoin, phenobarbital, corticosteroids, plicamycin)

- Signs and symptoms: muscular aches and/or pains; tingling sensation in feet, fingers, tongue, and lips; bronchospasm (leads respiratory problems); seizures; tetany; cardiac arrhythmias (can be life threatening)
- Goal of treatment: to correct and manage the underlying causes
- Treatment: Provide calcium supplements coupled with vitamin D.
- Complications: life-threatening cardiac arrhythmias
- Nursing interventions: Monitor cardiac and respiratory status; ensure client safety (client is at increased risk for bone fractures); initiate seizure precautions; administer calcium with vitamin D supplements after meals or at bedtime with a full glass of water.
- Prevention: Encourage the intake of foods high in calcium (Table 14.1): yogurt; sardines; cheese; spinach; collard greens; tofu; milk; rhubarb
- Magnesium
  - Magnesium plays an essential role in the body's enzyme activities, brain neuron activities, contraction of skeletal muscles, relaxation of respiratory smooth muscles, and in the metabolism of calcium, potassium, and sodium.
  - Normal range: between 1.7 and 2.2 mg/dL
  - Hypermagnesemia: magnesium level higher than 2.2 mg/dL
    - Possible causes: renal failure; diabetic acidosis; dehydration; hyperparathyroidism; Addison disease; excessive and/or prolonged use of magnesium-containing laxatives or antacids
    - Signs and symptoms: nausea and/or vomiting; weakness; cardiac arrhythmias; respiratory disturbances (possible respiratory paralysis); CNS depression; hypotension
    - Goal of treatment: to correct and manage the underlying causes
    - Treatment
      - Cessation of causative agents: magnesium-containing laxatives and renal dialysis
      - Administration of calcium gluconate, calcium chloride, and IV dextrose and insulin

TABLE 14.1	Calcium Content of Several Common Foods	
Food Item	**Serving Size**	**Calcium (mg)**
Plain yogurt, fat free	8 oz	452
American cheese	2 oz	593
Yogurt with fruit (low fat or fat free)	8 oz	383
Milk, low fat, (1%)	8 oz	305
Orange juice, calcium fortified	8 oz	349
Mustard spinach (tendergreen), raw	1 cup	315
Mozzarella cheese, part skim	1.5 oz	304
Ricotta cheese, part skim	½ cup	337
Sardines, canned in oil, drained	3 oz	325
Tofu, raw, regular, prepared with calcium sulfate	½ cup	434

From U.S. Department of Health and Human Services and U.S. Department of Agriculture. (2015). *Dietary guidelines for Americans 2015–2020*. (8th ed.). Available at http://health.gov/dietaryguidelines/2015/guidelines/.

- Complications: abnormal heart rhythms
- Nursing interventions
  - Monitor cardiac, respiratory, neuromuscular, renal, and GI status; watch for echocardiographic (ECG) changes.
  - Ensure client safety (client may be lethargic or drowsy).
- Prevention: Avoid magnesium antacids and laxatives in clients with renal failure, and avoid foods high in magnesium.
- Hypomagnesemia: magnesium level lower than 1.7 mg/dL
  - Possible causes: uncontrolled diabetes; prolonged use of diuretics; hypoparathyroidism; diarrhea; GI disorders (Crohn disease); severe burns; malnutrition; alcoholism; medications (cisplatin, cyclosporine, amphotericin, proton pump inhibitors [PPI], aminoglycoside antimicrobial drugs)
  - Signs and symptoms: muscular weakness; tingling and/or numbness; contusions; muscle spasms; cramps; fatigue; nystagmus (involuntary eye movement that may cause the eye to move rapidly)
  - Goal of treatment: to correct and manage the underlying causes
  - Treatment: Provide pain management, and administer IV fluids and magnesium.
  - Complications: pain and discomfort
  - Nursing interventions
    - Monitor cardiac, respiratory, neuromuscular, renal, and GI status.
    - Assess potassium levels.
      - ○ If potassium level is low, magnesium levels will be hard to increase.
      - ○ Closely monitor magnesium levels; the client can develop magnesium toxicity, causing depression and the loss of deep tendon reflexes
      - ○ Initiate seizure precautions.
  - Prevention: Encourage foods rich in magnesium: avocado; green leafy vegetables; peanut butter; pork; potatoes; oatmeal; nuts; oranges; milk.
- Phosphate
  - Phosphate is necessary for the formation of bone and teeth.
  - Phosphate plays an important role in the body to make protein for growth, maintenance, and repair of cells and tissues.
  - Normal range: between 0.81 and 1.45 molecules per liter
  - Hyperphosphatemia: phosphate level higher than 1.45 molecules per liter
    - Possible causes: severe and/or advanced renal disease; hypothyroidism; diabetic ketoacidosis; rhabdomyolysis (destruction of muscular tissue); systemic infections
    - Signs and symptoms: weakness; muscle spasms and/or cramping; tetany; crystal accumulations in the circulatory system and in the body's tissues (may lead to severe itching and palpable calcifications in the subcutaneous tissue)
    - Goal of treatment: to correct and manage the underlying causes
    - Treatment
      - Restrict dietary foods containing phosphates, such as milk and egg yolks.
      - Phosphate binders, such as lanthanum and sevelamer, make it hard for the body to absorb phosphates.
    - Complications: impaired circulation; cerebrovascular accident; myocardial infarction; atherosclerosis
    - Nursing interventions: Phosphate binders should be taken with or immediately after meals.
    - Prevention: Avoid the use of phosphate medications (laxatives, enema), and restrict foods high in phosphate.

- Hypophosphatemia: phosphate level lower than 0.81 molecules/L
  - Possible causes: severe burns; diarrhea; severe malnutrition; hyperparathyroidism; pronounced alcoholism; lymphoma; leukemia; hepatic failure; genetic predisposition; osteomalacia; prolonged use of certain diuretics; prolonged use of aluminum antacids; long-term use of theophylline
  - Signs and symptoms: respiratory alterations (respiratory alkalosis); irritability; cardiac dysrhythmias; confusion; coma; death
  - Goal of treatment: to correct and manage the underlying causes
  - Treatment: Administer oral and IV potassium phosphate, and increase the intake of foods high in phosphorous, such as milk and eggs.
  - Complications: Assess renal status (BUN, creatinine) before administering phosphorous. If kidneys are not functioning properly, the client will not be able to clear the phosphate.
  - Nursing interventions
    - Monitor cardiac, respiratory, neuromuscular, renal, and GI status.
    - Administer oral phosphorus with a vitamin D supplement. Vitamin D aids in the absorption of phosphate.
    - Initiate client safety (client is at risk of bone fractures).
  - Prevention: Encourage foods high in phosphate and low in calcium: fish; organ meats; nuts; chicken; pork; beef; whole grains.
- Chloride
  - Chloride is an essential part of the digestive juices that are needed to maintain proper balance of body fluids.
  - Normal range: between 97 and 107 mEq/L
  - Hyperchloremia: chloride level higher than 107 mEq/L
    - Possible causes: dehydration; renal disease; diabetes; certain medications (supplemental hormones, some diuretics); vomiting; diarrhea; hyponatremia; hyperparathyroidism
    - Signs and symptoms: pitting edema; extreme thirst; vomiting; diarrhea; dehydration; dyspnea; Kussmaul breathing (deep, labored breathing pattern); tachypnea; hypertension; decreased cognition; coma
    - Goal of treatment: to correct and manage the underlying causes
    - Treatment: Cautiously administer fluids, eliminate problematic medications, and correct any renal disease and hyperglycemia.
    - Complications: Can adversely affect the oxygen transportation in the body
    - Nursing interventions: Fluids must be administered with caution. Too rapid of rehydration may lead to cerebral edema and other complications.
  - Hypochloremia: chloride level lower than 97 mEq/L
    - Possible causes: vomiting; hypoventilation; metabolic alkalosis; respiratory acidosis; cystic fibrosis; hyponatremia; respiratory acidosis; high bicarbonate levels
    - Signs and symptoms: dehydration; muscular spasticity; nausea and/or vomiting; hyponatremia; tetany; muscular weakness and/or twitching; respiratory depression; diaphoresis; elevated temperature
    - Goal of treatment: to correct and manage the underlying causes
    - Treatment: Administer chloride replacements, and possibly administer hydrochloride acid and a carbonic anhydrase inhibitor (acetazolamide).
    - Complications: respiratory arrest; seizures; coma

- Nursing interventions: Monitor cardiac, respiratory, neuromuscular, renal, and GI status; and initiate client safety (the client may have increased agitation or irritability).
- Prevention: Offer foods high in chloride (table salt or sea salt, seaweed, rye, celery, olives, lettuce tomatoes); and use of dietary supplements.

APPLICATION AND REVIEW

11. Which medication is prescribed to lower a high serum potassium level?
    1. Lithium
    2. Kayexalate
    3. Plicamycin
    4. Phenobarbital
12. Which client statement should alert the nurse to further assess a client diagnosed with hypercalcemia?
    1. "I was diagnosed with bipolar disorder 15 years ago."
    2. "I've been on thyroid medication for several years."
    3. "I had a heart transplant last year."
    4. "I'm allergic to bee stings."
13. Which assessment question should the nurse ask a client diagnosed with hypocalcemia?
    1. "When did you begin anticonvulsive therapy?"
    2. "Have you been prescribed an antidiuretic medication?"
    3. "Are you currently on an antidepressant medication?"
    4. "How often do you take an antacid?"
14. Which conditions require regular assessment of a client with elevated serum magnesium levels? *(Select all that apply.)*
    1. Dehydration
    2. Crohn disease
    3. Diabetic alkalosis
    4. Addison disease
    5. Hypoparathyroidism
15. Which conditions require regular assessment of a client with decreased serum magnesium levels? *(Select all that apply.)*
    1. Obesity
    2. Alcoholism
    3. Renal failure
    4. Crohn disease
    5. Third-degree burns
16. Which conditions are the possible causes for a client's serum phosphate level of 1.49 molecules per liter? *(Select all that apply.)*
    1. Septicemia
    2. Hyperthyroidism
    3. Diabetic ketoacidosis
    4. Advanced renal failure
    5. Myocardial infarction
17. Which instructions concerning the timing of administering a medication should a nurse provide to a client for whom the phosphate binder, lanthanum, is prescribed?
    1. At bedtime
    2. Upon rising each morning
    3. On an empty stomach
    4. Immediately after a meal
18. Which intervention should the nurse implement to help minimize the risk of complications associated with a serum phosphorus level of 0.79 molecules per liter?
    1. Keeping the client's environment quiet and dimly lighted
    2. Helping the client make food selections that avoid whole grains
    3. Educating the client of the importance of taking a vitamin D supplement
    4. Suggesting the use of aluminum antacids to manage GI distress

19. An older adult client has a serum chloride level of 109 mEq/L. Which assessment finding is consistent with this result?
    1. +1 pitting edema noted bilaterally on the feet
    2. Serum sodium level of 133 mEq/L
    3. Oral temperature of 100.2° F
    4. Diaphoretic appearance

20. Which intervention should the nurse implement for a client with a serum chloride level of 94 mEq/L?
    1. Falls precautions
    2. Salt restrictive diet
    3. Cardiac monitoring
    4. Respiratory monitoring

See Answers on pages 256–259.

ANSWER KEY: REVIEW QUESTIONS

1. **4 A significant number of older adults (up to 85% over the age of 85 years) drinks less than 1 liter of fluid per day. Recommended fluid intake for this age group is 1500 mL (1.5 liters) a day.**
   1 Recommended fluid intake for this age group is 1500 mL (1.5 liters) a day. Without additional information, the assumption is incorrect. **2** The client's fluid intake demonstrates an understanding of the need for effective hydration. **3** Recommended fluid intake for this age group is 1500 mL (1.5 liters) a day. Without additional information, the assumption is incorrect.
   Client Need: Health Promotion and Maintenance; **Cognitive Level:** Understanding; **Nursing Process:** Assessment

2. **Answers: 2, 4, 5**
   2 Fluid balance relies on a client's ability to consume and use fluids effectively. Fulfillment of the older adult's nutritional needs, including fluids, is affected by numerous factors including chronic disease. **4** Fluid balance relies on a client's ability to consume and use fluids effectively. Fulfillment of the older adult's nutritional needs, including fluids, is affected by numerous factors including long-term eating habits. **5** Fluid balance relies on a client's ability to consume and use fluids effectively. Fulfillment of the older adult's nutritional needs, including fluids, is affected by numerous factors including socialization.
   1 Gender is not a risk factor of ineffective hydration since it does not affect a client's ability to consume and use fluids effectively. **3** History of pregnancies is not a risk factor of ineffective hydration since it does not affect a client's ability to consume and use fluids effectively.
   Client Need: Health Promotion and Maintenance; **Cognitive Level:** Analysis; **Nursing Process:** Assessment

3. **Answers: 1, 2, 3, 5**
   1 Factors that increase the risk for fluid loss include age-related and ineffective kidney function. **2** Factors that increase the risk for fluid loss include the physiological effects of using laxatives. **3** Factors that increase the risk for fluid loss include the physiological effects of diuretic therapy. **5** Thirst in older adults is not proportional to their metabolic needs, resulting in dehydration.
   4 A preference for salty foods is not relevant unless restrictions are otherwise prescribed.
   Client Need: Health Promotion and Maintenance; **Cognitive Level:** Analysis; **Nursing Process:** Assessment

4. **Answers: 1, 2, 4, 5**
   1 Dehydration presents a significant risk for falls. **2** Dehydration presents a significant risk for the development of constipation. **4** Dehydration presents a significant risk for the development of an infection-induced fever. **5** Dehydration presents a significant risk for the development of medication toxicity.
   3 Dehydration is not associated with the need for a low stimulus environment.
   Client Need: Physiological Integrity; **Cognitive Level:** Analysis; **Nursing Process:** Evaluation

5. **3 An initial assessment of the general condition of the skin for turgor, texture, and color will determine the risk for dehydration.**

   1 Cardiac-related clinical signs associated with dehydration might not show up until dehydration is well advanced. 2 Respiratory-related clinical signs associated with dehydration might not show up until dehydration is well advanced. 4 Gastrointestinal-related clinical signs associated with dehydration might not show up until dehydration is well advanced.

   Client Need: Physiological Integrity; **Cognitive Level:** Application; **Nursing Process:** Assessment

6. **1 Although typical signs and symptoms may not always be exhibited in older people, sunken eyeballs are a classic sign of dehydration.**

   2 A ruddy or reddened complexion is associated with an elevated temperature not dehydration. 3 Thrush exhibits white patches on the tongue. 4 Longitudinal furrows on the tongue, not around the mouth, are associated with dehydration.

   Client Need: Physiological Integrity; **Cognitive Level:** Understanding; **Nursing Process:** Assessment

7. **Answer: 1, 2, 3**

   1 A nurse-directed intervention is one over which the nurse has control of the desired outcome. Encouraging the ingestion of fluid in relationship to morning hygiene will allow the nurse to affect the client's fluid consumption directly. 2 A nurse-directed intervention is one over which the nurse has control of the desired outcome. Encouraging the ingestion of fluid in relationship to medication administration will allow the nurse to affect the client's fluid consumption directly. 3 A nurse-directed intervention is one over which the nurse has control of the desired outcome. Assessing the client's favorite beverages will allow the nurse to influence the fluid choices that are provided and will directly affect the client's fluid consumption.

   4 Although assessing the client's thirst drive is appropriate, doing so does not directly affect the client's fluid consumption. 5 Although providing the client with fresh water that is easily accessible is appropriate, doing so does not directly affect the client's fluid consumption since he or she is in control of whether and how much is consumed.

   Client Need: Health Promotion and Maintenance; **Cognitive Level:** Application; **Nursing Process:** Planning

8. **1 Hyponatremia is a sodium level lower than 135 mEq/L in an older adult.**

   2 The normal sodium range for older persons is between 135 and 145 mEq/L. 3 The normal sodium range for older persons is between 135 and 145 mEq/L. 4 Hypernatremia is a sodium level higher than 145 mEq/L in an older adult.

   Client Need: Physiological Integrity; **Cognitive Level:** Comprehension; **Nursing Process:** Assessment

9. **2 Normal serum potassium range for an older person is 3.7 to 5.2 mEq/L.**

   1 Normal serum magnesium range for an older person is 1.7 to 2.2 mg/dL. 3 Normal serum calcium range for an older person is 8.5 to 10.6 mg/dL. 4 Normal serum chloride range for an older person is 97 to 107 mEq/L.

   Client Need: Health Promotion and Maintenance; **Cognitive Level:** Knowing; **Nursing Process:** Assessment

10. **3 Normal serum potassium range for a pregnant woman during the third trimester is 3.3 to 5.1 mEq/L.**

    1 Normal serum phosphate range for a pregnant woman during the third trimester is 2.8 to 4.6 mg/dL. 2 Normal serum sodium range for a pregnant woman during the third trimester is 130 to 148 mEq/L. 4 Normal serum calcium range for a pregnant woman during the third trimester is 8.2 to 9.7 mg/dL.

    Client Need: Health Promotion and Maintenance; **Cognitive Level:** Knowing; **Nursing Process:** Assessment

11. **2 Kayexalate promotes GI sodium absorption, which causes potassium secretion.**

    1 Lithium has the potential to trigger hypercalcemia not treat hyperkalemia. 3 Plicamycin has the potential to trigger hypocalcemia not treat hyperkalemia. 4 Phenobarbital has the potential to trigger hypocalcemia not treat hyperkalemia.

    Client Need: Physiological Integrity; **Cognitive Level:** Understanding; **Integrated Process:** Teaching and Learning

12. **1 Possible causes of hypercalcemia include lithium medication therapy prescribed for the bipolar disorder.**

    2 Hypothyroid medication is not generally associated with causing hypercalcemia. **3** Neither cardiac medications nor antirejection medication therapy is generally associated with causing hypercalcemia. **4** Neither an allergy to bee venom nor the antidote, epinephrine, is generally associated with causing hypercalcemia.

    Client Need: Physiological Integrity; **Cognitive Level:** Analysis; **Nursing Process:** Assessment

13. **1 Anticonvulsive medications can trigger hypocalcemia.**

    2 Antidiuretic medications are not generally associated with causing hypocalcemia. **3** Antidepressant medications are not generally associated with causing hypocalcemia. **4** Antacids are not generally associated with causing hypocalcemia.

    Client Need: Physiological Integrity; **Cognitive Level:** Analysis; **Nursing Process:** Evaluation

14. **Answers: 1, 4**

    1 Possible causes for hypermagnesemia include dehydration. **4** Possible causes for hypermagnesemia include Addison disease.

    2 Crohn disease is not a known cause of hypermagnesemia. **3** Diabetic acidosis, not alkalosis, is a known cause of hypermagnesemia. **5** Hyperparathyroidism, not hypoparathyroidism, is a known cause of hypermagnesemia.

    Client Need: Physiological Integrity; **Cognitive Level:** Application; **Nursing Process:** Planning

15. **Answers: 2, 4, 5**

    2 Alcoholism is a possible cause of hypomagnesemia. **4** Possible causes for hypomagnesemia include Crohn disease. **5** Possible causes for hypermagnesemia include severe burns.

    1 Possible causes for hypomagnesemia include malnutrition, not obesity. **3** Possible causes for hypomagnesemia do not include renal failure.

    Client Need: Physiological Integrity; **Cognitive Level:** Application; **Nursing Process:** Planning

16. **Answers: 1, 3, 4**

    1 Hyperphosphatemia occurs when a phosphate level is higher than 1.45 molecules per liter. Systemic infections, such as septicemia, are triggers for this imbalance. **3** Hyperphosphatemia occurs when a phosphate level is higher than 1.45 molecules per liter . Diabetic ketoacidosis is a trigger for this imbalance. **4** Hyperphosphatemia occurs when a phosphate level is higher than 1.45 molecules per liter. Advanced renal failure is a trigger for this imbalance.

    2 Hyperphosphatemia occurs when a phosphate level is higher than 1.45 molecules per liter. Hypothyroidism is a trigger for this imbalance. **5** A myocardial infarction is a complication not a cause of hyperphosphatemia.

    Client Need: Physiological Integrity; **Cognitive Level:** Analysis; **Nursing Process:** Assessment

17. **4 Lanthanum is used to lower high blood phosphate levels and should be taken with or immediately after meals.**

    1 Phosphate binders, such as lanthanum, should be taken with or immediately after meals, not at bedtime. **2** Phosphate binders, such as lanthanum, should be taken with or immediately after meals, not upon rising each morning. **3** Phosphate binders, such as lanthanum, should be taken with or immediately after meals, not on an empty stomach.

    Client Need: Health Promotion and Maintenance; **Cognitive Level:** Application; **Integrated Process:** Teaching and Learning

18. **3 Hypophosphatemia exists when a phosphate level is lower than 0.81 molecules per liter. This imbalance puts the client at risk for bone fractures. Vitamin D aids in the absorption of phosphate, thus helping to minimize the risk.**

    1 Hypophosphatemia exists when a phosphate level is lower than 0.81 molecules per liter. This imbalance does not suggest the need for a low stimulus environment. **2** Hypophosphatemia exists when a phosphate level is lower than 0.81 molecules per liter. Ingestion of high phosphorus foods is therapeutic;

whole grains are high in phosphate. **4** Hypophosphatemia exists when a phosphate level is lower than 0.81 molecules per liter. This imbalance can be triggered by the effects of prolonged use of aluminum antacids.

Client Need: Physiological Integrity; **Cognitive Level:** Analysis; **Nursing Process:** Implementation

19. **1 Hyperchloremia exists when the chloride level is higher than 107 mEq/L. Pitting edema is a sign of hyperchloremia.**

    2 Hypochloremia exists when the chloride level is lower than 97 mEq/L. Hyponatremia (serum sodium level below 135 mEq/L) is a sign of hypochloremia. **3** Hypochloremia exists when the chloride level is lower than 97 mEq/L. Elevated temperature is a sign of hypochloremia. **4** Hypochloremia exists when the chloride level is lower than 97 mEq/L. Diaphoresis is a sign of hypochloremia.

    Client Need: Physiological Integrity; **Cognitive Level:** Analysis; **Nursing Process:** Evaluation

20. **4 A serum chloride level of 94 mEq/L is consistent with hypochloremia. A possible complication of this imbalance is respiratory arrest.**

    1 Although it may be appropriate for an individual client, falls precautions are not generally associated with hypochloremia interventions. **2** Foods high in salt (chloride) would be prescribed for this client. **3** Although it may be appropriate for an individual client, cardiac monitoring is not generally associated with hypochloremia interventions.

    Client Need: Physiological Integrity; **Cognitive Level:** Analysis; **Nursing Process:** Planning

15 Fluid Balance in Surgery and Trauma

FLUID BALANCE OVERVIEW

Shock

- The cardiovascular system consists of three components that are necessary for the regulation of adequate perfusion of oxygen and nutrients to tissues and vital organs.
- These three components are heart (pump), vascular system, and blood volume.
- Adequate perfusion is dependent on cardiac output, vascular tone, and total circulating blood volume.
- Shock may develop when a disruption occurs in any one of these components.
- The four primary types are cardiogenic shock, distributive shock, hypovolemic shock, and obstructive shock.
- Hypovolemic shock develops when a disruption occurs with the circulating blood volume.

Pathophysiological Characteristics of Shock

- The cardiovascular system is closed (i.e., blood is always enclosed in vessels and in the heart), continuous (i.e., blood is continuously circulating in the body), and is comprised of heart vessels and blood volume.
    - The cardiovascular system is balanced to provide adequate cardiac output for nourishment of the body by carrying essential oxygen and nutrients to every organ, tissue, and cell of the body.
    - The heart pumps the circulating blood volume into the vessels of the vascular system.
    - Shock is a disruption in one or more of three components: signs, symptoms, and effects.
    - In response to a disruption, the body's compensatory mechanisms are set in motion.
        - A cascade of events attempts to maintain cellular function and homeostasis (balance, state of equilibrium), as well as provide adequate perfusion (blood flow to provide nutrients and to remove waste from cells).
            - Perfusion is adequate when supply meets demand and when healthy tissue is maintained.
    - Shock is not caused by one specific event; rather, shock is the result of a combination of signs, symptoms, and effects.
        - Palpated signs: bounding pulse; thready pulse; moisture (fluid around the heart)
        - Auscultated signs: heart sounds; bowel sounds; lung sounds
        - Observed signs: abnormal vital signs; pallor; swelling
        - Symptoms: chills; vertigo (dizziness); nausea
        - Effects (result or outcome of a cause): compensatory changes; organ damage or failure; death
    - If the disruption in perfusion is not alleviated, death will occur.
    - With inadequate delivery of oxygen to tissues, poor perfusion develops, resulting in anaerobic (without oxygen) metabolism.
        - The body uses glucose for energy, resulting in lactic acid production and a decrease in body pH.
            - Normal arterial pH: between 7.35 and 7.45
            - Acidosis: less than 7.35
            - Blood pH less than 6.9: fatal

APPLICATION AND REVIEW

1. Which client is at risk for ineffective oxygen perfusion? *(Select all that apply.)*
   1. 3-month-old infant in cardiogenic shock
   2. 45-year-old with an insufficient ejection fraction
   3. 25-year-old diagnosed with exercise-induced asthma
   4. 62-year-old diagnosed with peripheral vascular disease (PVD)
   5. 15-year-old with severe blood loss attributable to a traumatic amputation
2. Which term is used to describe a state of physiological equilibrium in an individual?
   1. Homeostasis
   2. Perfusion
   3. Wellness
   4. Balance
3. Which physiological outcomes are the result of anaerobic metabolism? *(Select all that apply.)*
   1. Glucose is the primary source of energy.
   2. Arterial pH is between 7.35 and 7.45.
   3. Blood pH is more than 6.9.
   4. Tissue perfusion is poor.
   5. Body pH level is increased.
4. Which blood pressure assessments are most supportive of cardiogenic shock? *(Select all that apply.)*
   1. Systolic blood pressure above 180 mm Hg
   2. Systolic blood pressure below 90 mm Hg
   3. Diastolic blood pressure above 100 mm Hg
   4. Diastolic blood pressure below 60 mm Hg
   5. Diastolic blood pressure that is too low to record

See Answers on pages 276–278.

Types of Shock

- Cardiogenic shock
  - Cardiogenic shock is a disruption in the function of the heart itself.
  - Blood volume is not a contributing factor.
  - The vascular compartment is not a contributing factor.
  - Total body fluid volume remains normal.
  - The force of heart muscle contraction (myocardial contractility) decreases.
    - Decreased contractility causes a decrease in blood volume pumped with each contraction, which affects cardiac output.
      - Increased blood volume filling of the ventricles (primary pumping chambers)
      - Increased ventricular chamber size
      - Low cardiac output over time, causing hypotension (blood pressure lower than 90/60 mm Hg), pulmonary edema (fluid in the air spaces of the lung), decreased gas exchange, hypoxia (lack of oxygen), and respiratory failure
  - Causes of cardiogenic shock
    - Acute myocardial infarction (MI); heart attack
      - Between 5% and 10% of clients who experience an acute MI will develop cardiogenic shock.
      - Even with treatment, 70% of these cases are fatal.
    - Prior MI
    - Heart failure (HF)

- Arrhythmias: irregular or abnormal rhythm
  - Tachycardia: abnormally fast heart rate; greater than 100 beats per minute (bpm)
  - Bradycardia: abnormally slow heart rate; less than 60 bpm
- Aneurysm (weak, bulging area of the ventricular wall)
- Rupture of the septal wall that separates the ventricles
- Cardiomyopathy (enlarged heart muscle)
  - Myocarditis (inflammation of the heart muscle)
  - Heart valve disease
    - Stenosis (abnormal narrowing); valve is not able to open fully
      - Reduces the supply of oxygenated blood to the body
      - Causes: older age; congenital defect; illness; drug use
    - Regurgitation
      - Valve opens fully but does not close tightly.
      - Blood leaks back through the valve after it closes.
      - Reduction in oxygen-rich blood moving through the heart, resulting in fatigue, shortness of breath (SOB), fainting, dizziness, irregular heartbeat, and swelling of the ankles and feet
      - Regurgitation can be life threatening.
    - Complication related to heart valve disease: prolonged cardiac surgery using heart-lung bypass machine
- Distributive shock
  - Disruption of vascular wall tone occurs with distributive shock.
    - Vessel walls lose muscle tone and dilate, becoming more permeable to fluids.
    - Abnormal flow of fluids cross the vessel wall into the tissues.
    - An imbalance exists between the circulating blood volume and the fluid in the tissues.
    - The total body fluid volume is normal.
    - Fluid moves into the tissues and out of the circulating volume, which is known as third-spacing.
  - Heart function is not a contributing factor.
  - Possible causes of distributive shock
    - Septic shock (bacterial infection in the bloodstream)
      - Bacterial toxins are released.
      - The most common cause is gram-negative bacteria.
      - Most frequent source of infections: respiratory system (pneumonia); genitourinary system (urinary tract infections [UTIs])
      - Older adults are particularly susceptible to septic shock.
    - Anaphylaxis, a life-threatening allergic reaction affecting multiple organ systems
    - Dysregulation of vasculature tone
      - Neurologic impairment
      - Neurogenic shock, possibly caused by spinal cord injury, high spinal anesthesia, head trauma, or vasovagal response
    - Drug overdose
    - Severe adrenal gland insufficiency
      - Adrenal glands
        - Are located on top of the kidneys
        - Produce cortisol
        - Helps the body respond to stress
        - Controls blood sugar levels

- ○ Reduces inflammation
- ○ Helps control salt and water balance
- ○ Maintains blood pressure and heart function
  - ▪ Aldosterone
    - ○ Regulates the balance of blood pressure, water retention, salt (conservation of sodium), and potassium secretion
    - ○ Addison disease crisis, causing decreased levels of cortisol and aldosterone
      - ○ Kidneys are not able to maintain salt and water balance.
      - ○ Blood volume decreases.
      - ○ Blood pressure drops.
      - ○ Addison disease can be life threatening.
- Hypovolemic shock
  - Hypovolemic shock is defined as a disruption in the total circulating blood volume.
    - ▪ Decreased blood volume
    - ▪ Decreased oxygen and nutrients supplied to cells
  - Heart function is not a contributing factor.
  - Vascular compartment is not a contributing factor.
  - Blood volume and total body fluid volume are decreased.
  - Hypovolemic shock is the most common type of shock associated with surgery and trauma.
  - Hypovolemic shock is characterized by rapid fluid loss.
  - Effects of hypovolemic shock
    - ▪ Hemorrhage (excessive bleeding)
      - ▪ Trauma
      - ▪ Surgery
      - ▪ Ruptured aortic aneurysm
    - ▪ Deficit in fluid volume
      - ▪ Severe vomiting
        - ○ Inability to adequately hydrate with oral intake
        - ○ Disruption of electrolyte balance
      - ▪ Diarrhea
        - ○ Excessive water loss
      - ▪ Burns
        - ○ Skin is a barrier that regulates the passage of fluids to the outside of the body; when the skin is damaged by burns, fluids have free passage to the outside of the body, which causes a significant water loss.
      - ▪ Sweating
      - ▪ Diabetes insipidus
        - ○ Uncommon disorder
        - ○ Imbalance of water in the body
          - ○ Polyuria (excretion of large amounts of urine)
          - ○ Polydipsia (extreme thirst)
      - ▪ Diabetic ketoacidosis (DKA)
        - ○ Is life threatening
        - ○ Is a complication of diabetes
        - ○ Lacks insulin
          - ○ Cells are not able to access glucose for fuel.
          - ○ Body uses fat instead.

- ○ Ketones are produced, and fatty acids are released into the bloodstream, resulting in metabolic acidosis and/or ketoacidosis
- ○ Polyuria
- ○ Polydipsia (dehydration)
  - ▪ Third-spacing
- Obstructive shock
  - Disruption in cardiac output
    - ▪ Inability of sufficient blood volume entering the heart, attributable to an obstruction outside of the heart
      - ▪ Is an extracardiac condition
      - ▪ Prevents the heart muscle from effectively pumping
      - ▪ Results in inadequate filling
      - ▪ Decreased oxygen delivered to cells
  - Causes of obstructive shock
    - ▪ Pericardial tamponade; defined as a fluid buildup between the heart and the pericardial lining that surrounds the heart
      - ▪ Causes of pericardial tamponade
        - ○ Blood trauma
        - ○ Complication from a medical procedure or surgery
          - ○ Pericardiocentesis procedure: A needle is used to remove fluid from the pericardium (sac around the heart); the fluid is tested for infection, inflammation, cancer, and the presence of blood.
          - ○ Pericardial effusion; defined as fluid around the heart that is caused by an infection or a malignancy
      - ▪ The heart muscle is unable to relax to allow for adequate filling.
    - ▪ Massive pulmonary embolism; defined as a blockage of blood flow to the lungs
      - ▪ Causes of a massive pulmonary embolism
        - ○ Deep vein thrombosis (large blood clot) that forms in the upper or lower extremities and migrates to the lungs
        - ○ Piece of tissue, such as a fat droplet from a large bone fracture
        - ○ Gas bubble (air embolism)
        - ○ Amniotic fluid emboli after childbirth
    - ▪ Tension pneumothorax
      - ▪ Is defined as a collapsed lung caused by pressure from a misplaced collection of air (free air) that accumulates in the pleural space or thoracic cavity
      - ▪ Possible causes
        - ○ Disease process in the lungs
          - ○ Chronic obstructive pulmonary disease (COPD)
          - ○ Cystic fibrosis
          - ○ Pneumonia
        - ○ Trauma (rib fracture)
        - ○ Mechanical ventilation
        - ○ Opening in the pleura (lining around lungs) or chest wall
        - ○ Spontaneous or unknown cause
        - ○ Severe high blood pressure
          - ○ More difficult for the heart to pump against high pressure
  - Total body fluid volume is not a factor for obstructive shock.
  - Blood volume is normal.

- Vascular compartment is not a factor for obstructive shock.
- There is an inability of blood to enter the heart.

APPLICATION AND REVIEW

5. Which assessment findings increase a client's risk of developing cardiogenic shock? *(Select all that apply.)*
   1. Tachypnea
   2. Irregular heartbeat
   3. Heart rate of 58 bpm
   4. Heart rate of 110 bpm
   5. History of MI
6. Which term is used to describe the condition that results in fluid inappropriately collecting in the tissues?
   1. Edema
   2. Permeability
   3. Third-spacing
   4. Hemorrhage
7. Which client is at highest risk for the development of distributive shock, secondary to septic shock?
   1. 30-year-old with a history of type 1 diabetes
   2. 55-year-old 2 days after an MI
   3. 78-year-old with a newly inserted urinary catheter
   4. 12-year-old with a compound fracture of the left humerus
8. Which form of shock is the most direct result of a disruption in cardiac output caused by factors outside of the heart?
   1. Cardiogenic
   2. Obstructive
   3. Distributive
   4. Anaphylactic

See Answers on pages 276–278.

Stages of Shock

- Initial stage
  - Onset: Early signs and symptoms are exhibited.
- Nonprogressive stage
  - Compensatory mechanisms: is able to maintain balance and function
  - Oxygen supply is adequate for tissue perfusion.
- Progressive stage
  - Compensatory mechanisms: is not able to maintain oxygen supply adequately
- Refractory stage
  - Is irreversible
  - Is fatal

Signs and Symptoms of Shock

- There are many different causes of shock.
  - Signs and symptoms related to the initial and nonprogressive stages of shock
    - Compensatory mechanism: is able to maintain oxygenation to vital organs
  - Signs and symptoms related to the progressive and refractory stages of shock
    - Compensatory mechanism: is unable to maintain oxygenation to vital organs
- Signs and symptoms common to all types of shock
  - Altered mental status (AMS)
  - Level of consciousness (LOC)
    - Early stage: restlessness; agitation; anxiety; apprehension

- Progressive stage: confusion; lethargy; unresponsiveness; unconsciousness; coma (inadequate oxygenation to the brain)
- Skin
  - Pallor
  - Moist
  - Cool
- Heart rate
  - Increases in an early attempt to increase perfusion
- Electrocardiographic (ECG) changes
  - Myocardial ischemia: ST segment and T wave
  - Decreased pump function
- Respiratory rate
  - Increases
  - Normal resting respiratory rate: between 12 and 20 breaths per minute
- Respirations become deep in an attempt to increase available oxygen.
- Blood pressure changes
  - Early stage
    - The difference of the orthostatic blood pressure between the lying down position and the sitting position is 10 mm Hg or more.
    - Systolic blood pressure: less than 90 mm Hg
    - Diastolic blood pressure: less than 30 mm Hg below baseline
  - Progressive stage
    - Systolic blood pressure: less than 80 mm Hg
      - Peripheral pulses are weak or absent.
      - Blood is shunted to more vital organs than the skin or subcutaneous muscles.
    - Narrowing pulse pressure
      - Less than a 20 mm Hg difference exists between the systolic blood pressure and the diastolic blood pressure.
    - Changes in the arterial blood gases (ABGs)
      - Respiratory acidosis
        - Decrease in respirations (hypoventilation)
      - Decreased partial pressure of arterial oxygen (PaO_2)
        - Oxygen concentration in the arterial blood
        - Increased carbon dioxide concentration in the blood
        - Decrease in pH to less than 7.35 (acidosis)
    - Oliguria (low urine output)
      - Compensatory mechanism: to maintain enough circulating volume
    - Extreme thirst
      - Compensatory mechanism: in response to fluid volume imbalance
    - Nausea
    - Vomiting
    - Depressed central nervous system; due to hypoxia (lack of oxygen)
    - Decreased function of the gastrointestinal system
- Septic shock signs and symptoms
  - Initial signs and symptoms: fever; shaking; chills; flushed skin; bounding pulse; tachypnea (rapid respirations, greater than 20 respirations per minute)
  - Progressive symptoms:
    - Body temperature below normal (98.6° F [37° C])

- Body loses more heat through rapid respirations than it can absorb or maintain.
  - Weak and thready pulse
  - Skin: pale and cool

Nursing Care of the Client in Shock

- Assessment
  - Early detection of symptoms
  - Early diagnosis is essential for client survival.
  - Obtain a history to determine the cause.
  - Obtain a health history: comorbidities; diagnoses; current medications, including the dates of the last chemotherapy and/or radiation therapy; infections, including recent antibiotic treatments; exposure to others with illness; recent travel; exposure to pets
  - Head-to-toe assessment
    - Cognition: alert and oriented to person, place, and time
    - Demeanor: agitated; anxious; irritable
  - Frequent vital signs
    - Paying close attention: abnormal; trends
    - Temperature
    - Pulse rate
      - Palpate pulse to determine quality.
      - Assess peripheral pulses in all four extremities.
    - Capillary refill
      - Normal: less than 3 seconds
    - Respiratory rate
      - Auscultate respirations for distinction of sounds (crackles, rhonchi, diminished, absent); depth; air movement
      - An individual assessment of all lobes is important.
    - Blood pressure
      - Orthostatic blood pressure if the client is able to sit
      - Pulse pressure
      - Pulse oximetry
        - Determines the peripheral capillary oxygen saturation (SpO_2)
        - Measures oxygen concentration in the blood, including the percentage of red blood cells (RBCs) with oxygen-carrying hemoglobin (Hgb) molecules out of the total number of RBCs
    - Skin
      - Color
        - Bruising
        - Petechiae
      - Skin turgor test: Pinch the skin.
        - Does it snap back into place?
        - Does it sustain a peak?
          - Sign of dehydration
          - Indicates fluid loss
          - The skin turgor test is not a great indicator of dehydration in older adults because of the age-related loss of skin elasticity.
      - Moist or Dry
      - Intact: rashes; lesions; drainage

- Strict intake and output
- Bleeding
- Obvious deformities (broken bones)
- Reassessing and reassessing is very important to challenge the efficacy of treatments.
- Diagnostics
  - Blood chemistry panel including the basic metabolic panel
  - Complete blood count (CBC)
    - Decreased Hgb
      - Oxygen-carrying molecules on the RBCs
    - Decreased hematocrit (Hct):
      - Percentage of RBCs in the total blood volume
      - Low blood volume: ABGs; lactate level; blood glucose
  - Microbiology laboratory values: blood cultures; urine cultures; sputum cultures
  - Radiological tests
    - Chest x-ray (CXR) imaging
    - Computerized axial tomography (CAT); also known as computed tomography (CT)
  - Target diagnostic tests to client history and findings.
  - Invasive monitoring may be indicated.
    - Severe shock
    - No compensatory mechanisms
      - Central venous pressure (CVP) monitoring
        - A peripherally inserted central line in the vena cava near the right atrium measures the amount of blood returning to the heart and the preload for the right ventricle.
      - Arterial line (A-line)
        - Line inserted into an artery
        - Measures blood pressure directly and in real time
        - Easily obtains an ABG sample
- Goals of care: identify and treat the underlying cause; sustain life; maintain vital organ function; maintain homeostasis; alleviate symptoms
- Treatment: The cause of shock will guide treatment.
  - Life-supporting measures: airway, breathing, circulation (ABCs)
  - Focus of treatments
    - Cardiogenic shock
      - Coronary blood flow is improved.
      - Oxygen-rich blood perfuses the heart itself.
      - Workload on the heart is decreased by decreasing the oxygen demand and increasing the intravascular compartment fluid.
    - Distributive shock
      - Identification of the cause is key: infection; allergic reaction; neurological issue.
    - Hypovolemic shock
      - Source of the fluid loss is eliminated.
      - Fluids are replenished.
      - Circulating blood volume is restored.
    - Obstructive shock
      - Cardiac output is restored.
      - The obstruction is identified.
      - The size of the obstruction is either removed or decreased.

- Complications of shock
  - Fluid and electrolyte imbalances
  - Increased antidiuretic hormone (ADH)
    - Produced in the hypothalamus
    - Released by the pituitary gland; prevents diluted urine from being produced
    - Compensatory mechanism
    - Decrease of urinary output
  - Metabolic acidosis (Table 15.1)
    - Inadequate perfusion
    - Anaerobic metabolism
    - Increased lactic acid
  - Hyperkalemia
    - Increased potassium
    - Released from cell injury

TABLE 15.1 Summary of Acid-Base Imbalances

Type	Cause	Compensatory Mechanism
Respiratory acidosis (carbonic acid excess)	Chronic lung disease	Buffer system
	Surgery Airway obstructions Pneumonia	Renal system: excretes more hydrogen
Respiratory alkalosis (carbonic acid deficit)	Increased pulmonary ventilation	Buffer system
	Encephalitis Hypoxia Fever Salicylate poisoning Asthma Anxiety	Renal system: excretes more bicarbonate
Metabolic acidosis (base deficit)	Diabetic ketoacidosis	Buffer system
	Uremic acidosis	Respiratory system: rapid and deep breathing
	Diarrhea	Renal system: excretes more hydrogen; retains more bicarbonate
	Starvation Renal failure	
Metabolic alkalosis (base excess)	Excessive ingestion of base (antacids)	Buffer system
	Vomiting	Respiratory system: slow and shallow breathing
	Gastric suction	Renal system: retains more hydrogen; excretes more bicarbonate
	Excess aldosterone Steroids Diuretics	

From Speakman, E., Weldy, N. J. (2002). *Body fluids and electrolytes: A programmed presentation*, (8th ed.). St. Louis: Mosby.

- Decreased renal function
  - Potassium level: greater than 5.3 mEq/L
    - Muscle cramping: an early sign of hyperkalemia
    - Weakness: a late sign of hyperkalemia
    - Low blood pressure
    - Bradycardia
- Respiratory alkalosis
  - Compensatory mechanism and early complication
    - Reverse of metabolic acidosis
    - pH: greater than 7.45
    - Partial pressure of carbon dioxide ($PaCO_2$): less than 35 mm Hg
      - Tachypnea (hyperventilation)
      - Loss of carbon dioxide
- Respiratory acidosis
  - Respiratory failure
    - Decompensated
      - Late complication
      - Decreased respiratory rate
      - Decreased volume
      - Decreased oxygenation
      - pH: less than 7.35
      - $PaCO_2$: greater than 45 mm Hg
- Increased anion gap
  - Due to metabolic acidosis
  - Accumulation of acid
- Decreased pH
  - Acidosis
  - pH: less than 7.35
- Nursing interventions
  - Early recognition, intervention, and prevention
  - Treat the cause.
  - Focus on symptom management.
    - ALWAYS administer supplemental oxygen.
      - SpO_2 greater than 90% may require endotracheal intubation or mechanical ventilation.
    - Intravenous (IV) access
      - Use a 20-gauge needle or larger.
      - Infusion volume is dependent on the amount of fluid resuscitation indicated.
      - Fluids are infused for volume expansion.
      - Infusion may require a central line, providing IV access into a large vein in the neck, chest, groin, or arm that will allow large amounts of fluid to infuse at a rapid rate.
    - Administer, as ordered, IV fluids; antibiotics and other medications or infusions to correct the underlying problem and to prevent complications.
      - Vasopressors: dopamine; norepinephrine; epinephrine; vasopressin (vasoconstrictors to increase blood pressure); narcotics; sedatives; tranquilizers
      - Blood products to expand circulating blood volume
      - Sodium bicarbonate: reverses acidosis. Do NOT administer.
- Prevention
  - Early detection of shock symptoms

- Identification of risk factors in clients
  - Older adults are more susceptible to shock.
    - Less reserve to compensate when compromised
    - Decreased renal and respiratory function
    - Become more easily dehydrated
    - Tachycardia and hypovolemia may be initially masked in clients with a pacemaker and/or clients who are taking prescribed beta blockers and calcium channel blockers.
      - Heart failure is most common in the older adult population.
      - Increasing oral fluids as a response to thirst may hinder physical and neurological capabilities.
      - Older clients are more susceptible to bacterial infections.
  - Risk factors of cardiogenic shock
    - Heart failure
    - Diabetes
  - Risk factors of distributive shock
    - UTIs
    - Respiratory tract infections
    - Cancer
    - Immunocompromised system (difficulty fighting infections): chemotherapy; chronic use of steroids
    - Cerebrovascular accident (CVA)
    - Trauma
  - Risk factors of obstructive shock
    - Pulmonary hypertension
    - Pulmonary emboli
    - Tension pneumothorax
    - Cardiac tamponade (complication of cardiac surgery)
      - Thoracic tumors

APPLICATION AND REVIEW

9. Which assessment findings are commonly noted early in all types of shock? *(Select all that apply.)*
   1. Decreasing respiratory rate
   2. Orthostatic hypotension
   3. Agitation
   4. Pale skin
   5. Thirst

10. Which assessment data support the diagnosis of early-stage septic shock? *(Select all that apply.)*
    1. Fever
    2. Chills
    3. Flushed skin
    4. Thready pulse
    5. Rapid respirations

11. A client is diagnosed with early-stage septic shock. Which is the priority nursing assessment?
    1. Gradual increase in body temperature
    2. Respirations of 18 breaths per minute
    3. Client report of experiencing chills
    4. Slight body shaking

12. Which nursing intervention is the priority when caring for a client in shock?
    1. Effective head-to-toe assessment
    2. Effective monitoring of cardiac function
    3. Early identification of related symptoms
    4. Treatment of respiratory-related symptoms
13. The nurse assesses the skin turgor of a 30-year-old client experiencing hypovolemic shock. Which question is the most important for the nurse to address in this client?
    1. Does the skin quickly snap back into place?
    2. Are there any noticeable rashes?
    3. Is the skin easily bruised?
    4. Is the skin moist?
14. Which intervention should the nurse implement in a client diagnosed with cardiogenic shock?
    1. Regularly scheduling and monitoring the CBC
    2. Regularly scheduling and monitoring the ABG level
    3. Insertion and regular monitoring of the CVP
    4. Continuous monitoring of blood pressure with an external device
15. Which outcome is critical in the client diagnosed with cardiogenic shock?
    1. Restoration of adequate perfusion of the heart itself
    2. Identification of the causative factor
    3. Restoration of adequate cardiac output
    4. Replenishment of the blood volume
16. Which assessment data suggests that a client is experiencing shock-induced hyperkalemia? *(Select all that apply.)*
    1. Bilateral muscle cramping in the legs
    2. Gradual decrease in blood pressure
    3. Serum potassium level of 5 mEq/L
    4. Gradual decrease in the heart rate
    5. Serum pH level of 7.50
17. Which metabolic imbalance is a result of a compensatory mechanism for shock?
    1. Respiratory alkalosis
    2. Respiratory acidosis
    3. $PaCO_2$ of 49 mm Hg
    4. pH level of 7.43
18. Which nursing interventions are critical for a client in shock? *(Select all that apply.)*
    1. Supplemental oxygen
    2. Pain control with narcotics
    3. Large-vein IV access
    4. Agitation control with tranquilizers and sedatives
    5. Regular monitoring of peripheral capillary oxygen saturation (SpO^2)
19. Which is the purpose of prescribing IV sodium bicarbonate for a client diagnosed with shock?
    1. Reversing acidosis
    2. Expanding fluid volume
    3. Stimulating vasodilation
    4. Constricting the blood vessels

See Answers on pages 276–278.

Surgery

- Preoperative period
  - Maintain fluid and electrolyte balance.
    - Maintain daily requirements.
    - Replace lost fluids and electrolytes.

- Prevent dehydration.
  - Client has not had any hydration by mouth.
  - Replace lost fluids with specific IV fluids at the prescribed rate of infusion.
    - Several considerations affect the IV solution of choice.
      - Individual daily maintenance requirements
      - Current fluid and electrolyte imbalances
      - Clinical status of client
      - Kidney function
      - Comorbidities: diabetes; congestive heart failure (CHF)
- Check requested laboratory reports.
  - Chemistry panel
  - Replace electrolytes as ordered.
- Monitor vital signs.
- Monitor intake and output.
- Obtain client weight preoperatively.
- Importance and purpose of **not** orally administering solid and liquid medications (NPO; *nil per os* [nothing through the mouth]) 8 hours before surgery
  - Client is under the effects of anesthesia and is unable to protect the airway.
  - If vomiting occurs, aspiration, inadequate oxygen exchange (hypoxia), and/or pneumonia may occur.
  - Vomiting is less likely to occur with an empty stomach.
- Prevention of deep vein thrombosis (DVT) and pulmonary embolism (PE)
  - Identify the clients at risk: age; health history; diagnosis; length and type of surgical procedure
  - Initiate measures to prevent DVT
    - Minimize risk
    - Educate the client and family concerning the methods that increase circulation
      - Ankle pumps
      - Foot exercises
      - Frequent repositioning
      - Proper positioning to minimize pressure to bony areas
    - Enhance client outcomes with sequential compression devices (SCDs), if indicated.
    - Provide compression hose to promote blood circulation and venous return.
      - Contraindications include arteriosclerosis, infection (cellulitis), PVD (leg ulcers), and CHF (leg edema [swelling]).
    - Pharmacologic prophylaxis
      - Heparin
      - Enoxaparin
        - Contraindications to enoxaparin include trauma injuries; bleeding; recent surgery; and recent lumbar puncture, spinal anesthesia, or epidural anesthesia
- Operative period
  - Hypovolemic management
    - Anesthesiologist will manage fluids and electrolytes during surgery, based on the client's clinical status.
    - Fluid requirements are determined by many factors.
      - Number of hours the client has been under NPO orders
      - Ongoing maintenance requirements and surgical fluid loss
        - Anticipated extent of fluid loss adjustments
          - The greater the tissue trauma, the higher fluid replacement requirement

- ○ Unanticipated fluid loss adjustments
    - ○ Blood loss
    - ○ Complications
- Postoperative period
  - Shock management
    - ▪ Closely monitor vital signs for a drop in blood pressure, and monitor for early signs and symptoms of shock.
    - ▪ Prevent the progression of shock.
      - ▪ Stop blood loss.
      - ▪ Administer oxygen.
      - ▪ Assist breathing, if necessary.
      - ▪ Administer medications as prescribed to increase blood pressure.
    - ▪ Common causes of shock
      - ▪ Hemorrhage
        - ○ At the surgical site
        - ○ Inadvertent involvement of another organ
        - ○ Fluid replacement
          - ○ IV fluid
          - ○ Blood plasma
          - ○ RBCs
        - ○ Return to the surgical unit to stop the bleeding.
      - ▪ DVT and PE
        - ○ Immobility
        - ○ Trendelenburg positioning (head lower than feet); increases risk for venous stasis
          - ○ Decrease venous return.
          - ○ Decrease carbon dioxide level.
      - ▪ Cardiac issues: MI
      - ▪ Brain injury: hypoxia
      - ▪ Metabolic issues
      - ▪ Anaphylaxis

Trauma

- Trauma may result in different types of shock.
  - Types of injury: blunt force; crush; laceration; fracture; burns
  - Results of injury: pneumothorax; pericardial tamponade; PE; hemorrhage (rapid loss of blood that might result in hypovolemic shock)
- Trauma is the number one cause of hypovolemic shock.
  - Burns
    - ▪ Burns affect all age groups.
    - ▪ Fluid resuscitation is determined by the extent of the total body surface area (TBSA), the degree of burn, and the age and size of client.
    - ▪ Injury is a major cause of death in toddlers.
      - ▪ Burns are ranked as the second most common injury among girls as the cause of death.
      - ▪ Burns are ranked as the third most common injury among boys as the cause of death.
    - ▪ Classifications
      - ▪ First-degree burns
        - ○ Superficial, affecting the epidermis (top layer of skin)
        - ○ Reddened skin

- o Blanches
- o Dry to the touch (sunburn)
  - ▪ Second-degree burns
    - o Partial thickness, affecting the epidermis and dermis (middle layer of skin)
    - o Red with blisters
    - o Serous (clear) drainage
    - o Blanches
  - ▪ Third-degree burns
    - o Full thickness, affecting the epidermis, dermis, and subcutaneous tissue (fatty layer) beneath the skin
    - o Does not blanch
  - ▪ Fourth-degree burns
    - o Full thickness, involving all of the layers of skin, including muscle, fat, bone, and nerve endings
  - ▪ Third- and fourth-degree burns destroy the sweat glands.
    - o Results in dysfunction in body temperature regulation
    - o Major fluid loss results in hypovolemic shock.
- Hypovolemic shock management
  - The goal is to shift fluids into the intravascular space and to replace the fluid volume that has been lost.
  - Isotonic IV solutions are typically used.
    - ▪ 0.9% saline
    - ▪ Lactated Ringer solution
      - ▪ Is most similar to blood serum
      - ▪ Is not compatible with blood transfusion
  - Initial steps
    - ▪ Rapidly replacing the first 1 to 2 liters to restore tissue perfusion and to prevent irreversible progressive shock.
    - ▪ Reassessing after each intervention is essential.
  - Maintenance steps
    - ▪ Continuing fluid replacement at a rapid rate if hypotension persists
    - ▪ Decreasing the infusion rate if clinical signs are improving
      - ▪ Blood pressure
      - ▪ Mean arterial pressure (MAP): between 65 and 70 mm Hg (adequate perfusion)
      - ▪ Urine output
      - ▪ Mental status
      - ▪ Peripheral perfusion
      - ▪ Burn fluid replacement
    - ▪ Follow strict fluid resuscitation protocols.
    - ▪ Early fluid replacement in the first 24 hours after injury is critical to survival.

APPLICATION AND REVIEW

20. The nurse is caring for a client with a third-degree burn. For which situation should the nurse monitor in this client?
    1. Major fluid losses
    2. Risk for infection
    3. Destruction of nerve endings
    4. Loss of subcutaneous fatty tissue

See Answer on page 276–278.

ANSWER KEY: REVIEW QUESTIONS

1. **Answers: 1, 2, 4, 5**

   1 Adequate perfusion is dependent on cardiac output; cardiogenic shock diminishes cardiac output, vascular tone, and total circulating blood volume. **2** Adequate perfusion is dependent on cardiac output; an insufficient ejection fraction diminishes cardiac output. **4** Adequate perfusion is dependent on vascular tone; PVD affects vascular tone. **5** Adequate perfusion is dependent on total circulating blood volume; hemorrhage affects total circulating blood volume.

   3 Asthma affects respiratory function by diminishing oxygen intake, but asthma does not affect perfusion since it does not directly affect the perfusion of tissues and vital organs.
   Client Need: Physiological Integrity; **Cognitive Level:** Analysis; **Nursing Process:** Evaluation

2. **1 Homeostasis is the term used to denote a state of equilibrium in the body.**

   2 Whole perfusion, the delivery of oxygen to tissues, is a part of physiological equilibrium, it is not the term used to denote all the necessary components of this state of health. **3** Wellness is a term used to describe the quality or state of being healthy in body and mind, especially as the result of deliberate effort. **4** In general, the term balance can use used to denote equilibrium, but it is not the term generally used to denote physiological equilibrium in humans.
   Client Need: Health Promotion and Maintenance; **Cognitive Level:** Comprehension; **Integrated Process:** Teaching and Learning

3. **Answers: 1, 2**

   1 Anaerobic metabolism results in the body using glucose as its primary source of energy. **2** Anaerobic metabolism results in the body having a pH between 7.35 and 7.45.

   3 Anaerobic metabolism results in the body having a blood pH less than 6.9. **4** Poor tissue perfusion is the cause, not the outcome, of anaerobic metabolism. **5** Anaerobic metabolism results in the body experiencing a decrease in pH.
   Client Need: Physiological Integrity; **Cognitive Level:** Comprehension; **Integrated Process:** Teaching and Learning

4. **Answers: 2, 4**

   2 Cardiogenetic shock is characterized by a blood pressure reading less than 90/60 mm Hg. **4** Cardiogenetic shock is characterized by a blood pressure reading less than 90/60 mm Hg.

   1 Cardiogenetic shock is characterized by a systolic blood pressure less than 90 mm Hg. **3** Cardiogenetic shock is characterized by a diastolic blood pressure less than 60 mm Hg. **5** Cardiogenetic shock is characterized by a blood pressure reading less than 90/60 mm Hg.
   Client Need: Physiological Integrity; **Cognitive Level:** Comprehension; **Nursing Process:** Assessment

5. **Answers: 2, 3, 4, 5**

   2 Causes of cardiogenic shock include an irregular heartbeat. **3** Causes of cardiogenic shock include bradycardia. **4** Causes of cardiogenic shock include tachycardia. **5** Causes of cardiogenic shock include a history of MI.

   1 Shortness of breath is a potential trigger for cardiogenic shock.
   Client Need: Physiological Integrity; **Cognitive Level:** Application; **Nursing Process:** Evaluation

6. **3 As fluid moves into the tissues out of the circulating volume, a condition known as third-spacing occurs.**

   1 Edema is swelling caused by excess fluid trapped in the body's tissues as a result of insufficient venous return. **2** Permeability is the state or quality of a material or membrane that causes it to allow liquids or gases to pass through it. **4** Hemorrhage is a profuse escape of blood from a ruptured blood vessel.
   Client Need: Physiological Integrity; **Cognitive Level:** Comprehension; **Integrated Process:** Teaching and Learning

7. **3 Septic shock can be the cause of distributive shock; a common cause of septic shock is a UTI with the older adult being particularly susceptible. Urinary catheters are a risk factor for UTI development.**

   1 Hypovolemic shock can result from diabetic ketoacidosis. **2** Cardiogenic shock is a risk associated with an MI. **4** Although a bacterial infection can trigger septic shock, the risk is not as high as that of an older adult diagnosed with a UTI.
   Client Need: Physiological Integrity; **Cognitive Level:** Analysis; **Nursing Process:** Assessment

8. **2 Obstructive shock is the most direct result of a disruption in cardiac output, resulting in an insufficient blood volume entering the heart attributable to an obstruction outside of the heart itself.**
   1 Cardiogenic shock is caused by a disruption in the function of the heart itself. **3** Distributive shock results in an imbalance between circulating blood volume and the fluid in the tissues. **4** Anaphylactic shock is a hyperreaction to an allergen.
   Client Need: Physiological Integrity; **Cognitive Level:** Comprehension; **Integrated Process:** Teaching and Learning

9. **Answers: 2, 3, 4, 5**
   2 Early signs and symptoms common to all types of shock include orthostatic hypotension. **3** Early signs and symptoms common to all types of shock include agitation. **4** Early signs and symptoms common to all types of shock include pallor or pale skin. **5** Early signs and symptoms common to all types of shock include thirst.
   1 Early signs and symptoms common to all types of shock include an increase in respiratory rate to increase available oxygen.
   Client Need: Physiological Integrity; **Cognitive Level:** Application; **Nursing Process:** Assessment

10. **Answers: 1, 2, 3, 5**
    1 Initial signs and symptoms of septic shock include an infection-associated fever. **2** Initial signs and symptoms of septic shock include chills associated with fever. **3** Initial signs and symptoms of septic shock include flush skin associated with fever. **5** Initial signs and symptoms of septic shock include respirations greater than 20 breaths per minute to increase oxygen consumption.
    4 Initial signs and symptoms of septic shock include a bounding pulse to increase circulation.
    Client Need: Physiological Integrity; **Cognitive Level:** Application; **Nursing Process:** Assessment

11. **1 Fever is a characteristic of septic shock. An increase in body temperature would indicate a worsening of the fever.**
    2 Tachypnea of 20 or more breaths per minute is considered rapid and a possible indicator of shock. **3** Chills are associated with fever; the greater concern would be an increase in the chills. **4** Shaking is associated with chills; the greater concern would be an increase in the shaking.
    Client Need: Physiological Integrity; **Cognitive Level:** Analysis; **Nursing Process:** Assessment

12. **3 Early detection of shock symptoms is critical for early diagnosis, which is essential for client survival.**
    1 Although an effective head-to-toe assessment is important to treatment, early detection of shock symptoms is critical for early diagnosis, which is essential for client survival, and allows for effective treatment. **2** Although effective monitoring of cardiac function is important, early detection of shock symptoms is critical for early diagnosis, which is essential for client survival, and allows for effective treatment. **4** Although effective treatment of respiratory-related symptoms is important, early detection of shock symptoms is critical for early diagnosis, which is essential for client survival, and allows for effective treatment.
    Client Need: Physiological Integrity; **Cognitive Level:** Analysis; **Nursing Process:** Implementation

13. **1 Skin turgor is clinically used to determine the extent of dehydration, or fluid loss, in the body. Skin that quickly returns to its normal flat position after pinching is considered to have good turgor; therefore dehydration is unlikely.**
    2 Skin turgor is reflective of hydration; the presence of a rash is not relevant. **3** Skin turgor is reflective of hydration; the presence of bruising is not relevant; rather, a bruise might be related to ineffective blood clotting. **4** Skin turgor is reflective of hydration; the presence of moisture is not relevant; rather, moisture might be a possible sign of a fever.
    Client Need: Physiological Integrity; **Cognitive Level:** Application; **Nursing Process:** Assessment

14. **3 A peripherally inserted central line in the vena cava measures the CVP, the right ventricle preload, and the amount of blood returning to the heart available for circulation.**
    1 CBC provides information regarding the oxygen concentration of the blood, not the function of the heart itself. **2** An ABG test measures the oxygen and carbon dioxide levels in the blood, as well as the

body's acid-base (pH) level, not the function of the heart itself. **4** Although continuous monitoring of the peripheral blood pressure provides some information about heart function, it is not as definitive as the information provided by the inserted central line that measures the CVP.
Client Need: Physiological Integrity; **Cognitive Level:** Analysis; **Nursing Process:** Assessment

15. **1 The focus of treatment for cardiogenic shock is to improve coronary blood flow.**
2 The focus of treatment for distributive shock is to identify the underlying cause. **3** The focus of treatment for obstructive shock is restoring cardiac output. **4** The focus of treatment for hypovolemic shock is restoring circulating blood volume.
Client Need: Physiological Integrity; **Cognitive Level:** Analysis; **Nursing Process:** Evaluation

16. **Answers: 1, 2, 4**
1 An early sign of hyperkalemia is muscle cramping. **2** A gradual decrease of the blood pressure would alert the nurse to possible hypotension. Hypotension is a sign hyperkalemia. **4** A gradual decrease in the heart rate would alert the nurse to possible bradycardia. Bradycardia is a sign hyperkalemia.
3 Hyperkalemia is diagnosed when the serum potassium is greater than 5.3 mEq/L. **5** A serum pH level greater than 7.45 is associated with respiratory alkalosis not hyperkalemia.
Client Need: Physiological Integrity; **Cognitive Level:** Application; **Nursing Process:** Assessment

17. **1 Respiratory alkalosis is an early complication of shock as the body attempts to compensate and regain homeostatic balance.**
2 Respiratory acidosis is a late complication of shock and occurs when the body can no longer compensate for the resulting shock processes. **3** $PaCO_2$ of 49 mm Hg is associated with decompensation-induced respiratory acidosis. **4** A pH level of 7.43 is associated with decompensation-induced respiratory acidosis.
Client Need: Physiological Integrity; **Cognitive Level:** Analysis; **Nursing Process:** Assessment

18. **Answers: 1, 3, 5**
1 Symptom management of shock includes supplemental oxygen administration to support oxygen saturation of 90% or greater. **3** Symptom management of shock includes IV access into a large vein to support fluid resuscitation. **5** Symptom management of shock includes regular SpO_2 monitoring to evaluate the amount of oxygen in the blood.
2 Narcotic administration is contraindicated because of concerns related to respiratory failure. **4** Tranquilizers and sedatives are contraindicated because of concerns related to respiratory failure.
Client Need: Physiological Integrity; **Cognitive Level:** Application; **Nursing Process:** Implementation

19. **1 Sodium bicarbonate is prescribed and administered to facilitate the reversal of acidosis.**
2 Blood products are prescribed and administered to facilitate fluid volume expansion. **3** With a major complication of shock being hypotension, vasodilation would be contraindicated. **4** Vasopressors are prescribed to facilitate vasoconstriction to manage hypotension.
Client Need: Physiological Integrity; **Cognitive Level:** Comprehension; **Integrated Process:** Teaching and Learning

20. **1 A third-degree burn can damage blood vessels and cause major fluid loss. This loss results in a trigger for hypovolemic shock.**
2 Although the risk for infection is increased, this factor would tend to increase the risk for septic shock. **3** The destruction of nerve endings, although a factor in pain, does not contribute to hypovolemic shock. **4** Although loss of fatty tissue causes a dysfunction in temperature regulation, it does not contribute to hypovolemic shock.
Client Need: Physiological Integrity; **Cognitive Level:** Analysis; **Nursing Process:** Assessment

Fluids and Electrolytes in Congestive Heart Failure   16

CONGESTIVE HEART FAILURE OVERVIEW

Heart Failure

- Heart failure (HF) can be caused by any condition that interferes with the ability of the ventricles to fill or pump blood to the body.
- Congestive heart failure (CHF) is also referred to as simply HF.
- Not all HF involves pulmonary congestion; therefore HF is commonly classified as acute versus chronic.
- HF occurs when the heart is unable to pump adequately enough to supply the body's demand for oxygen and nutrients.
- HF is classified as right side, left side, or both.
- Regardless of where the HF originates, eventually the entire pump function of the heart will be affected.
- HF occurs most commonly in adults over the age of 60 years.
- The incidence of HF is greater in men than in women.
- HF is usually a chronic progressive condition.

Causes

- Myocardial infarction (MI)
  - Causes injured cardiac tissue
  - Has decreased ability to contract
  - Has difficulty pumping blood out
- Coronary artery disease (CAD)
  - Plaque buildup in the arteries of the heart (atherosclerosis) (Figure 16.1)
    - Cholesterol
    - Fat
- Heart muscle disease
  - Cardiomyopathy: enlarged heart muscle; becomes "floppy"
    - Has decreased contractility
- Infection
  - Myocarditis: infection of the heart muscle
  - Endocarditis: infection of the lining of the heart chambers and valves
- Heart valve disease
  - Increased workload on the heart in an attempt to pump adequate blood volume
  - Stenosis
    - Is defined as a narrowing
    - Valve is unable to open all of the way.
    - Reduced blood supply is delivered to the body.
    - Causes
      - Related to age
      - Congenital defect (from birth)
      - Acquired: Valves were once normal.

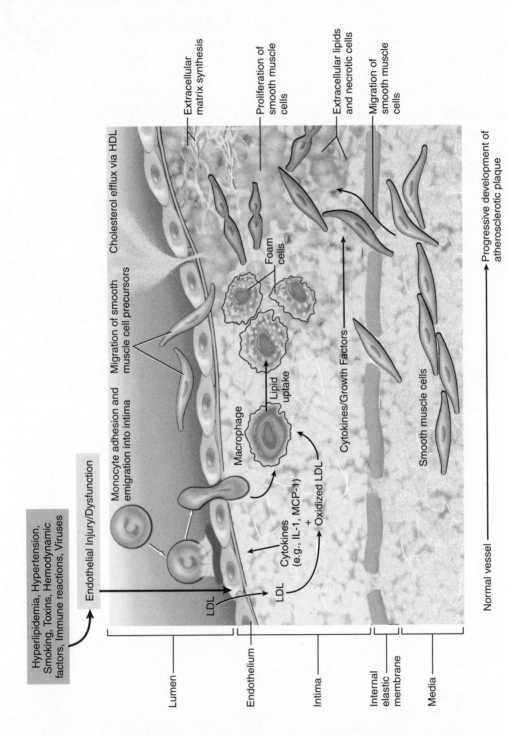

FIGURE 16.1 Sequence of events in atherosclerosis. (From Hovland, A., Jonasson, L., Garred, P., Yndestad, A., Aukrust, P., Lappegård, K. T., Espevik, T., & Mollnes, T. E. [2015]. The complement system and toll-like receptors as integrated players in the pathophysiology of atherosclerosis. *Atherosclerosis, 24*[2], 480–494.)

- ▪ Illness: rheumatic fever; streptococcal bacteria
  - ○ Scarring of the valve
- ▪ Drug use
  - ○ High-risk endocarditis
- • Regurgitation
  - ▪ Valve does not close tight.
    - ▪ Allows blood to leak back through after closing
    - ▪ Reduced oxygenated blood is pumped from the heart, resulting in symptoms that include fatigue, shortness of breath, and fainting
- • Uncontrolled hypertension (HTN)
  - • Is defined as consistent elevation in blood pressure (BP)
  - • Causes the heart to work harder
  - • Will result in the heart muscle becoming stiff and weak
- • Pulmonary HTN
  - • BP is high in the arteries of the lungs.
  - • The heart has to pump harder against pressure.

APPLICATION AND REVIEW

1. HF is caused by any condition that directly interferes with the function of which specific component of the cardiovascular system?
   1. Ventricles
   2. Atria
   3. Arteries
   4. Veins
2. Which risk factors are associated with the development of CHF? *(Select all that apply.)*
   1. Age
   2. Gender
   3. Ethnicity
   4. Occupation
   5. Family history
3. Which conditions dramatically increase the client's risk for CHF as a result of impaired cardiac muscle function? *(Select all that apply.)*
   1. Myocarditis
   2. Cardiomyopathy
   3. Heart valve stenosis
   4. MI
   5. CAD
4. The nurse notes that a client's medical history includes incompetent atrial valve. Which question should the nurse ask the client?
   1. "Are you being treated for a respiratory issue?"
   2. "Were you ever diagnosed with rheumatic fever?"
   3. "How old were you when you developed the valve problem?"
   4. "Do you have a family history of incompetent valve problems?"

See Answers on pages 297–299.

Pathophysiological Characteristics

- • Acute condition versus chronic condition
  - • Acute condition
    - ▪ Sudden onset
    - ▪ No compensatory mechanism

- Presentation may include acute pulmonary edema, low cardiac output, and/or cardiogenic shock.
- A chronic condition may become acute.
  - Dysrhythmias: abnormal heart rhythm
  - Ischemia: heart attack (MI); high altitude
  - Sudden onset of illness
  - Noncompliance with medications
- Chronic condition
  - Is ongoing
  - Is progressive
  - Symptoms are managed with medications, diet, and a reduction in activity levels.
    - Hypervolemic (fluid overload)
    - Sodium retention
    - Water retention
    - Heart chamber remodeling
      - Dilation
      - Hypertrophy of heart muscle wall
- Diastolic dysfunction
  - Defect of ventricular filling
  - Inability of the ventricle(s) to relax, stretch, and/or fill
  - Abnormality during diastole
  - Ejection fraction (EF) maintained at 40% to 50%
- Systolic dysfunction
  - Defect of ventricular ejection with a decreased EF below 40% to 50% (normal EF is 55%)
- Left-sided HF
  - Causes: HTN; CAD; valve disease
  - HF occurs most often in left side first.
  - Enlarged left atrium (upper chamber of the heart) receives blood from the lungs.
  - Enlarged left ventricle (lower chamber of the heart) pumps blood out through the body.
  - Oxygenated blood enters the heart from the lungs.
  - The heart is unable to effectively pump an oxygen-rich supply of blood to the body.
    - Blood backs up into the lungs.
    - Cardiac output is low.
      - Compensatory mechanism: peripheral artery vasoconstriction
        - Systemic vascular resistance (SVR) increases.
          - Creates pulmonary edema (congestion of fluid in the lungs)
        - Weak pulses
        - Cool and pale extremities
        - Cyanosis (bluish color of the skin) with progression, indicating low oxygenation
    - Elevated pulmonary pressures (pulmonary HTN)
      - Is a progressive condition
      - Results in right-sided HF
- Right-sided HF
  - Causes: left-sided HF; MI of the right ventricle; pulmonary embolism (blood clot in the lung); pulmonary HTN
  - Right ventricle
    - Receives deoxygenated blood from the body; the blood returns via veins
    - Pumps blood to the lungs

- Right ventricle does not completely empty.
  - Decreased blood supply is pumped to the lungs.
  - Venous congestion develops, and blood backs up in the veins.
- Compensatory mechanisms
  - Attempt is made to adequately supply perfusion to tissues.
    - Delivery of oxygen and nutrients
  - Heart rate (HR) increases.
    - An attempt is made to improve cardiac output, which works in the short term.
    - With an increase in the HR, ventricular filling time is less.
      - Cardiac output decreases.
  - Sympathetic nervous system is stimulated in response.
    - Contractility (force of contraction) increases.
    - Stroke volume (amount of blood pumped into left ventricle) increases.
    - Arteries constrict.
    - Kidneys retain sodium and water, which increases the blood volume returning to the heart.
    - The myocardium (heart wall muscle) thickens (hypertrophy) in attempt to increase force of contraction.

Diagnostic Factors

- Medical history
  - Presenting symptoms
  - Physical examination
- Echocardiogram (ultrasound of the heart)
  - Assesses the heart function
    - EF, represented by a percentage, measures the amount of blood pumped by the left ventricle with each contraction.
      - HF with a reduced EF is referred to as systolic dysfunction.
      - HF with a normal EF is referred to as diastolic dysfunction.
  - Assesses valvular function, myocardial thickness, and chamber size (ventricular remodeling)
- Electrocardiogram (ECG)
  - An ECG is a recording of the electrical conduction of the heart.
- Chest x-ray (CXR) image
  - A CXR radiographic image is used to diagnose conditions affecting the chest, such as heart size and fluid in the lungs.
- Laboratory tests
  - Serum chemistry panel
  - Cardiac markers
  - Brain natriuretic peptide (BNP)
    - BNP is the hormone that is released when the heart is overworked, over stretched, and/or stressed.
      - The higher the severity of the HF, the higher the BNP.
      - Normal BNP is less than 100 picograms per milliliter (pg/mL).
      - BNP greater than 200 pg/mL is required for HF diagnosis.
    - Liver function tests
    - Thyroid function tests
    - Complete blood cell count
    - Lipid profile

- Kidney function tests
- Urinalysis
- Arterial blood gases (ABGs)
- Exercise stress test to assess heart function with exertion
- Nuclear imaging studies
  - Small amount of a radioactive substance is injected to visualize the heart.
- Cardiac catheterization (also called a coronary angiogram)
  - A thin catheter is introduced into a large vessel in the groin, arm, or neck that then leads into the heart.
  - Diagnostic studies can be performed.

APPLICATION AND REVIEW

5. Which clinical signs serve to support a diagnosis of left-side HF? *(Select all that apply.)*
   1. Weak pulses
   2. Progressive cyanosis
   3. Cool, pale extremities
   4. Respiratory wheezing
   5. EF of 65%

6. Which condition increases the risk of right-sided HF?
   1. HTN
   2. Enlarged left atrium
   3. CAD
   4. Right ventricle MI

7. Which is a common compensatory mechanism observed in clients with right-sided HF?
   1. Increase in respiratory rate
   2. Increase in HR
   3. Atrophy of the heart muscle
   4. Vasodilation of coronary arteries

8. Which information can the nurse expect to find when reviewing the echocardiogram of a client diagnosed with possible HF? *(Select all that apply.)*
   1. EF
   2. Thickness of the heart muscle
   3. Degree of valvular dysfunction
   4. Presence of ventricular remodeling
   5. Status of the electrical conduction system

9. Which diagnostic laboratory test result confirms that the heart is under significant stress?
   1. Lipid profile
   2. Cardiac markers
   3. ABG test
   4. BNP

10. Assessing for possible allergies is especially important when preparing a client for which cardiac-focused diagnostic test?
    1. Stress test
    2. Echocardiogram
    3. Nuclear imaging studies
    4. ECG

See Answers on pages 297–299.

Signs and Symptoms

- Progression of disease is based on the severity of the symptoms and client activity level, resulting in the following symptoms.
  - Left-sided HF signs and symptoms
    - Decreased cardiac output (inadequate systemic circulation)
      - Pulmonary congestion: pulmonary edema; poor gas exchange in lungs; inspiratory and expiratory gurgling; increased pulmonary artery pressures
      - Hypoxia (lack of oxygen)
      - Cyanosis
      - Tachypnea

- Dyspnea (shortness of breath; exertional)
- Orthopnea (shortness of breath while lying flat)
- Persistent cough
- Hemoptysis (blood in sputum, frothy sputum)
- Tachycardia (rapid HR, greater than 100 beats per minute [bpm])
- Extra heart sounds (gallop)
- Fatigue (loss of energy)
- Dizziness
- Confusion
- Oliguria (low urine output)
- Paroxysmal nocturnal dyspnea (waking, sitting upright, needing more air)
- Right-sided HF signs and symptoms
  - Venous stasis (systemic venous congestion)
  - Increased blood volume
    - Edema (swelling in the feet, ankles, legs, abdomen, sacrum [dependent edema])
    - Unexplained weight gain
    - Distended neck veins (jugular vein distention, fluid volume overload)
    - Hepatomegaly (enlarged liver)
    - Liver tenderness
    - Jaundice
    - Ascites
    - Splenomegaly (enlarged spleen)
    - Gastrointestinal symptoms: anorexia (loss of appetite); nausea; vomiting; feeling of fullness
    - HTN (high BP)
    - Elevated CVP
    - Weakness

Goals of Care

- Early identification of the cause
  - Determine the abnormality that is creating ventricular dysfunction.
- Early correction of the cause
  - Reduce workload on the heart by decreasing the venous return.
  - Improve contractility.
- Decrease of symptoms
  - Shortness of breath
  - Fatigue
  - Peripheral edema
  - Increased exercise tolerance
- Compliance with plan of care
- No complications
- Prevent hospital admissions

Treatment

- Goals of treatment are symptom management.
  - Medication management
    - Angiotensin-converting enzyme (ACE) inhibitors
      - Enlarge (dilate) blood vessels, reducing BP

- Angiotensin-receptor blockers (ARBs)
  - Block the action of angiotensin.
  - Enlarge (dilate) blood vessels, reducing BP
- Diuretics (water pill)
  - Decrease total circulating blood volume by decreasing the workload on the heart
  - Act on the kidneys to remove salt and water from the blood; the fluid is then excreted through urination
- Beta blockers
  - Regulate heartbeat (prevent the heart from beating too fast)
  - Improve the force of contraction
- Digoxin
  - Increases the force of contraction
  - Slows electrical conduction in the myocardium, reducing the HR
- Behavioral changes
  - Maintain a healthy weight.
    - Adopt healthy eating habits
    - Eliminate tobacco
    - Limit alcohol consumption
    - Do not use illicit drugs
    - Increase physical activity
- Surgical interventions may be indicated.
  - Coronary artery bypass graft (CABG) to open blocked coronary arteries
  - Heart valve repair or replacement
  - Pacemaker
  - Automated implantable cardioverter defibrillator (AICD) to treat potentially fatal abnormal heart rhythms
  - Heart transplantation (as a last resort and after the failure of other treatments)

APPLICATION AND REVIEW

11. Which nursing interventions are directed at managing the signs and symptoms associated with left-sided HF? *(Select all that apply.)*
    1. Administering supplemental oxygen
    2. Encouraging deep breathing and coughing
    3. Placing the client in a high Fowler position
    4. Grouping interventions to conserve client strength
    5. Elevating the legs and feet to help manage dependent edema
12. Which interventions should the nurse include in the care plan of a client diagnosed with right-sided HF? *(Select all that apply.)*
    1. Assessment of respiratory function to identify the presence of inspiratory gurgling
    2. Monitoring the jugular vein for possible distention
    3. Regular assessment of cognitive function
    4. Monitoring for jaundice
    5. Recording client's weight daily

13. Which statement made by a client being treated for HF should have the greatest positive effect on the client's general health and wellness?
    1. "I sleep using two pillows, and it seems to help my breathing."
    2. "I haven't been sick enough to be hospitalized in 2 years."
    3. "I may not want to, but I follow my health care provider's instructions."
    4. "I elevate my legs and feet whenever I sit down to help minimize the swelling."
14. Which instruction provided by the nurse is an example of necessary behavioral modifications appropriate for a client diagnosed with HF? *(Select all that apply.)*
    1. "It is very important that you stop smoking tobacco products."
    2. "Walking each day is an excellent form of appropriate exercise."
    3. "Here is a weekly menu that will help you plan healthy meals."
    4. "It is important that you learn to meditate to manage stress."
    5. "Weighing yourself weekly will help you recognize any weight gain."

See Answers on pages 297–299.

Complications

- Pleural effusion (increased pressure in the capillaries in the lungs)
  - Causes fluid accumulation between the lung tissue and the lining around the lungs
- Enlarged (dilated) chambers of the heart
- Atrial fibrillation (rapid, irregular heart beat)
  - Risk of the formation of emboli (blood clots, air bubble, or piece of fatty deposit)
- Ventricular dysrhythmias
  - Ventricular tachycardia: greater than 100 bpm
  - Ventricular fibrillation: rapid, ventricle function that is not in sync with atrial function
  - Heart block
- High risk for thrombus formation in the left ventricle
  - Enlarged chamber
  - Decreased cardiac output; risk of stroke
- Hepatomegaly (venous congestion of blood)
  - May lead to cirrhosis
- Kidney injury
  - Decreased cardiac output
  - Inadequate perfusion to organs
- End-stage HF
  - HF becomes nonresponsive to treatments.

Assessment

- Vital signs
  - HR and rhythm
  - Respiratory rate, rhythm, and depth
  - BP
  - Oxygen (O_2) saturation
  - Temperature
- Orientation
  - Client may be confused.
    - Hypoxia

- Anxiety
  - Difficulty getting enough air
- Bloody or frothy sputum with pulmonary edema
- Heart sounds
  - Extra sounds: third heart sound (S_3); fourth heart sound (S_4)
- Neck veins
  - Flat or distended
- Pulses
  - Quality
  - Regularity
- Skin
  - Color
  - Dry or moist
- Edema
  - Nonpitting versus pitting
    - +1 to +4
    - Finger indentations remain after pressing.
  - How far up the legs or the abdomen does the edema go?
- Lung sounds
  - Clear
  - Crackles
  - Audible gurgling
- Abdomen
  - Distention
  - Tenderness
- Energy level
  - compared with reported baseline
- Urine output

Nursing Interventions

- Promote cardiopulmonary function.
- Provide comfort.
- Provide emotional support.
- Count and record calorie intake; encourage sufficient nutritional consumption.
- Provide supplemental oxygen; recommend high Fowler (upright) positioning
- Provide a low sodium diet.
- Strictly and accurately measure intake and output.
- Record daily weights.
- Trend vital signs.
- Monitor heart function; assess response of HR with exertion
- Monitor efficacy of prescribed medications.
  - Diuretics to reduce excess fluid
  - Digitalis to increase cardiac contractility and cardiac output
  - Vasodilators
  - Pay close attention to medication toxicity.
- Identify disease progression.
  - Vital signs
  - Heart sounds

- Lung sounds
- ABGs results
- Laboratory values
- Nutrition consultation
  - Sodium restriction
  - Fluid restriction
  - Sufficient calorie intake
  - High-potassium foods for electrolyte balance
- Palliative consultation, if indicated for chronic or progressive HF
- Restrict activity.
- Educate client and family.

Prevention

- Identify preexisting conditions: impaired renal function; impaired liver function; diseases of the lungs (chronic obstructive pulmonary disease [COPD])
- Identify risk factors: CAD; HTN; diabetes; metabolic syndrome; older age; tobacco use (smoking, chewing); vascular disease; male gender; alcohol and drug abuse; medications that can damage the heart (chemotherapy); arrhythmias; thyroid issues; anemia (low red blood cell [RBC] count; decreased oxygen-carrying capacity)

Calcium (Figure 16.2)

- Normal serum calcium level: between 8.5 and 10 mg/dL
- Calcium is essential for cardiac function.
  - Regulates cell membrane permeability
  - Maintains cell membrane stability
  - Initiates cardiac muscle contraction
  - Assists in nerve impulse transmission
  - Regulates HR and BP
  - Maintains contractility of the heart muscle
- Hypercalcemia related to HF
  - Serum calcium level: greater than 11 mg/dL
  - Causes: hyperparathyroidism; overdose of vitamin D; malignancies (break down of bone); immobility (bone loss)
  - Blocks effects of sodium
    - Decreased excitation of muscles and nerves
  - Cardiac symptoms of hypercalcemia
    - Arrhythmias
      - Most commonly bradycardia (slow HR)
      - Short QT interval
      - Short ST segment
      - Depressed T wave
      - Increase in the force of contraction
      - Heart block
    - Cardiac arrest
  - Goals of treatment
    - Identify cause
    - Increase excretion through urination
    - Decrease reabsorption from bone

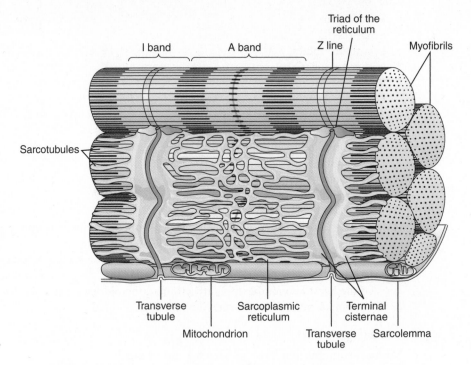

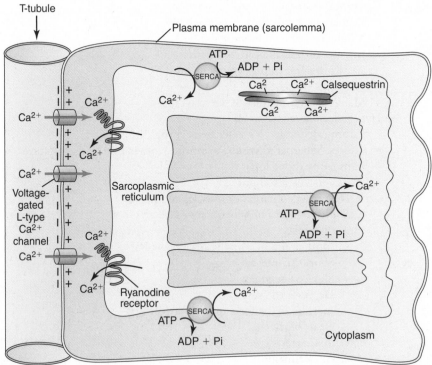

FIGURE 16.2   Calcium Ions. (From Banasik, J. L., & Copstead, L. E. C. [2019]. *Pathophysiology* [6th ed.]. St. Louis: Elsevier.)

- Nursing interventions
  - Review medications that may cause hypercalcemia.
  - Calcium and sodium are excreted together; administer IV fluids with saline; and administer prescribed loop diuretics after saline.
  - Administer calcitonin (synthetic medication) to lower calcium levels and bisphosphonates to reduce bone absorption.
  - Complete hydration to increase renal blood flow (results in increased excretion).
  - Closely monitor vital signs, cardiac monitoring, signs of HF, and signs of pulmonary edema.
  - Increase mobility with weight-bearing exercises.
  - Limit the intake of high calcium foods: dairy; dark green, leafy vegetables; "fortified" juices; canned oysters, sardines, and salmon.
  - Increase oral fluid intake.
- Hypocalcemia related to HF
  - Serum calcium level: greater than 8.5 mg/dL
  - Causes
    - Certain diuretics can lower calcium levels.
    - Inadequate calcium consumption
    - Inadequate absorption
    - Too much phosphorus will bind with calcium.
    - Lack of vitamin D
  - Cardiac symptoms
    - Arrhythmias
      - Heart block
      - Ventricular fibrillation
      - Prolonged QT interval: greater than 0.48 seconds
        - Ventricular tachycardia
          - Rapid ventricular rate (greater than 100 bpm) not in sync with atrial beats
          - Torsades de pointes
    - Palpitations
    - Decreased BP
    - Decreased contractility
  - Goals of treatment: Identify and treat the underlying cause.
  - Nursing interventions
    - Nonacute
      - Asymptomatic
      - Administer prescribed calcium by mouth; administer with vitamin D for better absorption.
      - High calcium diet
    - Acute
      - Emergency
      - Monitor for heart dysrhythmias.
      - Monitor ECG changes.
      - Trend vital signs: decrease in BP
      - IV calcium gluconate: closely monitor the IV site; infiltration into tissues can cause necrosis
      - Monitor the serum calcium level every 4 to 6 hours.
      - Goal: between 7 mg/dL and 8.5 mg/dL

Sodium

- Located in the extracellular fluid (ECF)
- Is the most abundant electrolyte
- Functions: determines ECF volume; regulates water balance; maintains BP
  - Regulates neuromuscular nerve impulses (muscle fibers)
  - Is necessary to initiate heart contraction
- Normal serum sodium levels
  - Adult: between 135 and 145 mEq/L
  - Child: between 138 and 145 mEq/L
  - Infant: between 139 and 146 mEq/L
- Is absorbed in the gastrointestinal tract
- Is excreted in the urine
  - An abnormality in renal function causes a sodium imbalance.
- Hypernatremia related to HF
  - Serum sodium level: greater than 147 mEq/L
    - Water retention
    - Increased BP
  - Causes: high sodium intake; excess water loss (diuretics); dehydration; saline IV fluids
  - Signs and symptoms related to clients with CHF
    - Hypervolemic hypernatremia
      - Retention of sodium, causing oliguria (decreased urine output)
      - HTN
      - Bounding pulses
      - Dyspnea (difficulty breathing)
  - Goal of treatment: treat underlying cause, gradually correcting the fluid imbalance and avoiding complications
  - Nursing interventions
    - Monitor vital signs. BP will increase with fluid volume overload.
    - Strictly monitor, measure, and record fluids (intake and output [I&O])
    - Record daily weights.
    - Assess edema.
      - Nonpitting
      - Pitting
        - 1+ mild pitting: no visible swelling; slight indentation
        - 2+ moderate pitting: indentations quickly disappear
        - 3+ deep pitting: visible swelling; indentations remain for a short period
        - 4+ deeper pitting: excess swelling; indentations remain for a long period
- Hyponatremia related to CHF
  - Serum sodium levels: less than 135 mEq/L
  - Critical low serum sodium levels: less than 110 mEq/L
  - Causes in reference to clients with CHF: excess excretion (diuretics); dilutional effect; volume excess
  - Delayed neuromuscular impulse
  - Signs and symptoms related to CHF: rapid HR; HTN; elevated central venous pressure; distended neck veins
  - Goals of treatment
    - Restore sodium levels.
    - Identify causes: hypovolemic hyponatremia; hypervolemic hyponatremia

- Nursing interventions
  - Strictly monitor, measure, and record fluids (I&O)
  - Record daily weights.
  - Monitor laboratory values.
  - Administer IV fluids if the client is hypovolemic.
  - Increase dietary sodium intake.

Potassium

- Normal serum potassium levels: between 3.5 mEq/L and 5 mEq/L
- Regulates fluid balance in the cells
- Maintains normal cardiac rhythms and contractions
- Abnormal levels can be life threatening.
- Hyperkalemia related to HF
  - Serum potassium level: greater than 5.5 mEq/L
  - Signs and symptoms
    - ECG abnormalities: decreased contractility of the myocardium; peaked T wave; wide QRS; absent P waves; short QT interval; depressed ST segment; prolonged PR interval
    - Bradycardia
    - Hypotension
    - Dysrhythmias: ventricular fibrillation; cardiac arrest
  - Causes
    - Excess intake of potassium
    - Decreased excretion of potassium
    - Medications: angiotensin-converting enzyme (ACE) inhibitors; nonsteriodal antiinflammatory drugs (NSAIDs)
  - Goal of treatment: Restore normal potassium levels.
    - Stop potassium intake.
    - Promote potassium excretion.
      - Administer diuretics.
      - Dialysis may be necessary for renal failure.
  - Nursing interventions
    - Provide a potassium-free diet.
    - Monitor renal function.
    - Educate the client on medications that increase serum potassium levels.
    - Monitor ECG changes and abnormalities.
- Hypokalemia related to HF
  - Serum potassium level: less than 3.5 mEq/L
  - Signs and symptoms
    - Irregular pulse
    - Weak pulse
    - Bradycardia
    - ECG changes: flat T wave; presence of U wave; depressed ST segment; peaked P wave; peripheral vascular diseases (PVCs)
  - Goals of treatment: Restore serum potassium levels, and prevent cardiac arrhythmias.
  - Nursing interventions
    - Provide oral replacement with food high in potassium.
    - Increase potassium intake if the client is taking diuretics.

- NEVER administer potassium IV push (fast).
  - Fatal
  - Replace with 10 to 20 mEq/L over 1 hour. Faster replacement can cause cardiac arrest.

Magnesium

- Magnesium initiates the sodium-potassium pump and affects muscular contractions and irritability.
- Affects potassium levels in the cell
- Is essential for cardiac conduction
- Can be misinterpreted for calcium or potassium imbalance
- Normal serum magnesium level: between 1.3 mEq/L and 2.1 mEq/L
  - 1% serum magnesium is found in the ECF.
  - Serum levels may be normal when intracellular fluid (ICF) levels of magnesium are low.
- Hypermagnesemia in reference to HF
  - Serum magnesium level: greater than 2.1 mEq/L
  - Causes: renal failure; excess ingestion of antacids containing magnesium
  - Signs and symptoms: delayed nerve function; skeletal muscle contraction; muscle weakness; hypotension; bradycardia; respiratory depression; severely elevated serum levels, which can result in a state of deep unconsciousness (coma); cardiac arrest, if left untreated
  - Goal of treatment: Correct the magnesium level; the treatment is based on kidney function.
  - Nursing interventions
    - Administer IV fluids.
      - Promote excretion of magnesium through the kidneys to decrease serum levels.
      - IV calcium may be administered to counteract the effects of magnesium on the myocardium.
    - Monitor serum levels.
    - Monitor ECG abnormalities: prolonged QT; wide QRS complex; atrioventricular (AV) block
    - Monitor cardiac function.
    - Administer diuretics with normal renal function.
    - Dialysis may be indicated with poor renal function.
    - Strictly monitor, measure, and record fluids (I&O)
    - Monitor vital signs for bradycardia and hypotension.
- Hypomagnesemia in reference to HF
  - Serum magnesium level: less than 1.3 mEq/L
  - Calcium and potassium levels may also be decreased.
  - Signs and symptoms: cardiac dysrhythmias (atrial fibrillation; premature ventricular contractions [PVCs])
  - Goal of treatment: Replace lost magnesium.
  - Nursing interventions
    - Oral magnesium replacement
    - IV magnesium replacement; NEVER give magnesium as a bolus; can cause cardiac arrest.
    - Monitor laboratory values.
      - Low magnesium levels exhibit symptoms similar to the signs of low calcium levels.

15. To best maintain normal cardiac rhythm and contractions in an adult, which serum blood level is necessary? *(Select all that apply.)*
    1. Potassium between 3.5 and 5 mEq/L
    2. Calcium between 8.5 and 10 mg/dl
    3. Sodium between 135 and 145 mEq/L
    4. Magnesium between 1.3 and 2.1 mEg/L
    5. Chloride between 95 and 110 mEq/L

16. Which electrocardiographic results suggest a possible depletion of potassium, secondary to HF? *(Select all that apply.)*
    1. Flat T wave
    2. Flat P wave
    3. Depressed ST segment
    4. Absence of a U wave
    5. Presence of PVCs

17. Implementing which focused assessments demonstrates the nurse's understanding of the signs and symptoms associated with a magnesium imbalance secondary to HF? *(Select all that apply.)*
    1. HR
    2. Bowel sounds
    3. Grip strength
    4. BP
    5. Pupil reactions

18. Which statement made by a nurse demonstrates a need for further instruction regarding the administration of magnesium prescribed for a client diagnosed with HF?
    1. "Magnesium can be prescribed both intravenously and orally."
    2. "Magnesium should be rapidly infused to minimize cardiac complications."
    3. "A serum magnesium level of less than 1.3 mEg/L may result in magnesium therapy."
    4. "Magnesium is very important for the normal functioning of cells, nerves, muscles, bones, and the heart."

See Answers on pages 297–299.

Chloride

- Primary functions, along with sodium, include regulating osmotic pressure, which is the pressure necessary to keep water from diffusing through the semipermeable membrane (water balance), and maintaining the electroneutrality in the ECF.
- Anion: negative-charged chloride ion
- Works closely with sodium
- Normal serum chloride levels
  - Newborn: between 98 and 104 mEq/L
  - Infant: between 95 and 110 mEq/L
  - Child: between 101 and 105 mEq/L
  - Adult: between 95 and 110 mEq/L
- Hyperchloremia related to HF
  - Serum chloride level: greater than 110 mEq/L
  - Critical chloride level: greater than 115 mEq/L
  - Commonly occurs with hypernatremia (elevated sodium)
  - Is associated with hypervolemia (fluid overload)
  - Can exacerbate CHF
  - Signs and symptoms: tachypnea (hyperventilation); decreased cardiac output; tachycardia; agitation; HTN; edema; elevated serum chloride level; elevated serum sodium level; metabolic acidosis (low pH); elevated bicarbonate level

- Goals of treatment: Correct the fluid imbalance, increase blood pH, and increase the bicarbonate level.
- Nursing interventions: Administer IV hydration; monitor mental status and respirations; and monitor laboratory values for elevated chloride, elevated sodium, serum acidosis, and low bicarbonate levels.
- Hypochloremia related to HF
  - Serum chloride level: less than 95 mEq/L
  - Critical serum chloride level: less than 80 mEq/L
  - Hypochloremia can be caused by chloride excretion through the gastrointestinal tract, perspiration, and/or kidneys.
  - Conditions that cause low sodium and potassium will also cause low chloride.
  - Conditions that cause altered fluid balance can cause a decrease in the chloride level.
    - CHF
    - Fluid overload
  - Goals of treatment: Treat the underlying cause of hypochloremia, and replace chloride with IV fluids and oral intake.
  - Nursing interventions: Assess laboratory values for low chloride, low sodium, and/or low calcium levels; provide a salty diet with high-sodium chloride foods; discontinue diuretic medications; and closely monitor clients with CHF.

Phosphorous

- Assists with the production of adenosine triphosphate (ATP) for muscle contractions in mitochondria.
- Phosphorus is essential to RBC function.
- Phosphorus requires vitamin D for absorption.
- Normal serum phosphorus level: between 2.7 and 4.5 mg/dL
- Hyperphosphatemia related to HF
  - Serum phosphorus level: greater than 4.5 mg/dL
  - Excess phosphorus is deposited in the joints, arteries, skin, kidneys, and corneas.
  - Signs and symptoms in reference to HF
    - Phosphorus and calcium relationship: they react opposite to each other.
    - High phosphate equals low calcium, which causes neuromuscular irritability, tachycardia, dysrhythmias, and conduction issues.
  - Goals of treatment: Identify the cause, and restore both the phosphorus level and the calcium level.
  - Nursing interventions: Provide a phosphate-restricted diet (dairy free, egg yolk, meat, nuts); increase fluids; monitor cardiac status; and assess serum calcium and phosphate levels.
- Hypophosphatemia related to HF
  - Serum phosphorus level: less than 2 mg/dL
  - Critical serum phosphorus level: less than 1 mg/dL
  - Low phosphorus equals high calcium, which causes a disruption in the transport of oxygen by the RBCs and decreased contractility of the heart, resulting in decreased cardiac output and decreased BP.
  - Goal of treatment: Replenish the phosphorus level.
  - Nursing interventions: Provide a high phosphorus diet; treat with oral phosphorus supplements; initiate an IV infusion with phosphate supplements; monitor the calcium drop with the increased phosphorus for dysrhythmias; monitor cardiac function.

APPLICATION AND REVIEW

19. Which diagnostic laboratory result supports the resolution of a phosphorous imbalance related to HF?
    1. 0.7 mg/dL
    2. 3.1 mg/dL
    3. 4.8 mg/dL
    4. 8.1 mg/dL
20. A client has hyperphosphatemia secondary to HF. Which diagnostic laboratory value reflects the client's condition?
    1. Serum calcium level of 7.9 mg/dL
    2. Serum chloride level of 85 mEq/L
    3. Serum potassium level of 5.8 mEg/L
    4. Serum magnesium level of 2.9 mEq/L

See Answers on pages 297–299.

ANSWER KEY: REVIEW QUESTIONS

1. **1 HF can be caused by any condition that interferes directly with the ability of the ventricles to fill or pump blood to the body.**
   2 Although HF indirectly affects the function of the atria, it can be caused by any condition that interferes with the ability of the ventricles to fill or pump blood to the body. 3 Although HF indirectly affects the function of the arteries, it can be caused by any condition that interferes with the ability of the ventricles to fill or pump blood to the body. 4 Although HF indirectly affects the function of the veins, it can be caused by any condition that interferes with the ability of the ventricles to fill or pump blood to the body.
   Client Need: Physiological Integrity; **Cognitive Level:** Comprehension; **Integrated Process:** Teaching and Learning

2. **Answers: 1, 2**
   1 CHF is associated with age 60 years and older. 2 CHF is associated with the male gender.
   3 CHF is not associated with any specific ethnicity. 4 CHF is not associated with any specific occupation. 5 CHF is not associated with a family history of the disorder.
   Client Need: Health Promotion and Maintenance; **Cognitive Level:** Knowledge; **Integrated Process:** Teaching and Learning

3. **Answers: 1, 2, 4**
   1 Myocarditis involves an infection of the heart muscle, which results in impaired contractibility. 2 Cardiomyopathy is the enlargement of the heart muscle, which results in impaired contractibility. 4 MI causes injured cardiac tissue, which results in the decreased ability of the heart muscle to contract.
   3 Stenosis causes the narrowing of the valves, which result in reducing the blood supply. 5 CAD involves the buildup of plaque in the arteries of the heart, which affects blood supply.
   Client Need: Physiological Integrity; **Cognitive Level:** Analysis; **Integrated Process:** Teaching and Learning

4. **2 Rheumatic fever is a trigger for the development of valve scarring and the resulting valve stenosis.**
   1 Respiratory issues are not directly associated with valve incompetency and its resulting signs and symptoms. 3 Although an appropriate assessment question, the age when the diagnosis was made is not as relevant as a possible cause. 4 Although an appropriate assessment question, family history is not as relevant as a possible cause.
   Client Need: Health Promotion and Maintenance; **Cognitive Level:** Analysis; **Nursing Process:** Assessment

5. **Answers: 1, 2, 3, 4**
   1 Weak pulses are a clinical sign of left-sided HF. 2 Progressive cyanosis is a clinical sign of left-sided HF. 3 Cool, pale extremities are a clinical sign of left-sided HF. 4 Respiratory congestion resulting in wheezing is a clinical sign of left-sided HF.
   5 A 65% EF is within normal limits; left-sided HF results in an EF below normal (55% to 70%).
   Client Need: Physiological Integrity; **Cognitive Level:** Application; **Nursing Process:** Assessment

6. **4 Possible causes of right-sided HF include a right ventricle MI.**
   1 HTN is a known cause of left-sided HF. 2 An enlarged left atrium is a known cause of left-sided HF. 3 CAD is a known cause of left-sided HF.
   Client Need: Physiological Integrity; **Cognitive Level:** Comprehension; **Integrated Process:** Teaching and Learning

7. **2 An increased HR improves cardiac output.**

   1 Alteration of respiratory rate is not a common compensatory mechanism for right-sided HF. **3** Hypertrophy, not atrophy, of the myocardium is a common compensatory mechanism for right-sided HF. **4** Vasoconstriction of the coronary arteries is a common compensatory mechanism for left-sided HF.
   Client Need: Physiology Integrity; **Cognitive Level:** Comprehension; **Integrated Process:** Teaching and Learning

8. **Answers: 1, 2, 3, 4**

   1 An echocardiogram is an ultrasound image of the heart that assesses various aspects of heart function, including the EF. **2** An echocardiogram is an ultrasound image of the heart that assesses various aspects of heart function, including myocardial thickness. **3** An echocardiogram is an ultrasound image of the heart that assesses various aspects of heart function, including valvular function. **4** An echocardiogram is an ultrasound image of the heart that assessed various aspects of heart function, including alterations in chamber size attributable to remodeling.
   5 An ECG assesses the conduction system of the heart.
   Client Need: Health Promotion and Maintenance; **Cognitive Level:** Application; **Nursing Process:** Assessment

9. **4 BNP is a hormone that is released when the heart is overworked, overstretched, or in some fashion stressed.**

   1 Lipid profile identifies levels of cholesterol and triglycerides in the blood. **2** Cardiac markers are biomarkers measured to evaluate heart function. **3** An ABG is a blood test that measures the acidity, or pH level, and the levels of oxygen (O_2) and carbon dioxide (CO_2) from an artery.
   Client Need: Health Promotion and Maintenance; **Cognitive Level:** Comprehension; **Integrated Process:** Teaching and Learning

10. **3 Nuclear imaging studies use small amounts of radioactive material (dye) to diagnose and determine the severity of or treat a variety of diseases, including many types of heart disease. Clients can be allergic to the dye; therefore assessment for allergies is vital.**

    1 A stress test assesses heart function when under physical stress; it does not require the injection of a dye. **2** Echocardiogram is an ultrasound test; it does not require the injection of a dye. **4** An ECG assesses the electrical conduction system of the heart; it does not require the injection of a dye.
    Client Need: Health Promotion and Maintenance; **Cognitive Level:** Application; **Nursing Process:** Assessment

11. **Answers: 1, 2, 3, 4**

    1 Left-sided HF results in decreased cardiac output, which causes hypoxia and the resulting lack of oxygen. **2** Left-sided HF results in decreased cardiac output, which causes pulmonary congestion and the resulting cough and shortness of breath. **3** Left-sided HF results in decreased cardiac output, which causes hypoxia and the resulting dyspnea that is lessened with upright sitting positions. **4** Left-sided HF results in decreased cardiac output, which causes hypoxia and the resulting fatigue; energy is conserved by grouping care interventions.
    5 Right-sided HF is associated with increased blood volume that results in edema.
    Client Need: Health Promotion and Maintenance; **Cognitive Level:** Application; **Nursing Process:** Implementation

12. **Answers: 2, 4, 5**

    2 Right-sided HF results in a distention of the jugular vein, requiring regular monitoring. **4** Right-sided HF results in the development of jaundice, requiring regular monitoring. **5** Right-sided HF results in edema and the resulting unexplained weight gain.
    1 Left-sided HF results in pulmonary congestion and the resulting inspiratory and expiratory gurgling. **3** Left-sided HF results in confusion.
    Client Need: Health Promotion and Maintenance; **Cognitive Level:** Analysis; **Nursing Process:** Planning

13. **3 Adherence to the plan of care will have the greatest overall positive effect on the health of a client diagnosed with HF.**

    1 Sleeping while elevated on pillows will help with orthopnea, but it has no effect on the other signs and symptoms of HF. **2** Minimizing hospitalizations is certainly a positive outcome, but it is a goal that will be increasingly more difficult to achieve without adherence to the plan of care. **4** Elevating the legs and feet will help manage edema, but it will have no effect on the other signs and symptoms of HF.

Client Need: Health Promotion and Maintenance; **Cognitive Level:** Analysis; **Nursing Process:** Evaluation

14. **Answers: 1, 2, 3, 5**

    1 Behavioral changes appropriate for HF management include eliminating tobacco use because of its vasoconstriction properties. **2** Walking is an excellent form of cardio-friendly exercise. **3** Healthy eating is especially important to the management of fats, sugars, and carbohydrates. **5** Being aware of changes in weight is important in weight management.

    4 Although stress management is suggested, there are a variety of methods from which a client can choose in addition to meditation.

    Client Need: Health Promotion and Maintenance; **Cognitive Level:** Analysis; **Nursing Process:** Implementation

15. **1 Potassium is vital in maintaining normal cardiac rhythms and contractions.**

    2 Calcium initiates cardiac muscle contractions. **3** Sodium is necessary to initiate heart contractions. **4** Magnesium affects muscular contractions and irritability. **5** Chloride is associated with maintaining effective osmotic pressure to keep effective semipermeable in the blood vessels.

    Client Need: Health Promotion and Maintenance; **Cognitive Level:** Analysis; **Integrated Process:** Teaching and Learning

16. **Answers: 1, 3, 5**

    1 Electrocardiographic changes associated with hypokalemia include a flat T wave. **3** Electrocardiographic changes associated with hypokalemia include a depressed ST segment. **5** PVCs are associated with hypokalemia.

    2 Electrocardiographic changes associated with hypokalemia include a peaked P wave. **4** Electrocardiographic changes associated with hypokalemia include the presence of a U wave.

    Client Need: Physiological Integrity; **Cognitive Level:** Application; **Integrated Process:** Assessment

17. **Answers: 1, 3, 4**

    1 Hypermagnesemia is associated with bradycardia. **3** Hypermagnesemia is associated with muscle weakness. **4** Hypermagnesemia is associated with hypotension.

    2 Bowel sounds are not significantly altered by a magnesium imbalance. **5** Pupil reactions are not significantly altered by a magnesium imbalance.

    Client Need: Health Promotion and Maintenance; **Cognitive Level:** Analysis; **Nursing Process:** Evaluation

18. **2 IV magnesium replacement should NEVER be rapidly administered or in the form of a bolus; doing so can cause cardiac arrest.**

    1 Magnesium may be prescribed both orally and intravenously. **3** Serum magnesium levels less than 1.3 mEg/L indicate a deficit in magnesium that may require supplement therapy. **4** Magnesium is vital to the normal functioning of cells, nerves, muscles, bones, and the heart.

    Client Need: Health Promotion and Maintenance; **Cognitive Level:** Analysis; **Nursing Process:** Evaluation

19. **2 Normal serum phosphorus levels range between 2.7 and 4.5 mg/dL and would indicate the resolution of a phosphorus imbalance.**

    1 Normal serum phosphorus levels range between 2.7 and 4.5 mg/dL; 0.7 mg/dL reflects hypophosphatemia. **3** Normal serum phosphorus levels range between 2.7 and 4.5 mg/dL; 4.8 mg/dL would indicate hyperphosphatemia. **4** Normal serum phosphorus levels range between 2.7 and 4.5 mg/dL; 8.1 mg/dL would indicate hyperphosphatemia.

    Client Need: Health Promotion and Maintenance; **Cognitive Level:** Application; **Nursing Process:** Evaluation

20. **1 Phosphorus and calcium react opposite to each other; high phosphate equals low calcium; hypocalcemia is in response to hyperphosphatemia.**

    2 Hypochloremia related to HF has serum chloride levels less than 95 mEq/L, but chloride and phosphate do not react opposite to each other. **3** Hyperkalemia related to HF has serum potassium levels greater than 5.5 mEq/L, but potassium and phosphate do not react opposite of each other. **4** Hypermagnesemia related to HF has serum magnesium levels greater than 2.1 mEq/L, but magnesium and phosphate do not react opposite of each other.

    Client Need: Health Promotion and Maintenance; **Cognitive Level:** Analysis; **Nursing Process:** Assessment

17 Fluids and Electrolytes in Renal Failure

RENAL FAILURE OVERVIEW

Fluids and Electrolytes

- Renal refers to the kidneys.
- The kidneys are complex organs with multiple functions responsible for maintaining homeostasis.
  - Removal of wastes by the formation of urine
  - Maintenance of fluid and electrolyte imbalance
  - Acid-base balance
  - Blood pressure control
  - Bone formation
  - Red blood cell (RBC) production
- Renal dysfunction or failure results when one or more of these functions is disrupted, causing an imbalance in homeostasis of the body.
- Renal failure is classified as either acute or chronic.
- Kidneys are made up of approximately 1 million nephrons per kidney.
- Nephrons are the functional units that are able to perform all functions of the kidney individually.
- Thousands of nephrons can be damaged or destroyed before kidney function is affected.
- Older adults are at higher risk for kidney failure as kidney function declines with age.

Renal Failure Pathophysiological Factors

- Acute kidney injury (AKI)
  - Mild-to-severe impairment
  - Rapid deterioration in kidney function
  - Rapid decrease in glomerular filtration rate (GFR)
  - Elevated serum creatinine levels: product of muscle metabolism; normally completely excreted by kidneys; decrease in GFR
  - Decreased urine output (oliguria)
  - Azotemia
    - Elevated blood urea nitrogen (BUN)
    - Waste products (BUN, creatinine) accumulated in the blood
    - Leads to electrolyte imbalance, acid-base imbalance, and a disruption in fluid volume balance
  - May be potentially reversible
  - Has a high mortality rate
  - Often develops with other life-threatening conditions
    - Respiratory failure
    - Heart failure
    - Shock
    - Sepsis
    - Severe and/or prolonged hypotension
    - Hypovolemia (low circulatory volume), resulting in dehydration and low cardiac output

- Exposure to toxic substances (nephrotoxic) to the kidneys
  - Medications: antibiotics; nonsteroidal antiinflammatory drugs (NSAIDs); angiotensin-converting enzyme (ACE) inhibitors, which decrease perfusion pressure and may cause hyperkalemia
  - Intravenous (IV) contrast dye for imaging
  - Illicit drug use
- Three categories of AKI
  - Prerenal (before)
    - External factors affect the kidneys.
      - Reduced blood flow to the kidneys, resulting in decreased glomerular perfusion and decreased GFR (azotemia, oliguria)
    - Kidney tissue (parenchyma) is not damaged.
    - Prerenal AKI is reversible if treated in a timely manner.
    - Intrarenal disease may occur if not treated.
      - Prolonged hypotension: sepsis; vasodilation
      - Prolonged decreased cardiac output: heart failure; cardiogenic shock
      - Prolonged hypovolemia: rapid blood loss; dehydration
      - Vascular obstruction: renal thrombus
  - Intrarenal (intrinsic, within)
    - Tissue of the kidney is directly damaged, affecting nephron function
    - Causes
      - Prolonged ischemia (lack of oxygen)
      - Progression of prerenal AKI
      - Nephrotoxins
      - Muscle cell necrosis
        - Release of myoglobin, the by-product of muscle breakdown
        - Rhabdomyolysis: tissue destruction; rapid release of myoglobin
      - RBC hemolysis
        - Release of hemoglobin, the protein that carries oxygen and carbon dioxide
      - Primary renal diseases: infection (most common cause of intrarenal AKI); systemic lupus erythematosus; acute tubular necrosis
  - Postrenal (after)
    - Postrenal AKI is due to a mechanical obstruction of the urinary flow.
      - Urethra
      - Prostate
      - Bladder
        - Urinary reflux (urine flows back into the renal pelvis, resulting in decreased renal function)
    - Causes: benign prostatic hyperplasia (BPH); prostate cancer; urinary stones (calculi); trauma; extrarenal tumors; obstruction of the ureters (tubes connecting the kidneys to the bladder), resulting in hydronephrosis (dilation of the kidney); increased hydrostatic pressure
    - Kidneys may fully recover if obstruction is treated within 48 hours.
    - Phases of AKI progression
      - Oliguric AKI (low urine output)
        - Urine output less than 400 mL/day
        - Occurs 1 to 7 days after kidney injury
        - Ischemia causes oliguria to develop within 24 hours

- Has a nephrotoxic effect
- May be delayed for up to 1 week
- Lasts 14 days to months
- The longer the duration, the poorer the prognosis
- Nonoliguric AKI
  - Harder to diagnose
  - Urine output greater than 400 mL/day
  - Use of diuretics: urine output up to 5 L/day with large loss of fluids and electrolytes, requiring monitoring for hyponatremia, hypokalemia, and dehydration
  - Kidneys have recovered to excrete waste but are not yet concentrating urine, a condition that may last 1 to 3 weeks.
  - Recovery may take up to 12 months for full recovery: GFR increases; BUN decreases; serum creatinine level decreases.
- Kidney dysfunction may become permanent.
  - Chronic kidney disease (CKD)
  - End-stage renal disease (ESRD)
- Infection is the most common cause of death in AKI.
  - Types of infection
  - Sepsis
    - Infection enters the bloodstream.
    - Cascade of events causes multisystem complications: hypoxemia; hypotension; decreased perfusion
  - Pyelonephritis (Table 17.1): bacterial kidney infection
  - Glomerulonephritis: inflammation of the glomeruli
    - Glomeruli are clusters of capillaries in the kidneys that filter the blood.
  - Interstitial nephritis: inflammation between renal tubules
  - Prostatitis: inflammation of the prostate
  - Cystitis: bladder infection

TABLE 17.1 Common Causes of Pyelonephritis

Predisposing Factor	Pathologic Mechanisms
Kidney stones	Obstruction and stasis of urine, contributing to bacteriuria and hydronephrosis; irritation of epithelial lining with entrapment of bacteria
Vesicoureteral reflux	Chronic reflux of urine up the ureter and into the kidneys during micturition, contributing to a bacterial infection
Pregnancy	Dilation and relaxation of the ureter with hydroureter and hydronephrosis; partly caused by an obstruction from an enlarged uterus and partly from ureteral relaxation caused by higher progesterone levels
Neurogenic bladder	Neurological impairment interfering with normal bladder contraction with residual urine and ascending infection
Instrumentation	Introduction of organisms into the urethra and bladder by catheters and endoscopes introduced into the urinary tract for diagnostic purposes
Female sexual trauma	Movement of organisms from the urethra into the bladder with infection and retrograde spread to the kidneys

From Huether, S. E., McCance, K. L., Brashers, V. L., & Rote, S. R. (2017). *Understanding pathophysiology* (6th ed.). St. Louis: Elsevier.

- Causes of infection
  - Any condition that blocks the flow of urine out of the body
  - Any condition that does not allow the bladder to empty completely, which increases risk of bacteria entering the urinary system
  - *Escherichia coli (E. coli)* is the most common bacteria.
  - Catheter insertion into the urethra to drain the bladder may be a conduit for introducing bacteria.
  - Signs and symptoms of a urinary tract infection (UTI): pelvic pain; abdominal pain; flank pain; burning with urination; cloudy urine; sediment in urine; blood in urine; purulent drainage mixed with urine; strong odor; swelling; vomiting; fever; hypertension
- Chronic kidney disease (CKD)
  - CKD is progressive and irreversible.
  - That causes damage to kidney tissue and decreases GFR.
  - CKD stages
    - Stage 1: minimal loss of kidney function; estimated GFR greater than 90
    - Stage 2: mild-to-moderate loss of kidney function; estimated GFR between 60 and 89
    - Stage 3: moderate-to-severe loss of kidney function; estimated GFR between 30 and 59
    - Stage 4: severe loss of kidney function; estimated GFR between 15 and 30
    - Stage 5: complete kidney failure; estimated GFR less than 15, progressing to ESRD
  - Causes
    - Diabetes mellitus: 50% of cases and the leading cause of CKD
    - Hypertension: 25% of cases
  - Clients are often asymptomatic until the disease has progressed.
    - Loss of more nephrons
    - Not diagnosed early
    - Lack of early treatment
      - Uremia: urine in the blood
      - Azotemia: build-up of nitrogen-containing substances: urea, creatinine, phenols, hormones, water, electrolytes, and other nitrogen-rich compounds in the blood
    - Affects all body systems
      - Urinary system
        - Fluid retention, requiring diuretic therapy
        - Anuria (no urine production)
        - Metabolic imbalances: increases in BUN and serum creatinine levels
        - Electrolyte imbalances
          - Acid-base imbalances
          - Hyperkalemia: decreased excretion of potassium
          - Hypernatremia: sodium retention, resulting in edema, hypertension, and heart failure
          - Metabolic acidosis: unable to excrete acids; unable to use bicarbonate effectively
        - Insulin dysregulation
          - Kidneys are unable to excrete insulin.
          - Clients with diabetes may require less insulin to maintain blood glucose levels.
      - Hematologic system
        - Anemia: decreased erythropoietin, which is necessary for RBC production
        - Platelet dysfunction: risk of bleeding
        - Immunosuppression: risk of infections

- Cardiovascular system
  - Cardiovascular disease is the most common cause of death in those with CKD.
  - Hypertension
    - Cause of CKD
    - Complication of CKD
  - Cardiac effusions
- Pulmonary system
  - Pulmonary edema
  - Pleural effusions
- Musculoskeletal system
  - Slows the rate of bone remodeling
- Central nervous system
  - Peripheral neuropathy: numbness and tingling of the hands and feet
  - Altered mental status
- Gastrointestinal system
  - Constipation
- Integumentary system
  - Pruritus: unpleasant sensation of the skin that provokes the urge to scratch
- Reproductive system
  - Infertility
- Prognosis is dependent on the cause of CKD, age of the patient, comorbidities, and medical follow up.

APPLICATION AND REVIEW

1. Which components of homoeostasis are addressed by a functioning renal system? *(Select all that apply.)*
   1. White blood cell (WBC) formation
   2. Blood pressure control
   3. Formation of urine
   4. Acid-base balance
   5. Bone formation
2. Which client is at greatest risk for kidney failure?
   1. 5-year-old child diagnosed with the flu
   2. 20-year-old woman recovering from mononucleosis
   3. 40-year-old man recovering from knee replacement surgery
   4. 70-year-old man diagnosed with chronic Lewy body dementia
3. Which factors characterize acute renal injury and resulting kidney failure? *(Select all that apply.)*
   1. Decrease in serum creatinine
   2. Decrease in urine production
   3. Decrease in the BUN level
   4. Decrease in GFR
   5. Rapid onset of kidney function deterioration
4. A nurse is providing information to a client diagnosed with a prerenal form of AKI. Which information should be included in the discussion? *(Select all that apply.)*
   1. AKI may involve decreased blood flow to the kidneys.
   2. There is no significant damage to kidney tissue.
   3. AKI is seldom the cause of intrarenal kidney failure.
   4. AKI is often the result of exposure to a nephrotoxic substance.
   5. AKI triggers urinary reflux.

5. Which client is at risk for developing postrenal AKI?
   1. 15-year-old girl being aggressively treated for sepsis
   2. 70-year-old man with a diagnosis of BPH
   3. 50-year old woman diagnosed with right-sided congestive heart failure
   4. 30-year-old athlete who experienced a significant blood loss attributable to a compound fractured femur

6. Which assessment data suggest that the client is experiencing a UTI? *(Select all that apply.)*
   1. Fever
   2. Vomiting
   3. Flank pain
   4. Hypotension
   5. Blood in the urine

7. Which condition substantially increases the client's risk for developing CKD?
   1. Congestive heart failure
   2. Diabetes mellitus
   3. Chronic hypotension
   4. Anemia

8. A client diagnosed with CKD requires regular monitoring for which comorbid conditions? *(Select all that apply.)*
   1. Edema
   2. Anemia
   3. Hyponatremia
   4. Hypertension
   5. Hypokalemia

9. Which client's recovery should be most negatively affected by an existing diagnosis of CKD?
   1. 45-year-old woman recovering from a pacemaker implant
   2. 30-year-old man recovering from a fractured femur
   3. 15-year-old girl in treatment for anorexia nervosa
   4. 5-year old boy being treated for amblyopia

See Answers on pages 318–320.

Assessment for Renal Failure

- Mental status
- Vital signs
- Respiratory status
  - Lung sounds: crackles
  - Shortness of breath with little exertion (dyspnea on exertion)
  - Orthopnea (inability to breath adequately while lying flat)
  - Paroxysmal nocturnal dyspnea (sleep interrupted by periods of dyspnea)
  - Oxygenation
  - Rate of respirations
  - Depth of respirations
- Cardiac status
  - Auscultation
    - Third intercostal space
    - Left of sternum
    - Client leans slightly forward
      - Friction rub may indicate pericarditis
      - May indicate uremia from kidney failure
    - Extra (S_3 and S_4) heart sounds; may indicate fluid overload
  - Heart rate and rhythm
  - Hemodynamic monitoring
    - Fluid volume available for the heart to pump

- Central venous pressure (CVP)
  - Preload (fluid volume available to right ventricle)
    - Normal: between 2 and 5 mm Hg
    - Volume depletion: less that 2 mm Hg
    - Volume overload: greater than 5 mm Hg
  - Mean arterial pressure (MAP): average blood pressure in the arteries
    - Regulated by cardiac output and systemic vascular resistance (SVR)
    - Decreased MAP
      - Inadequate kidney perfusion, resulting in decreased blood flow and decreased oxygen supply
- Signs and symptoms of hypervolemia
  - Oliguric phase in AKI
  - Neck vein distention greater than 2 cm above the sternal notch
    - Raise the head of the bed 45 to 90 degrees.
  - Ascites (excess fluid accumulation in the abdomen)
  - Peripheral edema
    - Swelling does not diminish with the elevation of the extremity.
    - Pitting edema
      - Apply fingertip pressure to the swollen area.
      - If the indentation does not quickly return to normal, pitting edema is present.
      - Pitting edema scale
        - +1: between 1- and 2-mm indent depth, rebounding immediately
        - +2: between 3- and 4-mm indent depth, lasting up to 15 seconds before rebounding
        - +3: between 5- and 6 -mm indent depth, lasting up to 30 seconds before rebounding
        - +4: between 7- and 8-mm indent depth, lasting longer than 30 seconds before rebounding
- Signs and symptoms of hypovolemia
  - Diuretic phase AKI
  - Orthostatic hypotension
    - Blood loss
    - Dehydration
    - Inadequate preload when changing positions from lying to sitting to standing positions
  - Flat neck veins in the supine position
  - Skin turgor
    - Skin does not immediately return to its normal shape when pinched on the forearm.
    - The skin turgor test is not the best indicator in older adults attributable to lost elasticity of the skin.
  - Dry mucous membranes
  - Electrolyte imbalances
  - Skin assessment
    - Discoloration in the flank area
      - Grey Turner sign, which may indicate kidney trauma
  - Pain in the area of the kidneys
  - Auscultation above, left, and right of the umbilicus
    - Bruit may indicate vascular dysfunction.
      - Swishing sound
      - Abnormal blood flow to kidney

Diagnostics for Renal Failure

- History
  - Frequent UTIs
  - History of urinary obstruction
  - Possible causes
    - Recent use of over-the-counter medications (NSAIDs)
    - Recent infections requiring antibiotics
    - Antihypertensive medications (ACE inhibitors) and diuretics
    - IV contrast dye used for diagnostic imaging
  - Change in sleep habits: sleeping on extra pillows; sleeping upright in a chair
  - Family history: hypertension; diabetes mellitus; polycystic kidney disease; kidney disease; peripheral edema
- Urine output totals
  - May not be an accurate indicator of kidney function in the early stages
    - Nonoliguric AKI; excretes water but not solute component
- Intake and output
  - Intake exceeds output.
    - Positive fluid balance
      - Excess IV fluids
      - Decreased urine output
  - Kidney dysfunction and positive fluid balance
    - Fluid volume overload
  - Output exceeds intake.
    - Negative fluid balance
    - Volume deficit
      - Fever
      - Tachypnea (rapid respirations)
      - Excess sweating
      - Vomiting
      - Diarrhea
      - Suctioning of gastric contents
      - Diuretics
- Urinalysis
  - Needs to be a sterile collection if ruling out an infectious process.
  - Urine should be tested soon after its collection.
    - Urine will become alkaline
    - Lysis of cells
    - Casts will dissolve
  - Urine pH
    - Normal range: between 4.5 and 8
    - Indicates acidity or alkalinity of urine
    - Kidneys regulate acid-base balance.
    - Increase in urine acidity results in a decreased pH level, which indicates sodium retention and intrarenal AKI.
  - Urine sediment
    - Epithelial cells

- Urinary casts (cylindrical structures)
  - Made up of mucoprotein
  - Secreted by the epithelial cells of the Henle loop, distal tubules, and collecting ducts
  - Are formed when epithelial cells, RBCs, and WBCs are present in the tubules
  - Can help identify specific underlying disease processes
  - Prerenal AKI
    - No damage to kidney tissue
    - No urine sediment
  - Intrarenal AKI
    - Glomeruli or tubules are damaged.
    - Permeability of sediment into urine
- Hematuria (blood in the urine)
  - Small amounts of RBCs in the urine is normal.
  - Large amounts of RBCs in the urine indicate urinary tract trauma, UTI, and/or kidney damage.
  - Myoglobin (protein present with skeletal muscle damage or breakdown)
    - Crush injury
    - Rhabdomyolysis, caused by trauma, cocaine use, status epilepticus, and/or overheating
    - Myoglobin can obstruct tubules in intrarenal AKI.
- Pyuria (presence of pus in urine)
- Crystals, an indication of an infection
- Urine osmolality
  - Normal value: greater than 350 milliosmoles per kilogram (mOsm/kg)
  - Oliguria: less than 300 mOsm/kg
  - Oliguria to anuria: between 300 and 400 mOsm/kg
  - Reabsorption or excretion of water from the kidney tubules
  - Increased urine osmolality
    - Deficient fluid volume
      - Compensatory fluid retention
      - Decreased urine output
  - Decreased urine osmolality
    - Excessive fluid volume
      - Increased urine output
- Urine protein
  - No protein should be found in the urine.
  - Glomerular capillaries are impermeable to protein.
  - Protein spills into the urine when glomerular capillary membrane dysfunction is present, such as with intrarenal AKI.
- Specific gravity of urine
  - Weight of urine, compared with distilled water (solute)
  - Reflects fluid volume status
  - Indicates the kidneys' ability to dilute or concentrate urine
    - Low specific gravity: kidneys are unable to excrete solute to concentrate urine
    - High specific gravity: more concentrated with dehydration
      - Diabetes: glucose in urine
      - Glomerular dysfunction: protein in urine
  - Normal value of specific gravity of urine: greater than 1.020

- Specific gravity of urine with oliguria: 1.010
- Specific gravity of urine with oliguria to anuria (limited passage of urine): between 1.000 and 1.010
- Electrocardiogram (ECG)
  - Electrolyte imbalances
- Complete blood count (CBC)
  - Increased WBCs related to an infectious process (leukocytosis)
  - Decreased serum sodium
  - Increased serum sodium
- Hemoglobin and hematocrit (H&H)
  - Can be indicators of intravascular fluid volume
  - Normal hemoglobin (Hgb) values
    - Men: between 13.5 and 17.5 g/dL
    - Women: between 12 and 16 g/dL
  - Hgb transports oxygen and carbon dioxide.
  - Hgb is essential in acid-base balance.
  - Normal hematocrit (Hct) values
    - Is approximately three times the Hgb level
    - Is expressed in percentages
  - Hct is the RBC concentration in whole blood.
  - Decreased Hct may indicate fluid overload by dilution.
    - Hgb remains constant.
    - Anemia, caused by kidney failure
  - Increased Hct may indicate fluid volume deficit.
- Arterial blood gases (ABGs) indicate metabolic acidosis.
- Anion gap
  - Difference between extracellular cations and anions
    - Cations
      - Sodium (Na^+)
      - Extracellular potassium (K^+) is very low and not included in the calculation
    - Anions
      - Chloride (Cl^-)
      - Bicarbonate (HCO_3-)
  - Normal value: between 8 and 16 mEq/L
  - $Na^+ - (Cl^- + HCO_3-)$
  - The "gap" is a representation of the ions in the extracellular fluid (ECF) that are unmeasured: phosphates; sulfates; ketones; lactate
  - Increase in the anion gap
    - Overproduction of acid products
    - Decreased excretion of acid products in acute kidney disease and in CKD
- Decreased serum bicarbonate
- Increased BUN
  - Normal range: between 5 and 20 mg/dL
  - BUN increases as kidney function worsens, resulting in decreased GFR and decreased excretion of urea.
  - Uremia symptoms increase with increased BUN.
  - Is a product of protein and amino acid metabolism
  - Increased nitrogen waste products

- BUN may also be elevated by other factors: hematoma reabsorption; gastrointestinal bleed; licorice ingestion (excess); excess protein intake
- Increased serum creatinine
  - Normal range: between 0.5 and 1.2 mg/dL
  - Is proportional to muscle mass
  - The normal range for serum creatinine is slightly higher in men than in women.
  - Is a product of muscle and cell metabolism
  - Is a more reliable indicator of kidney function than BUN; it is affected by fewer factors
- Normal BUN-to-creatinine ratio: 10:1
  - Prerenal AKI
    - Increased ratio
    - Creatinine is excreted through functioning tubules.
    - BUN is retained; GFR is decreased.
    - Ratio is more accurate for prerenal than BUN and creatinine separately.
- Creatinine clearance
  - Indicates how effective the kidneys are at clearing the creatinine from the blood (clearance)
  - Indicates how well the glomeruli and tubules are working and how well the GFR and kidneys are functioning
  - Normal laboratory creatinine value: between 110 and 120 mL/min
  - Kidney impairment: less than 50 mL/min
  - A 24-hour urine collection and blood sample checks the amount of waste products in the urine and checks kidney function.
- Albumin
  - Normal value: between 3.5 and 5 g/dL
  - Makes up 50% of total plasma protein
  - Colloid osmotic pressure, which is exerted by albumin, keeps fluid in the vascular space.
  - Plasma proteins are not able to permeate the vessel walls.
  - Clinical conditions
    - Nephrotic syndrome
      - Glomerular capillary permeability increases, allowing proteins to pass and albumin to spill into the urine.
    - Severe burns
      - Cell membranes are damaged.
  - If fluid is not kept in intravascular space, it flows to the interstitial space, which causes peripheral edema.
- Kidney, ureter, and bladder (KUB)
  - X-ray study
  - Visualizes the position and size of the kidneys and identifies calculi (kidney or ureteral stones) and masses
  - Abnormal findings are usually followed by additional tests.
- Renal ultrasound
  - Visualizes the size and shape of the kidneys, masses or cysts, renal blood flow and renal artery stenosis, tubular function, and the collection system
- Computed tomography (CT)
  - Visualizes obstructions, abnormalities of the vascular system, and tumors and masses
- Magnetic resonance imaging (MRI)
  - Provides three-dimensional imaging with excellent clarity

- IV contrast imaging
  - Radiographic contrast dye is intravenously injected; many dyes are nephrotoxic.
  - Visualizes internal kidney tissues
- Angiography
  - A contrast medium is directly injected into the renal artery.
  - Visualizes renal blood flow stenosis, cysts, thrombi, traumatic damage to tissues, and infarctions (tissue death)
- Renal biopsy (definitive for diagnosing CKD)
  - Percutaneous needle biopsy
    - A needle is inserted through the flank to obtain tissue (cortical, medullary, specific mass) from the kidney.
  - Open biopsy
    - Surgical procedure (the last resort). The risks include bleeding, hematoma, and infection.

APPLICATION AND REVIEW

10. The nurse assesses a client experiencing hypervolemia in the oliguric phase of AKI. Which nursing intervention should the nurse implement?
    1. Implement falls precautions to help manage the risks related to orthostatic hypotension.
    2. Elevate the head of bed from 45 to 90 degrees to assess for neck vein distention.
    3. Monitor skin turgor for indications of dehydration.
    4. Auscultate the umbilical area for an indication of a bruit.
11. Which urine pH level is consistent with the intrarenal stage of AKI?
    1. 4.1
    2. 5.2
    3. 7.0
    4. 8.2
12. Which characteristic of a urinalysis is consistent with the results expected during the intrarenal stage of AKI?
    1. pH of 8.2
    2. Sediment present
    3. No RBCs noted
    4. No protein noted
13. Which urine osmolality and output results are reflective of fluid volume deficit and compensatory fluid retention?
    1. Output decreases and osmolality increases
    2. Output increases and osmolality increases
    3. Output decreases and osmolality decreases
    4. Output increases and osmolality decreases
14. Which is the definitive diagnostic tool to confirm the diagnosis of CKD?
    1. Percutaneous needle biopsy
    2. Renal ultrasound
    3. Angiography
    4. KUB x-ray study

See Answers on pages 318–320.

Signs and Symptoms of Renal Failure

- Altered mental status
- Bounding pulse
- Coma
- Decrease in cognitive function
- Dependent edema
  - Peripheral (lower legs) swelling
- Dyspnea (shortness of breath)

- Fatigue
- Fluid retention
- Headache
- Hypertension
- Itching
- Kussmaul respirations
  - Rapid and deep; compensatory mechanism to excrete carbon dioxide
- Loss of appetite
- Metallic taste
- Nausea
- Neck vein distention
- Nocturia (increased urination at night)
- Rapid weight gain
  - Fluid volume overload
  - Greater than 2 pounds per day (1 liter of fluid = 2.2 pounds = 1 kilogram)
- Seizures
- Weakness

Goals of Care for Renal Failure

- Preserve kidney function.
- Delay progression.
- Identify the cause.
- Treat the cause.
  - Early treatment may potentially reverse AKI.
  - Stages 1 through 4 of CKD
    - Treat the underlying cause.
      - Hypertension
      - Hyperparathyroidism
        - An enlarged parathyroid and elevated hormone calcitonin result in hypercalcemia (high calcium content in blood).
      - Anemia
      - Hyperglycemia (high blood sugar)
      - Dyslipidemia (elevated triglycerides in the blood)
- Maintain fluid and electrolyte balance.
- Decrease anxiety levels
- Compliance with follow-up care

Treatment of Renal Failure

- Manage the symptoms.
- Prevent complications during recovery.
- Provide adequate tissue perfusion, including adequate intravascular volume and adequate cardiac output.
- Provide diuretic therapy (loop diuretics) during the early stages.
- Strictly monitor and accurately measure intake and output (I&O).
- Replace fluids, if indicated.
  - Rapid blood loss
  - Burns
  - Long surgeries

- Restrict fluids, if indicated.
- Provide adequate nutrition.
- Replace electrolytes.
- Administer antibiotics to treat infection.
  - Pay close attention to the type, dosing, and frequency.
  - Many antibiotics are excreted by the kidneys.
- A client may need renal replacement therapy (RRT).
  - Dialysis
    - Indications: fluid overload affecting cardiac or pulmonary function; increased serum potassium level; metabolic acidosis; increased BUN level greater than 120 mg/dL; altered mental status; pericarditis; pericardial effusion; cardiac tamponade
    - Types of dialysis
      - Peritoneal dialysis (PD)
        - Is not commonly used
        - Can be performed at home
        - A PD catheter is inserted into the abdomen or peritoneal space.
        - A cleaning solution, called dialysate, is infused by gravity into the abdomen and acts as a filter, absorbing the waste and fluid from the blood and cleans the blood.
      - Hemodialysis (HD)
        - Cannot be performed at home
        - A special filter, called an artificial kidney or a dialyzer, filters the blood, removes excess fluid, and maintains electrolyte balance.
        - Clients with ESRD will require HD for the rest of their lives unless they undergo a kidney transplant.
        - HD is usually required three times a week.
  - Renal transplant
    - There is a shortage of donors.
    - Renal transplantation is a limited option.

Treatment Complications

- Fluid overload may lead to heart failure, pulmonary edema, pericardial effusions, or pleural effusions.
- Hyperkalemia
  - Can cause cardiac dysrhythmias
    - Lower with medication and HD
- Infections
- Fatigue
- Anxiety
- Drug toxicity
  - Accumulation of medications normally excreted by kidneys: digoxin; oral diabetic medications; antibiotics; opioids; NSAIDs

Nursing Interventions

- Strictly monitor and accurately measure I&O.
- Record daily weights.
- Replace fluids with prerenal AKI to prevent further loss.
  - Decreased perfusion
- Monitor serum electrolytes.
- Monitor for signs and symptoms of electrolyte imbalances.

- Monitor cardiac functions.
- Monitor electrocardiographic changes.
- Monitor kidney function, including serum creatinine and BUN levels and GFR.
- Educate the client and family on diet restrictions of foods high in protein, sodium, potassium, phosphate, and fluids.
- Maintain calorie counts.
- Prevent infection using the aseptic technique.
- Prevent skin breakdown caused by immobility.

Prevention of Renal Failure

- Identify clients with risk factors and health histories that make them at high risk for renal failure: older age; severe trauma; severe burn; cardiac failure; obstetric emergencies and complications; CKD diagnosis; frequent UTIs; diabetes mellitus; hypertension; smokers.
- Become knowledgeable of nephrotoxic agents.
- Prevent hypovolemia.
- Prevent prolonged hypoxemia.
- Prevent prolonged hypotension.

APPLICATION AND REVIEW

15. Dialysis is indicated when kidney failure causes which complication? *(Select all that apply.)*
    1. Cardiac tamponade
    2. Altered mental state
    3. Metabolic alkalosis
    4. Impaired respiratory function
    5. Impaired gastrointestinal function
16. Which is the primary reason that renal transplantation is a limited option for the treatment of kidney failure?
    1. Expense of the procedure
    2. Shortage of organ donors
    3. Reluctance on the part of clients
    4. Need for life-long medication therapy
17. Which clients are at risk for developing AKI related to the ingestion of a nephrotoxin? *(Select all that apply.)*
    1. Client taking ibuprofen for chronic neck pain
    2. Client currently being treated for fentanyl abuse
    3. Client being treated for diabetes with metformin
    4. Client prescribed Neomycin drops for a chronic ear infection
    5. Client with a medication history that includes five different prescriptions
18. Which statements made by a client diagnosed with CKD demonstrate an understanding of the dietary restrictions required of the plan of care? *(Select all that apply.)*
    1. "I eat several small meals a day."
    2. "It's hard, but I limit my fluid intake."
    3. "I eat a potassium source with each meal."
    4. "I'm very careful about the amount of protein I eat."
    5. "I love salty food, but I don't eat pretzels or chips now."
19. Which information should the nurse include when educating an older adult client about preventive measures of AKI?
    1. Measures to prevent UTIs
    2. Need to avoid prolonged exposure to the sun
    3. Recognition of the signs of hypotension
    4. Need to eat a well-balanced diet

See Answers on pages 318–320.

Electrolytes and Renal Failure

- Serum electrolytes are most commonly measured.
- Information can be gained regarding kidney function by measuring the electrolytes in a 24-hour urine specimen.
- Sodium and potassium can be randomly sampled.
  - Urine sodium
    - Indicates retention or excretion of sodium in the renal tubules
    - Maintains fluid balance
    - Hypovolemia can result due to urine sodium changes.
      - Tubules retain sodium and water
      - Low level of urine sodium
    - Hypervolemia can result due to urine sodium changes.
    - Intrarenal AKI can result due to urine sodium changes.
    - CKD can result due to urine sodium changes.
      - Sodium loss
      - High level of urine sodium
    - Prerenal AKI can result due to urine sodium changes.
      - Inadequate circulation to kidneys
      - Low level of urine sodium
  - Serum sodium
    - Is the most abundant electrolyte found in ECF
    - Calcium balance is regulated by the kidneys.
      - Adrenal glands secrete aldosterone.
      - Posterior pituitary gland secretes antidiuretic hormone (ADH).
    - Aldosterone influences the sodium reabsorption by the nephron.
      - Diuretics inhibit reabsorption, and sodium is excreted in the urine.
    - Normal range: between 135 and 145 mEq/L
    - Functions: fluid balance; water retention and excretion by the kidneys; nerve conduction; acid-base balance; enzyme functions
    - Hyponatremia: sodium level less than 135 mEq/dL
      - AKI: tubules are unable to conserve sodium; sodium is excreted in the urine, resulting in a low level of serum sodium
      - Signs and symptoms: disorientation; seizures; tachycardia; oliguria; headache; dizziness; nausea; vomiting; muscle twitching
    - Hypernatremia: sodium level greater than 145 mEq/dL
      - Signs and symptoms: excessive thirst; dry mucous membranes; altered mental status; seizures
- Calcium
  - Normal range: between 8.5 and 10.5 mg/dL
  - Is the most abundant electrolyte found in the body
  - 99% of the calcium is stored in bones.
    - Is the inactive form
    - May be reabsorbed if the serum calcium level is low
  - 1% of the calcium is found in the ECF and in the vascular space.
    - Calcium is found in three forms.
      - Ionized calcium
        - Is the active form
        - If the ionized calcium is not used, it will be reabsorbed by bone.

- ▪ Protein-bound calcium
  - ○ Ionizes faster than calcium in bone
  - ○ Converts to the active form
- ▪ Complexed calcium
  - ○ Is combined with other anions for the excretion of chloride, citrate, and phosphate
- • Hypocalcemia: calcium level less than 8.5 mg/dL
  - ▪ Signs and symptoms: irritability; muscle contractions (cramps, tetany, positive Chvostek or Trousseau sign); decreased cardiac contractility; bleeding (decreased coagulopathy); electrocardiographic changes
- • Hypercalcemia: calcium level greater than 10.5 mg/dL
  - ▪ Signs and symptoms: bone pain; excessive thirst; lethargy; weak muscles; anorexia
  - ▪ Functions: bone strength; heart muscle contractility; skeletal muscle contractions; blood clotting; cellular membrane permeability
- • Potassium
  - • Normal range: between 3.5 and 4.5 mEq/L
  - • Kidneys are the major regulators of potassium stores.
    - ▪ Potassium is normally reabsorbed by the proximal tubules and secreted by the distal tubules to maintain homeostasis.
    - ▪ AKI: Potassium levels increase and are not excreted; cardiac complications may occur.
  - • Hypokalemia: potassium level less than 3.5 mEq/L
    - ▪ Signs and symptoms: muscle weakness; electrocardiographic abnormalities; abdominal distention; paresthesia (numbness, tingling); decreased reflexes; anorexia; altered mental status
  - • Hyperkalemia: potassium level greater than 4.5 mEq/L
    - ▪ Signs and symptoms: irritability; anxiety; restlessness; nausea; vomiting; weakness; paresthesia
    - ▪ Electrocardiographic abnormalities (Figure 17.1): peaked T wave; widening QRS interval; ventricular tachycardia; ventricular fibrillation
  - • Interventions: Stop administering potassium supplements if the levels of potassium are elevated; administer IV diuretics, if urine is being effectively produced.
- • Magnesium
  - • Normal range: between 1.5 and 2.5 mEq/L
  - • 60% of magnesium is found in bone.
  - • 1% of magnesium is found in the ECF.
  - • 39% of magnesium is found in the intracellular fluid (ICF).
  - • Magnesium effects the ICF levels of calcium and potassium.
  - • Functions: active transport of sodium and potassium across cell membranes; essential for intracellular enzyme actions; neuromuscular activity; synthesis of proteins; energy production within the cell; heart muscle contractility; transmission of genetic information
  - • Hypomagnesemia: magnesium level less than 1.4 mEq/L
    - ▪ Signs and symptoms: facial tics; spasticity; cardiac rhythm abnormalities
  - • Hypermagnesemia: magnesium level greater than 2.5 mEq/L
    - ▪ Signs and symptoms: central nervous system depression; respiratory depression; lethargy; coma; bradycardia; electrocardiographic abnormalities
- • Phosphorus
  - • Normal range: between 2.7 and 4.5 mg/dL
  - • 80% of body phosphorus is found in bone.
  - • Most of the remaining phosphorus is found in the ICF.

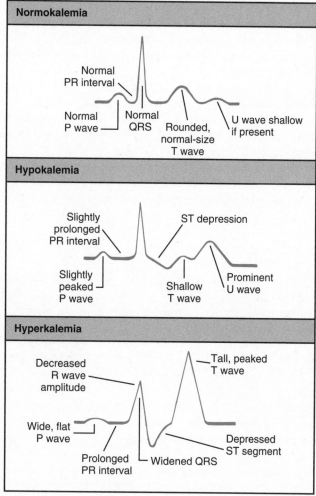

FIGURE 17.1 Electrocardiogram changes with potassium imbalance. (From Huether, S. E., McCance, K. L., Brashers, V. L., & Rote, S. R. [2017]. *Understanding pathophysiology* [6th ed.]. St. Louis: Elsevier.)

- Elevated phosphorus levels occur early in kidney failure.
- Functions: adenosine triphosphate (ATP) production for intracellular energy (active transport across cell membranes); structure of cell membranes; acid-base balance; bone strength; immunity; oxygen delivery to tissues
- Excreted by the kidneys (glomeruli)
- Reabsorbed by the kidneys (proximal tubules); is necessary when body phosphorus levels are low
- Combines with sodium and hydrogen to maintain acid-base balance
- Hypophosphatemia: phosphorus level less than 3.0 mg/dL
  - Signs and symptoms: anemia; immunity suppression (WBC depression); bleeding; nausea; vomiting; anorexia
- Hyperphosphatemia: phosphorus level greater than 4.5 mg/dL
  - Signs and symptoms: tachycardia; nausea; diarrhea; abdominal cramping; muscle weakness; paralysis; hyper reflexes

- Chloride
  - Normal value: between 98 and 108 mEq/L
  - Chloride is found predominantly in the ECF.
  - Changes in chloride levels indicate changes with other electrolytes and changes in the acid-base balance.
  - Excreted by the kidneys (proximal tubules)
  - Reabsorbed by the kidneys (proximal tubules)
  - Functions: serum osmolality balance in conjunction with sodium; fluid balance in conjunction with sodium; acid-base balance; gastric fluid acidity
  - Hypochloremia: chloride level less than 98 mEq/L
    - Signs and symptoms: irritability; muscle excitability; tetany; bradypnea (slow respirations)
  - Hyperchloremia: chloride level greater than 108 mEq/L
    - Signs and symptoms: muscle breakdown; peripheral edema; immunosuppression; poor wound healing

APPLICATION AND REVIEW

20. Which serum sodium result indicates normal kidney function?
    1. 94 mEq/L
    2. 130 mEq/L
    3. 143 mEq/L
    4. 168 mEq/L

See Answers on pages 318–320.

ANSWER KEY: REVIEW QUESTIONS

1. **Answers: 2, 3, 4, 5**
   2 Functions maintained by a functioning renal system include blood pressure control. **3** Functions maintained by a functioning renal system include the formation of urine. **4** Functions maintained by a functioning renal system include regulating acid-base balance. **5** Functions maintained by a functioning renal system include bone formation.
   1 Functions maintained by a functioning renal system include RBC formation.
   Client Need: Health Promotion and Maintenance; **Cognitive Level:** Comprehension; **Integrated Process:** Teaching and Learning

2. **4 Older adults are at the greatest risk for kidney failure; renal function declines with age.**
   1, 2, 3 In these situations, age is the greatest risk factor; the risk for kidney failure increases as renal function declines with age.
   Client Need: Health Promotion and Maintenance; **Cognitive Level:** Analysis; **Nursing Process:** Assessment

3. **Answers: 2, 4, 5**
   2 AKI results in a decrease in urine production. **4** AKI results in a decrease in GFR. **5** AKI results in rapid deterioration of kidney function.
   1 AKI results in an increase in serum creatinine. **3** AKI results in an increase in the BUN level.
   Client Need: Health Promotion and Maintenance; **Cognitive Level:** Comprehension; **Integrated Process:** Teaching and Learning

4. **Answers: 1, 2**
   1 Reduced blood flow to the kidneys is a common cause of AKI. **2** Kidney tissue is not damaged if the cause of the failure is related to prerenal issues.
   3 Prerenal AKI, if left untreated, can lead to intrarenal failure. **4** Intrarenal AKI is triggered by exposure to a nephrotoxin. **5** Urinary reflux, back flow into the renal pelvis, is a result of postrenal AKI or kidney failure.
   Client Need: Physiological Integrity; **Cognitive Level:** Comprehension; **Nursing Process:** Teaching and Learning

5. **2 Postrenal AKI is caused by an obstruction to urine flow such as that caused by BPH.**

   1 Prolonged hypotension resulting from sepsis triggers prerenal AKI. **3** Prolonged decrease in cardiac output resulting from heart failure triggers prerenal AKI. **4** Prolonged hypovolemia resulting from hemorrhaging triggers prerenal AKI.

   Client Need: Physiological Integrity; **Cognitive Level:** Analysis; **Nursing Process:** Assessment

6. **Answers: 1, 2, 3, 5**

   1 Signs and symptoms of a UTI include fever. **2** Signs and symptoms of a UTI include vomiting. **3** Signs and symptoms of a UTI include flank or side pain. **5** Signs and symptoms of a UTI include blood in the urine.

   4 Signs and symptoms of a UTI include hypertension.

   Client Need: Physiological Integrity; **Cognitive Level:** Comprehension; **Nursing Process:** Assessment

7. **2 Diabetes mellitus is the leading cause of CKD, accounting for 50% of the cases.**

   1 Congestive heart failure is not considered a leading cause of CKD. **3** Although chronic hypertension is considered a significant cause of CKD, it is not as significant a trigger as is diabetes mellitus. **4** Anemia is not considered a leading cause of CKD.

   Client Need: Physiological Integrity; **Cognitive Level:** Comprehension; **Integrated Process:** Teaching and Learning

8. **Answers: 1, 2, 4**

   1 CKD causes hypernatremia, which triggers edema. **2** CKD causes a decrease in erythropoietin, which triggers anemia. **4** CKD causes hypernatremia, which triggers hypertension.

   3 CKD causes hypernatremia. **5** CKD causes hyperkalemia.

   Client Need: Physiological Integrity; **Cognitive Level:** Analysis; **Nursing Process:** Assessment

9. **2 Recovery from a bone fracture will be impeded because of CKD's effect on bone remodeling.**

   1 CKD will have no specific negative effect on the recovery plan from a pacemaker implant. **3** CKD will have no specific negative effect on the recovery plan for anorexia nervosa. **4** CKD will have no specific negative effect on the recovery plan from such an eye surgery.

   Client Need: Physiological Integrity; **Cognitive Level:** Analysis; **Nursing Process:** Evaluation

10. **2 Neck vein distention is a sign associated with AKI-triggered hypervolemia and should be assessed for the client in a 45- to 90-degree sitting position.**

    1 Orthostatic hypotension is associated with hypovolemia during the diuretic phase of AKI. **3** Dehydration and the associated poor skin turgor are associated with hypovolemia during the diuretic phase of AKI. **4** The umbilical area may be auscultated for a bruit during the diuretic phase of AKI.

    Client Need: Physiological Integrity; **Cognitive Level:** Application; **Nursing Process:** Implementation

11. **1 The normal range for urine pH is between 4.5 and 8. Intrarenal AKI is associated with a decrease in pH.**

    2, 3, 4 The normal range for urine pH is between 4.5 and 8. Intrarenal AKI is associated with a decrease in pH.

    Client Need: Health Promotion and Maintenance; **Cognitive Level:** Analysis; **Nursing Process:** Assessment

12. **2 Sediment is found in urine sampled during the intrarenal stage of AKI.**

    1 A pH of 8.2 shows a slight increase above normal. During the intrarenal stage of AKI, pH demonstrates a decrease and is below normal. **3** RBCs are noted during the intrarenal stage of AKI. **4** Protein is noted during the intrarenal stage of AKI.

    Client Need: Physiological Integrity; **Cognitive Level:** Application; **Nursing Process:** Assessment

13. **1 Under these situations, output decreases and osmolality increases.**

    2, 3, 4 Under these situations, output decreases and osmolality increases.

    Client Need: Health Promotion and Maintenance; **Cognitive Level:** Analysis; **Integrated Process:** Teaching and Learning

14. **1 A renal biopsy is the definitive diagnostic tool for confirming CKD.**

    2 Although a renal ultrasound is an appropriate diagnostic tool in this situation, it is not used to definitively confirm the diagnosis of CKD. **3** Although an angiogram is an appropriate diagnostic tool in this situation, it is not used to definitively confirm the diagnosis of CKD. **4** Although a KUB

x-ray study is an appropriate diagnostic tool in this situation, it is not used to definitively confirm the diagnosis of CKD.
Client Need: Physiological Integrity; **Cognitive Level:** Application; **Integrated Process:** Teaching and Learning

15. **Answers: 1, 2, 4**

    1 Indications for dialysis include cardiac tamponade. **2** Indications for dialysis include an altered mental status. **4** Indications for dialysis include impaired respiratory function.

    3 Indications for dialysis include metabolic acidosis, not metabolic alkalosis. **5** Indications for dialysis do not include impaired gastrointestinal function
    Client Need: Health Promotion and Maintenance; **Cognitive Level:** Application; **Integrated Process:** Teaching and Learning

16. **2 The shortage of organ donors is the primary reason that renal transplantation is a limited option for those diagnosed with kidney failure.**

    1 Although expense can be a barrier, donor shortage is the primary reason that kidney transplantation is a limited option for the treatment of kidney failure. **3** Although client reluctance can be a barrier, donor shortage is the primary reason that kidney transplantation is a limited option for the treatment of kidney failure. **4** Although life-long medication therapy to manage organ rejection can be a barrier, donor shortage is the primary reason that kidney transplantation is a limited option for the treatment of kidney failure.
    Client Need: Health Promotion and Maintenance; **Cognitive Level:** Analysis; **Integrated Process:** Teaching and Learning

17. **Answers: 1, 2, 3, 4**

    1 NSAIDs, such as ibuprofen, pose a risk for nephrotoxicity. **2** Opioids, such as fentanyl, pose a risk for nephrotoxicity. **3** Oral diabetic medications, such as metformin, pose a risk for nephrotoxicity. **4** Antibiotics, such as Neomycin, pose a risk for nephrotoxicity.

    5 The type of medication is a greater risk factor than the number of prescriptions.
    Client Need: Health Promotion and Maintenance; **Cognitive Level:** Analysis; **Nursing Process:** Assessment

18. **Answers: 2, 4, 5**

    2 Restrictions required of a diet appropriate for this client would include fluids. **4** Restrictions required of a diet appropriate for this client would include protein. **5** Restrictions required of a diet appropriate for this client would include sodium.

    1 A client on this diet would not be required to eat several small meals. **3** Restrictions required of a diet appropriate for this client would include potassium.
    Client Need: Health Promotion and Maintenance; **Cognitive Level:** Analysis; **Nursing Process:** Evaluation

19. **1 Frequent UTIs increase the risk for AKI.**

    2 Although an appropriate general health–promotion topic, sun exposure is not directly associated with AKI. **3** Although an appropriate general health–promotion topic, hypertension, not hypotension, is directly associated with AKI. **4** Although an appropriate general health–promotion topic, diet is not directly associated with triggering AKI.
    Client Need: Health Promotion and Maintenance; **Cognitive Level:** Application; **Integrated Process:** Teaching and Learning

20. **3 Normal serum sodium range is between 135 and 145 mEq/L; 143 mEq/L would fall within that range.**

    1 Normal serum sodium range is between 135 and 145 mEq/L; 94 mEq/L would indicate hyponatremia.

    2 Normal serum sodium range is between 135 and 145 mEq/L; 130 mEq/L would indicate hyponatremia.

    4 Normal serum sodium range is between 135 and 145 mEq/L; 168 mEq/L would indicate hypernatremia.
    Client Need: Health Promotion and Maintenance; **Cognitive Level:** Comprehension; **Nursing Process:** Assessment

Fluids and Electrolytes in Brain Injuries 18

BRAIN INJURY OVERVIEW

Significance of Fluids and Electrolytes in Brain Injuries

- Brain injury is commonly referred to as a traumatic brain injury (TBI).
- TBIs can be caused by a congenital anomaly, heredity abnormalities, degenerative processes, or by birth trauma.
- Acquired TBIs are brain injuries that have occurred after birth and are not linked to any kind of congenital defect.
- There are several different types and causes of TBIs.
- Many symptoms are common to individuals with brain injuries, regardless of the mechanism of injury.
- Deficits resulting from a TBI correlate with the area of the brain that has been damaged.
- Sodium, potassium, and calcium are the primary electrolyte imbalances that are the result of TBIs.
- Maintaining fluid and electrolyte balance is essential for improving morbidity and mortality associated with TBIs.

Pathophysiological Characteristics of Brain Injuries

- The brain controls every function of the body.
- Damage from a TBI ranges from mild to severe.
- Damage may result in temporary symptoms or a permanent impairment.
- It may be difficult to identify the brain injury based on the appearance of the individual.
  - A TBI is referred to as an invisible injury because the resulting problems deal with thinking and with emotions.
- Results of the damage may be inconsistent, unpredictable, and can be frustrating to the individual with the injury and others associating with the injured person.
- Brain function is altered due to an external factor, such as a motor vehicle accident, a fall, an athletic injury, or violence.
- TBIs are classified by the mechanism (contact, acceleration-deceleration, rotational), the location of the impact to the brain, the severity of the injury (mild, moderate, severe), and the extent of the injury.
- Two categories of TBIs
  - Primary TBI
    - The injury occurs at the moment of impact.
    - Severity and prognosis is dependent on whether the injury is localized (limited area of the brain) or diffuse (affecting large area or areas of the brain).
    - Damage directly impacts the functional brain tissue (parenchyma).
    - Types of primary injury include contusion, laceration, shearing, and hemorrhage.
    - Cellular response to the injury starts immediately.

- Major catecholamines (epinephrine, norepinephrine, dopamine) are released after a TBI and are the indicators of the severity of the injury.
- Secondary TBI
  - A secondary TBI is a cellular chemical response to the initial injury that potentiates the primary TBI.
    - Increases the damage to the brain tissue
    - Affects recovery
  - Causes of secondary TBIs
    - Ischemia
      - Decreased or lack of perfusion (hypoxia, hypotension)
      - Edematous issues
      - Vasodilation of cerebral vessels occurs in an attempt to perfuse oxygen and nutrients to the tissues, increase blood volume in brain, and elevate the intracranial pressure (ICP; pressure inside cranium).
      - Hypertension initially occurs in an attempt to perfuse brain tissue and to increase both the blood volume and the ICP.
    - Hypotension
      - Hypotension is usually not directly associated with a TBI unless the medulla is injured.
      - Trauma may be the result of other injuries to the body, causing low blood pressure.
      - Assess for internal injuries.
    - Hypercapnia
      - Elevated carbon dioxide (CO_2)
      - Hypoventilation: lack of oxygen on inhalation; not exhaling CO_2
      - Causes vasodilation of the cerebral vasculature, which increases both blood flow and ICP
    - Cerebral edema
      - Is initially an attempt to perfuse brain tissue
        - ICP is increased.
        - Space is limited inside the skull (cranial vault).
        - Equilibrium: brain; blood volume; cerebral spinal fluid
        - Imbalance occurs if one increases or decreases.
      - Compensatory perfusion decrease
        - Further damage
      - Is localized around the site of injury
      - Is either diffuse or global
        - Hypoxia
        - Hypotension
      - Minimize cascade
        - Manage oxygenation.
        - Support ventilation.
        - Maintain perfusion.
    - Metabolic imbalance
      - Respiratory acidosis
      - Decreased respirations, resulting in an increase in CO_2
- A specific alteration in function is determined by the affected area of the brain.
- No injury is the same among individuals.

- Many of the effects of TBIs are typical or similar among individuals.
  - Individuals with a brain injury may describe a cloudy mind.
    - Feeling constantly hung over
    - Feeling of weightlessness
    - Disoriented to surroundings
  - Individuals with a brain injury may experience a lack of energy.
    - Need frequent naps
    - Tire easily from typical daily routines and from thinking
  - Individuals with a brain injury may experience a change in sleeping patterns.
    - Sleep too much
    - Sleep too little
    - Difficulty falling asleep
  - Individuals with a brain injury may experience many signs and symptoms.
    - Frequent and/or constant headaches
    - Chronic pain in different parts of the body
    - Ringing in ears (tinnitus)
    - Changes in vision (blurred vision, loss of visual fields, sensitivity to light)
    - Changes in the sense of smell (heightened, diminished)
    - Changes in the sense of taste (heightened, diminished)
    - Changes in hearing (sensitivity to noise, tinnitus)
    - Changes in appetite (decreased, not reaching a sense of fullness)
    - Fluctuation in body temperature
    - Difficulty swallowing (coughing, choking)
    - Speech abnormalities (mixing up words, a new stutter)
    - Uncoordinated balance (falls, stumbles when walking)
    - Weakness in the arms and legs
    - Numbness and tingling in the arms and legs
    - Muscle spasms
    - Changes in cognition (difficulty focusing, forgetfulness, slow thought processes)
      - Brain is overwhelmed
      - Difficulty understanding, especially with abstract concepts
      - Needs black-and-white instruction
    - Changes with social behavior
      - Self-awareness: inability to see own issues honestly; focus on self not others
      - Emotions: intense; labile; do not always match the situation; depression; anxiety not associated with any particular situation; irritable (anger, quick temper); impulsive (acts with no thought of the consequences); loss of coping; decreased motivation; misperception of situations; relationship problems with family, friends, and/or co-workers; difficulty with employment
- Causes of TBI (Table 18.1)
  - Anoxia (absence of oxygen)
    - Brain cells start to become damaged after 3 minutes without oxygen.
    - Near drowning
    - Asphyxiation by strangling
    - Cardiac arrest
    - Respiratory arrest
    - Rapid, extensive loss of blood

TABLE 18.1	Causes of Brain Injury
Type of Injury	**Mechanism**
Focal Brain Injury	Localized injury from direct impact
Blunt trauma	Closed injury
Coup	Injury directly below the site of the forceful impact
Contrecoup	Injury on opposite side of brain from the site of the forceful impact
Extradural (epidural) hematoma	Vehicular accidents, minor falls, sporting accidents
Subdural hematoma	Vehicular accidents or falls, especially in older adults or persons with chronic alcohol abuse
Intracerebral hemorrhage; subarachnoid hemorrhage	Contusions caused by a forceful impact, usually vehicular accidents or long-distance falls
Compound fracture	Objects strike the head with great force or the head forcefully strikes the object; temporal blows, occipital blows, upward impact of cervical vertebrae (basilar skull fracture)
Penetrating trauma	Open injury
	Missiles (bullets) or sharp projectiles (knives, ice picks, axes, screwdrivers)
Diffuse brain injury (diffuse axonal injury)	Traumatic shearing forces; tearing of axons from twisting and rotational forces with injury over widespread area
	Moving head strikes hard, unyielding surface or moving object strikes stationary head; vehicular accidents (occupant or pedestrian); torsional head motion

From Huether, S. E., McCance, K. L., Brashers, V. L., & Rote, S. R. (2012). *Understanding pathophysiology* (5th ed.). St. Louis: Mosby.

- Infection
  - Encephalitis (infection of the brain tissue)
  - Abscess
  - Meningitis (infection of the membrane surrounding the brain)
- Stroke
  - Ischemic
    - Lack of oxygen
    - Blocked artery by a blood clot or plaque
    - Transient ischemic attack (TIA)
      - Is a nonsustained hypoxic event
      - Does not cause permanent damage
  - Hemorrhage (bleeding in the brain)
    - Aneurysm (weak spot in a vessel wall that breaks)
    - Blood, itself, damages tissue.
    - Pressure on surrounding tissues
- Surgery
  - Cutting of nerve fibers
  - Removal of brain tissue
- Trauma
  - Crush: The skull and brain are injured between two hard surfaces.

- Penetration: The skull and brain are injured by a penetrating object.
  - Bullet shot from a gun
  - Knife
  - High-velocity impact
    - Object may ricochet within the skull, causing damage to brain tissue with each pass.
    - May cause shockwaves through the brain tissue, causing further damage
  - Penetration injury
    - Fragments of bone, skin, and hair introduced into the brain tissue
  - Low-velocity injury
    - Knife
  - High risk of infection
    - Abscess
    - Foreign objects left in brain tissue
- Closed trauma
  - The brain remains enclosed by the skull.
    - The skull may be fractured.
    - The dura mater, the membrane covering the brain and spinal cord, remains intact.
- Open trauma
  - The skull is open, causing exposure of the brain to the outside environment.
  - The dura mater is torn.
- Tumor
  - A tumor causes damage in two ways.
    - Pressure to the surrounding brain tissue
    - Tumor growth destroys brain cells.
- Types of brain injury
  - Anoxic brain injury
    - Anemic (inadequate supply of oxygen is carried by the blood)
    - Anoxia (no oxygen)
    - Hypoxic
      - Ischemic
      - Some oxygen but not enough, resulting in a lack of blood flow and severe hypotension (low blood pressure)
    - Toxic
      - Prevention of oxygen in the blood from being used by the cells
      - Exposure to a toxic substance from illicit drugs, common cleaning products, or some pharmaceutical agents
  - Closed brain injury
    - Impact of an outside force to the head
    - Some brain injuries occur in the absence of skull fracture.
    - Some brain injuries occur in the presence of skull fracture.
      - Nondisplaced (parts of the skull remain aligned)
      - Intact dura mater
    - Concern for cerebral edema (swelling of the brain)
      - No room for the brain to expand
        - Increased ICP
        - Compression of brain tissue, resulting in damage to the cells

- Brain tissue attempts to move through available space or openings.
  - Eye sockets
    - Pressure on cranial nerve III
    - Dilated pupils
  - Base of the brain
    - Passage for the brainstem
    - Swelling through the base of the brain (herniation)
    - Usually fatal: brain death; absent brainstem function (apnea, nonreactive pupils, flat electroencephalogram [EEG])
- Concussion
  - Direct impact to the head or body
  - Impaired neurological function
  - Mild to severe
  - May last seconds to hours
  - With or without a loss of consciousness
  - May have amnesia
    - Loss of memories before the injury (retrograde)
    - Loss of memories after the injury (anterograde)
    - Microscopic damage
      - Stretching of the blood vessels in the brain
      - Cranial nerve damage
      - Is not usually detected on imaging
    - Damage may be temporary or permanent.
  - Is diagnosed by history and symptoms
- Contusion
  - Bruising of the brain tissue
  - Superficial bleeding spreads into the parenchyma.
  - Clinical symptoms correspond with the area of the brain injury.
  - Types of hematomas
    - Epidural hematoma (EDH)
      - Bleeding between the dura mater and the skull
      - Extraparenchymal (outside of the parenchyma)
      - Increased ICP
      - Displaced brain tissue
    - Subdural hematoma (SDH)
      - Bleeding between the dura mater and the arachnoid mater (middle layer of the membrane surrounding brain and spinal cord)
      - Extraparenchymal
      - Increased ICP
      - Displaced brain tissue
      - Three types of SDH are distinguished by the injury-to-bleed time and clinical symptoms.
        - Acute SDH: bleeds at the onset of injury; rapid progression
        - Subacute SDH: bleeds 4 days to 3 weeks after the injury; slow progression
        - Chronic SDH: bleeds 3 weeks or longer after the injury; older adults at greater risk; balance issues; anticoagulation issues; often an unknown cause

- Intracerebral hematoma (ICH)
  - Bleeding within the brain tissue itself
    - Intraparenchymal (within the parenchyma)
  - Directly damages the neural tissue
  - No space exists in cranial vault for additional blood.
    - Increased ICP
    - Displaces brain tissue
- Diagnosed with computed tomography (CT) scan
  - Severity of the contusion
    - Small
      - Localized neurological damage
      - Treat medically with frequent neurological assessments
      - Treat the symptoms
    - Large
      - May take several days to know the full extent of tissue involvement, edema, and continued bleeding
      - Mass effect, involving more of the brain; increased ICP
      - May require surgical intervention
      - Frequent neurological assessments; changes may be subtle
- Coup contrecoup injury (Figure 18.1)
  - Is frequently caused by acceleration-deceleration impact
  - Contusion occurs on one side of the brain from a direct impact.
  - The brain then moves in the opposite direction, impacting the skull and causing a contusion on the opposite side of the brain that was hit.
  - Coup contrecoup injury is caused by one incident.
- Diffuse axonal injury
  - Refers to damage of the axons, which are nerve fibers that transmit impulses
  - Tearing and stretching of nerve fibers
    - Acceleration-deceleration
    - Rotational injury
    - The brain does not normally move inside the skull.

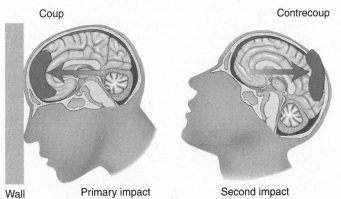

Coup   Contrecoup

Wall   Primary impact   Second impact

FIGURE 18.1 Coup contrecoup injury. (From Lewis, S. L., Bucher, L., Heitkemper, M. M., Harding, M. M., Kwong, J., & Roberts, D. [2017]. *Medical-surgical nursing: Assessment and management of clinical problems* [10th ed.]. St. Louis: Elsevier.)

- The skull moves quickly, but the brain does not move at the same speed.
  - Motor vehicle accidents
  - Shaken baby syndrome (rotation)
- Disruption in the nerve impulses, causing the release of chemicals that are toxic to tissues
- Hypoxic injury
  - Infection is a cause.
  - Open injury is a cause.
    - Is a penetrating injury
    - Dura mater is open.
    - Skull fracture
      - Is not the cause of the brain injury alone
      - Is a good indicator of the potential for ICH
        - Significant force is required to fracture the skull.
      - May require surgical intervention
- Second impact syndrome
  - A second impact to the head occurs after an initial impact that caused the first injury.
    - Causes a concussion
    - First injury has not yet healed
    - May occur days to weeks after the initial injury
  - A second impact is more likely to cause cerebral edema, large area of damage, and permanent damage, including muscle spasticity, increase in muscle tone, labile emotions, difficulty learning, and difficulty thinking.
  - The second impact syndrome can be fatal if not treated immediately.
- Shaken baby syndrome
  - Is an abusive activity
  - Involves violently shaking a baby
  - Whiplash type of movement, resulting in coup contrecoup brain injury
    - Blood vessels between brain and skull tear and bleed.
    - Brain tissues swell.
  - Shaken baby syndrome is an emergency if symptoms are present: irritability; sleepy; lethargic; breathing difficulties; change in eating habits; pupil changes (dilated); headache; seizure; coma; death
  - Permanent brain damage includes life-long disabilities.
- Stroke
  - Ischemic
  - Hemorrhagic
- Toxicity
  - Toxic encephalopathy
  - Brain tissue exposed to a toxic substance, causing an altered mental status, memory loss, and visual disturbances
    - Usually causes permanent damage
    - Treat the symptoms.
- Tumor
- Various tumors can cause injury to brain tissue.
- Symptoms of brain injury
  - Symptoms correlate with the anatomical area of the brain injury.
  - Brain injuries have a wide variety of physical and cognitive symptoms.

- Functions of the brain by location
  - Frontal lobe (forehead): reasoning; organization; planning; movement; facial expression; behavior; self-control; emotions
  - Parietal lobe (upper back portion of the brain): higher thought; senses (vision, touch); spatial awareness; distinguishing right and left; understanding language; comprehension of numbers; objects and relation
  - Occipital lobe (back of the brain): visual center (recognition, processing, perception)
  - Temporal lobe (side of the brain near the ear): auditory (perception, recognition); understanding the spoken language; language (word recall, speaking)
  - Cerebellum (back of brain below the occipital lobe): movement; coordination; balance; posture; cardiac; respiratory
  - Brainstem
    - Is vital for life
      - Vital signs: heart rate; blood pressure; respirations
      - Swallowing
  - Any function can be disrupted.
  - Frontal lobe
    - Paralysis: loss of simple movement
      - May be expressed in different parts of the body
    - Expressive aphasia: inability to express thoughts through speech
    - Executive functioning impairment: disruption in sequencing
      - Unable to complete tasks requiring multiple steps
      - Inability to form a plan
      - Inability to sequence complex movements to accomplish a task
        - Laundry
        - Making coffee
      - Difficulty solving problems
      - Loss of flexibility: rigid thinking
      - Loss of spontaneity
      - Perseveration (fixed on a task or thought)
      - Attention deficit: inability to focus on a task for a period
      - Labile emotions (moody)
      - Notable changes in personality
      - Notable changes in social behavior
  - Parietal lobe
    - Anomia: inability to name common objects
    - Difficulty drawing objects
    - Can focus only on one object at a time
    - Agraphia: word recall for writing is hindered
    - Alexia: difficulty reading
    - Difficulty identifying left and right
    - Disruption with hand-eye coordination
    - Dyscalculia: difficulty with mathematics
    - Lack of awareness of surrounding space and body parts
    - Apraxia: inability to execute or carry out skilled movements and gestures
    - Inability to care for oneself
    - Visual focus attention deficit: inability to focus

- Occipital lobes
  - Visual field deficits
    - Peripheral vision deficit
  - Inability to find objects in the environment
  - Color agnosia: difficulty identifying colors
  - Visual illusions: not accurately seeing objects
  - Hallucinations
  - Word blindness: inability to recognize written words
  - Inability to recognize objects drawn on a paper
  - Movement agnosia: inability to identify movement of objects
  - Difficulty with reading
  - Difficulty with writing
- Temporal lobes
  - Prosopagnosia: impaired facial recognition
  - Wernicke aphasia: difficulty with understanding speech
  - Right temporal lobe damage
    - Persistent talking
  - Short-term memory loss
  - Difficulty with identifying objects through speech
  - Categorization: difficulty categorizing objects
  - Disconnected long-term memory
  - Sexual drive (reduction or heightened)
  - Increased aggressive behavior
  - Tinnitus
- Brainstem
  - Impaired breathing capacity
    - Necessary for speech
  - Dysphasia: impaired ability to swallow
  - Inability to organize the surrounding environment
    - Difficulty perceiving the environment
  - Impaired balance
  - Impaired movement
  - Vertigo: dizziness
  - Nausea
  - Insomnia: difficulty sleeping
  - Sleep apnea: periods of not breathing during sleep
    - Obstructed airway attributable to obesity or tissues in the back of the throat
- Cerebellum
  - Fine motor coordination deficits
  - Loss of the ability to walk
  - Tremors
  - Vertigo
  - Slurred speech
  - Difficulty reaching and grabbing for objects
- May mimic other sources that cause dysfunction
  - Ruling out other causes is important.
  - Migraine headaches

- Pain
- Medications
- Depression
- Stress
- Signs and symptoms may decrease over time with brain healing.

APPLICATION AND REVIEW

1. Which event increases the risk for secondary TBI?
   1. Strangulation-induced brain ischemia
   2. Cerebral hemorrhagic stroke
   3. Frontal cerebral contusion
   4. Blunt force brain trauma
2. Which client statements support a diagnosis of TBI? *(Select all that apply.)*
   1. "My mind seems to always be in a fog."
   2. "I really have trouble getting enough sleep."
   3. "I've been depressed; I've never been depressed before."
   4. "My partner says that nothing seems to upset me anymore."
   5. "Remembering numbers and names has become a problem for me."
3. Which safety issues in a client diagnosed with TBI are of primary concern to the nurse? *(Select all that apply.)*
   1. Dysphasia
   2. Concrete thinking
   3. Impaired balance
   4. Impaired anger control
   5. Impaired concentration
4. How long of a period of impaired oxygenation can the brain cells tolerate before they become damaged?
   1. 30 seconds
   2. 3 minutes
   3. 10 minutes
   4. 30 minutes
5. Which factor indicates a TIA is a common stroke?
   1. It involves a sustained period of cerebral hypoxia.
   2. It is most commonly a result of past brain trauma.
   3. It does not result in permanent cell damage.
   4. It is primarily treated with surgery.
6. What is the primary effect of a toxic brain injury on the cells of the brain?
   1. Swelling of the brain
   2. Insufficient oxygen supply
   3. Ineffective use of oxygen
   4. Microscopic damage to the cerebral vessels
7. Which type of brain injury results from violently shaking an infant?
   1. Open
   2. Concussion
   3. Coup contrecoup
   4. ICH
8. The nurse is caring for a client who sustained an open head injury. For which complication should the nurse monitor?
   1. Cerebral edema
   2. Coup contrecoup
   3. ICH
   4. ICP
9. The nurse assesses a client diagnosed with an acceleration-deceleration head injury. Which is the nurse's priority assessment? *(Select all that apply.)*
   1. Urinary
   2. Cardiac
   3. Respiratory
   4. Neurological
   5. Gastrointestinal

10. Which assessment data support the diagnosis of a parietal lobe brain injury?
    1. Unable to demonstrate effective hand-to-mouth coordination
    2. Demonstrating behaviors associated with receptive aphasia
    3. Experiencing problems related to balance
    4. Demonstrating dysphagia

See Answers on pages 338-340.

Goals of Care

- Maintaining cerebral perfusion
- Preventing and reducing increasing ICP
- Preventing a secondary injury
- Maintaining hemodynamic balance
  - Oxygenation
  - Fluid and electrolyte balance
  - Vital signs
- Preservation of neurological function

Assessment

- Emergency assessment
  - Airway
  - Breathing
  - Circulation
- Vital signs
  - Glasgow coma scale (GCS) used to assess
    - Severity of brain injury
    - Loss of consciousness: eye opening; motor movement; verbal response
    - Minimum score: 3
    - Maximum score: 15
    - Mild TBI
      - GCS score: 13 to 15
      - Possible loss of consciousness for up to 15 minutes
      - No hospitalization is required unless symptoms worsen.
      - Caregiver is taught the signs and symptoms to assess.
    - Moderate TBI
      - GCS score: 9 to 12
      - Loss of consciousness for up to 6 hours
      - Hospital admission is required.
      - High risk for a rapid decline in clinical status, cerebral edema, and ICP
        - Complete frequent assessments.
        - Perform a baseline CT scan.
        - Repeat the CT scan if changes in the neurological status occur.
    - Severe TBI
      - GCS score: 8 or less
      - Loss of consciousness for several hours
      - Critical care admission
        - Provide mechanical ventilation.
        - Monitor ICP.
        - Provide hemodynamic monitoring.

- ○ Prevent hypercapnia, hypoxia, and hypotension.
- ○ Assess alertness, orientation (person, place, and time), and arousable to verbal and painful stimuli.
  - Ability to move extremities
  - Pupils equal, round, react to light, and accommodation (PERRLA)
    - Pupils equal and reactive to light
    - Pupillary asymmetry
    - Pupillary reaction to light: slow, a parasympathetic response, indicating a brainstem injury
    - Pupillary dilation: fully dilated (blown pupil, cranial nerve III compression [herniation]); a sympathetic response

Diagnostics

- CT scan
  - Gold standard for acute injury
    - To identify the type, location, and extent of the brain damage
      - Mass lesions
      - Hemorrhage
      - Cerebral edema
      - Midline shift (a shift of the brain past its center line)
  - Easy to compare scans for changes
- Magnetic resonance imaging (MRI)
  - Is primarily used for subacute and chronic TBIs
  - Is not used for unstable acute TBI
- EEG
  - To demonstrate abnormal brain electrical activity attributable to a brain injury
- ICP monitoring
- GCS assessment tool
- Cerebrospinal fluid (CSF) studies
  - To identify an infection
- Postinjury neuropsychological testing
  - To evaluate the extent of the dysfunction
  - To identify the specific area of brain damage

Treatments

- Surgical interventions may be indicated.
  - Shift of brain to one side (displaced)
  - Increasing ICP
    - Decompressive craniectomy: neurosurgical procedure to decrease ICP
      - A piece of the skull is removed to allow room for the swelling brain to expand.
    - Craniotomy: neurosurgical procedure during which a piece of the skull is temporarily removed
      - Hematoma evacuation is often required to treat EDH, SDH, and ICH.
      - The piece of skull is replaced once the surgical procedure is completed.
    - Burr hole evacuation
      - Holes are drilled through the skull to relieve pressure, drain blood, or remove a clot.
      - Can be performed under local anesthesia

- Hypertonic intravenous (IV) solutions
  - Draws water from the brain tissue to decrease cerebral edema and ICP
  - Uses hypertonic saline or mannitol (osmotic diuretic)

Nursing Interventions

- Hemodynamic monitoring
  - Management: heart rate; blood pressure; mean arterial pressure (MAP)
    - MAP less than 60 mm Hg (normal range: between 70 and 100 mm Hg)
    - MAP is an indicator of perfusion to the vital organs.
  - Arterial blood pressure line (A-line)
    - Is the most accurate tool for measuring partial pressure of carbon dioxide ($PaCO_2$)
      - An increase in $PaCO_2$ results in increased compensatory blood volume and increased ICP.
- Administer vasopressors as prescribed to maintain MAP and to prevent hypotension.
- ICP monitoring
  - Management: Ventricular drain may be placed to drain the CSF from the ventricles and to maintain a safe ICP level.
    - Normal ICP range: between 5 and 15 mm Hg
- Cerebral perfusion pressure (CPP)
  - $MAP - ICP = CPP$
    - Pressure that drives blood flow
      - Oxygen perfusion
- Administer IV fluids as prescribed.
- Pulmonary monitoring
  - Management: respiratory rate; quality of respirations
- Maintain acid-base balance.
  - Monitor arterial blood gases.
- Maintain body temperature.
  - Between 36° and 37° C
  - Cerebral oxygen requirements increase with fever.
- Control the environment.
  - Low light
  - Quiet
  - Limited activities
    - Plan interventions to decrease stimulation.
    - Distribute the interventions throughout the shift.
    - Limit visitations.
- Monitor for infections.
  - Meningitis
  - Encephalitis: fever; chills; lethargy; neck and back stiffness; severe neck pain; sensitivity to light
  - Monitor for CSF leaks.
    - Indicates skull fracture
      - Is an open pathway for bacteria to enter
      - Is a high risk for meningitis
      - Can lead to encephalitis
    - Clear fluid draining
      - Nose
      - Ears

- Insertion of lines and monitors increase the risk for infection
  - ICP monitor
  - A-line
  - IV line
- Immunosuppression attributable to trauma
  - Stress to the body
  - Results in a decreased ability to fight infection
- Surgery

APPLICATION AND REVIEW

11. The nurse is caring for a client with a GCS score of 8. Which intervention should the nurse implement?
    1. ICP monitoring
    2. Neurological assessment
    3. Mechanical ventilation
    4. Hospitalization
12. Which pupil response to light serves to help confirm a diagnosis of brainstem injury?
    1. Brisk
    2. Sluggish
    3. Full dilation
    4. Unilaterally fixed
13. A client is being evaluated for the cause of an acute brain injury. To determine the type, location, and extent of the injury, the nurse should anticipate preparing the client for which diagnostic test?
    1. CT scan
    2. MRI
    3. CSF scan
    4. EEG
14. Which condition makes a client a candidate for a burr hole evacuation procedure?
    1. Temporal lobe injury
    2. SDH
    3. Increasing cerebral edema
    4. GCS score of 11
15. Which factors should the nurse assess when monitoring a client's hemodynamic status post head injury? *(Select all that apply.)*
    1. Body temperature: 100° F
    2. Blood pressure: 110/74 mm Hg
    3. Respiratory rate: 20 breaths per minute
    4. Heart rate: 100 beats per minute
    5. MAP: 60 mm Hg
16. Which ICP results are considered within normal limits? *(Select all that apply.)*
    1. 0 mm Hg
    2. 7 mm Hg
    3. 12 mm Hg
    4. 17 mm Hg
    5. 19 mm Hg
17. Which environmental controls should be included in the plan of care of a client who is being treated for acute TBI? *(Select all that apply.)*
    1. Keep the room cool.
    2. Limit visitations.
    3. Keep the room dimly lighted.
    4. Provide for noise management.
    5. Space nursing interventions throughout the day.
18. Which is the primary symptom of a CSF leak?
    1. Headache
    2. Encephalitis
    3. Photosensitivity
    4. Decreased ICP

See Answers on pages 338-340.

Prevention

- Brain injury is the leading cause of disability in the world.
- Wear a seat belt in a motor vehicle.
- Use the correct car seat for a child.
- Wear a helmet when riding on a motorcycle.
- Avoid driving while under the influence of alcohol or drugs.
- Wear appropriate protective gear.
  - Athletics in sporting events
  - Leisure activities (riding bicycles)

Fluids and Electrolytes in Brain Injury

- Maintaining fluid and electrolyte balance is extremely important for maintaining the best outcomes after a brain injury.
- Many symptoms of electrolyte imbalance are similar to those symptoms of brain injury.
- Sodium, potassium, and calcium are the primary electrolyte imbalances resulting from a TBI.
  - Causes
    - Trauma to the cell membrane from the injury itself
    - Autoregulation impairment: syndrome of inappropriate antidiuretic hormone secretion (SIADH)
    - Cerebral salt washing (often mistaken for SIADH)
    - Diabetes insipidus
- Central nervous system (CNS) plays a major role in water-sodium balance.
  - Autoregulation
    - Is driven by thirst and salt appetite
    - Is disrupted with a brain injury
  - Sodium
    - Extracellular and intracellular sodium concentrations
      - Sodium-potassium adenosine triphosphatase (ATPase) pump
    - Total sodium concentration in body
      - Excretion by the kidneys
    - Hyponatremia (low serum sodium): less than 135 millimoles per liter (mmol/L)
      - Hypotonic fluid administration
      - Increased antidiuretic hormone (ADH) levels
        - Stress response
        - Made by the hypothalamus
        - Is stored in the posterior pituitary gland
        - Regulation of water conservation
      - SIADH
        - ADH is released.
        - Water conservation: excess water; hypotonic (low osmotic pressure); no dehydration
        - Hyponatremia: diluted urine test; the level is not low as a result of a deficiency
        - TBI: SAH; brain tumor; encephalitis; meningitis
        - SIADH reverses on its own without treatment.
          - Treat if the client is symptomatic.
          - If the serum and sodium levels continue to decrease, treat with water restriction to result in a slow rise of sodium.

- Cerebral salt wasting
  - TBI: tumor; ischemic stroke; meningitis
  - CNS impairment
  - Renal loss of sodium: hyponatremia; loss of water
  - Is self-limiting after 2 to 4 weeks. Treat with fluids and sodium replacements.
  - Symptoms of hyponatremia: nausea and vomiting; headache; confusion; fatigue; muscle weakness and spasms; irritability; seizures; coma
- Hypernatremia
  - Indicator of brain injury severity
  - Caused by diabetes insipidus
    - CNS impairment
      - TBI: SAH; intracerebral hemorrhage; pituitary damage (severe cerebral edema); brainstem death
    - Impairment of ADH release
      - Unable to concentrate urine
      - Large volume of water output (diluted urine)
      - High serum sodium
      - Dehydration
    - Excess osmotic diuretic administration
  - Symptoms of hypernatremia: thirst (dehydration); muscle twitching; altered mental status; seizure; coma; death
- Ischemia and injury damage to cell membranes
  - Dysfunction of the sodium-potassium pump
  - Dysfunction of the calcium pump
    - Causes water, sodium, and calcium to rush into the cells
    - Cellular edema
    - Influx of calcium
    - Cell membrane breakdown
    - Toxic enzymatic reactions
    - Cell death
    - Hypercalcemia symptoms affecting the CNS include weakness, lethargy, altered mental status, and coma.
    - Causes potassium to rush out of the cells
    - Hyperkalemia
      - Can be life threatening
      - Symptoms include lethargy, weakness, numbness and tingling, cardiac dysrhythmias, and paralysis
      - Acidosis results
        - Ionic influx and outflow
        - Anaerobic metabolism

APPLICATION AND REVIEW

19. Which statement supports a client's diagnosis of hypernatremia?

1. "I'm so thirsty; I can't seem to drink enough."
2. "I'm nauseated again; I feel like vomiting."
3. "I've got a horrible headache."
4. "I'm too weak to hold a cup."

See Answer on page 338-340.

1. **1 Secondary TBI is a result of a cellular response to an initial injury; hypoxia triggered by strangulation is an example of such an event.**

   2 Primary TBI is a result of direct damage to the brain tissue; hemorrhage is an example of such damage. **3** Primary TBI is a result of direct damage to the brain tissue; a brain contusion is an example of such damage. **4** Primary TBI is a result of direct damage to the brain tissue; blunt force to the brain is an example of such damage.

   Client Need: Physiological Integrity; **Cognitive Level:** Application; **Integrated Process:** Teaching and Learning

2. **Answers: 1, 2, 3, 5**

   1 TBI is often described as having a cloudy or foggy mind. **2** TBI often causes changes in sleep patterns. **3** TBI is often associated with depression. **5** TBI is often associated with cognitive problems.

   4 TBI is often associated with irritability, anger, and a quick temper.

   Client Need: Physiological Integrity; **Cognitive Level:** Analysis; **Nursing Process:** Assessment

3. **Answers: 3, 4**

   3 Impaired balance is a risk factor for falls, which is a common source of physical injury. **4** Poor anger control is a risk factor for injury resulting from harming one's self and/or attempting to harm others.

   1 Although speech issues can exist, they do not present the increased risk for injury that the correct options create. **2** Although concrete thinking can exist, it does not present the increased risk for injury that the correct options create. **5** Although concentration issues can exist, they do not present the increased risk for injury that the correct options create.

   Client Need: Health Promotion and Maintenance; **Cognitive Level:** Analysis; **Nursing Process:** Assessment

4. **2 Brain cells start to become damaged after 3 minutes without oxygen.**

   1, 3, 4 Brain cells start to become damaged after 3 minutes without oxygen.

   Client Need: Physiological Integrity; **Cognitive Level:** Knowledge; **Integrated Process:** Teaching and Learning

5. **3 A TIA does not cause permanent damage to the brain cells.**

   1 A TIA is a nonsustained hypoxic event that usually lasts minutes to hours. **2** A TIA has similar causes as other forms of ischemic strokes. **4** A TIA can be treated with medication and lifestyle changes.

   Client Need: Health Promotion and Maintenance; **Cognitive Level:** Comprehension; **Integrated Process:** Teaching and Learning

6. **3 A toxic brain injury causes the ineffective use of oxygen in the blood by the brain cells.**

   1 The impact of a closed brain injury results in brain swelling. **2** A hypoxic brain injury greatly minimizes the amount of oxygen in the blood. **4** A concussion (closed brain injury) can result in the microscopic damage to the blood vessels in the brain.

   Client Need: Physiological Integrity; **Cognitive Level:** Comprehension; **Integrated Process:** Teaching and Learning

7. **3 Coup contrecoup results in two contusions; one contusion is caused by the direct impact, and the other contusion is on the other side of the brain as it comes into forceful contact with the skull.**

   1 Open injuries require the opening of the dura mater; the dual impact sites are not present. **2** A concussion is the result of the direct impact to the head; the second site of impact is not present. **4** An ICH involves bleeding from within the brain tissue itself; the dual impact sites are not present.

   Client Need: Physiological Integrity; **Cognitive Level:** Application; **Integrated Process:** Teaching and Learning

8. **3 An open head injury exposes the dura mater because of significant applied direct force that results in a contusion with associated bleeding.**

   1 Cerebral edema is associated with a closed head injury that has traumatized the brain causing swelling. **2** Coup contrecoup results in dual contusions on the brain from an acceleration-deceleration closed head injury. **4** Increased ICP is associated with closed head injuries resulting in brain swelling.

   Client Need: Physiological Integrity; **Cognitive Level:** Analysis; **Nursing Process:** Assessment

9. **Answers: 3, 4**

    3 Due to the possibility of dyspnea, a respiratory assessment and monitoring is a priority. **4** Due to the possibility of changes to the level of consciousness and pupils, a neurological assessment and monitoring is a priority.

    1 Although appropriate, a urinary assessment is not as critical as the respiratory and neurological assessments. **2** Although appropriate, a cardiac assessment is not as critical as the respiratory and neurological assessments. **5** Although appropriate, a gastrointestinal assessment is not as critical as the respiratory and neurological assessments.

    Client Need: Physiological Integrity; **Cognitive Level:** Analysis; **Nursing Process:** Planning

10. **2 Receptive aphasia involves difficulty understanding the spoken or written language.**

    1 Poor coordination is associated with damage to the cerebellum. **3** Poor balance is associated with damage to the cerebellum. **4** Difficulty swallowing is associated with damage to the brainstem.

    Client Need: Physiological Integrity; **Cognitive Level:** Application; **Nursing Process:** Assessment

11. **3 A GCS score of 8 or less indicates severe TBI and requires admission to a critical care unit where mechanical ventilation is available.**

    1 Hospitalization and ICP monitoring is required for any client with a GCS score of 12 or lower. **2** Neurological assessment is required for any client suspected of a TBI. **4** Hospitalization is required for any client with a GCS score of 12 or lower.

    Client Need: Physiological Integrity; **Cognitive Level:** Application; **Nursing Process:** Implementation

12. **2 In response to a brainstem injury, pupils bilaterally react sluggishly.**

    1, 3, 4 In response to a brainstem injury, pupils bilaterally react sluggishly.

    Client Need: Physiological Integrity; **Cognitive Level:** Comprehension; **Nursing Process:** Assessment

13. **1 A CT scan is the gold standard for acute TBI diagnosis and can identify the type, location, and extent of the injury.**

    2 An MRI is primarily used for diagnosing subacute and chronic TBIs. **3** A CSF scan is used to identify a possible infection and abnormal flow of spinal fluid. **4** An EEG demonstrates the brain's electrical activity.

    Client Need: Health Promotion and Maintenance; **Cognitive Level:** Application; **Nursing Process:** Planning

14. **2 The burr hole evacuation procedure is used to drain a collection of blood associated with an SDH.**

    1 Temporal lobe injury is not necessarily a criterion for this procedure. **3** Hypertonic IV solution would be used to help decrease cerebral edema. **4** A GCS sore of 11 would not necessarily be a criterion for this procedure.

    Client Need: Physiological Integrity; **Cognitive Level:** Application; **Nursing Process:** Planning

15. **Answers: 2, 4, 5**

    2 Hemodynamic monitoring includes blood pressure. **4** Hemodynamic monitoring includes heart rate. **5** Hemodynamic monitoring includes MAP.

    1 Hemodynamic monitoring does not include body temperature. **3** Hemodynamic monitoring does not include respiratory rate.

    Client Need: Physiological Integrity; **Cognitive Level:** Application; **Integrated Process:** Communication and Documentation

16. **Answers: 1, 2, 3**

    1 Normal ICP is between 0 and 15 mm Hg. **2** Normal ICP is between 0 and 15 mm Hg. **3** Normal ICP is between 0 and 15 mm Hg.

    4, 5 Normal ICP is between 0 and 15 mm Hg.

    Client Need: Health Promotion and Maintenance; **Cognitive Level:** Knowledge; **Integrated Process:** Teaching and Learning

17. **Answers: 2, 3, 4, 5**

    2 Environmental control should include limiting stimulation in its various forms; visitors should be limited and spaced out over time. **3** Environmental control should include limiting stimulation in its various forms; rooms should be dimly lighted. **4** Environmental control should include limiting stimulation in its various forms; noise levels should be kept low. **5** Environmental control should include limiting stimulation in its various forms; activities should be evenly distributed throughout the day.

1 Keeping the room cool does not provide environmental control that limits stimulation in its various forms.

Client Need: Health Promotion and Maintenance; **Cognitive Level:** Application; **Nursing Process:** Planning

18. **2 The primary risk associated with a CSF leakage is infection; encephalitis is an associated infection.**

1 Although a positional headache is possible, the primary risk is infection. **3** Although photosensitivity is possible, the primary risk is infection. **4** Although decreased ICP is possible, the primary risk is infection.

Client Need: Health Promotion and Maintenance; **Cognitive Level:** Analysis; **Nursing Process:** Assessment

19. **1 Hypernatremia is characterized by extreme thirst.**

2 Hyponatremia is characterized by nausea and vomiting. **3** Hyponatremia is characterized by headaches. **4** Hyponatremia is characterized by muscle weakness.

Client Need: Physiological Integrity; **Cognitive Level:** Analysis; **Nursing Process:** Assessment

Fluids and Electrolytes in Diabetic Ketoacidosis and Hyperglycemic Hyperosmolar State

19

DIABETIC KETOACIDOSIS AND HYPERGLYCEMIC HYPEROSMOLAR SYNDROME OVERVIEW

Diabetic Ketoacidosis and Hyperglycemic Hyperosmolar Syndrome

- Diabetic ketoacidosis (DKA) and hyperglycemic hyperosmolar syndrome (HHS) are two acute complications of diabetes.
- Many differences exist between the two complications; however, the underlying mechanism is a reduction in the net effective concentration of circulating insulin, coupled with a concomitant increase of counterregulatory hormones.
- Counterregulatory hormones
  - A counterregulatory hormone is a hormone that opposes the actions of another.
    - Released during hypoglycemia and under stress conditions
    - Affects the liver and peripheral tissues
  - The action of insulin is counter regulated by
    - Glucagon
    - Catecholamines
      - Epinephrine (adrenaline)
      - Norepinephrine (noradrenaline)
    - Cortisol
    - Growth hormone
- DKA and HHS are the leading causes of morbidity and mortality among clients with diabetes.
  - The cause of death in clients with DKA and HHS is rarely a result of a metabolic complication; rather, it is related to the underlying medical illness that precipitated the metabolic decompensation.
    - Treatment requires quick recognition of the precipitating causes (Box 19.1).

Diabetic Ketoacidosis

- Most clients with DKA have type I diabetes.
  - Clients with type 2 diabetes are also at risk during catabolic stress stages of acute illness.
- DKA is more common in adults than in children.
  - Initial manifestation of diabetes is 20% of adult clients.
- DKA is the most common cause of mortality in children and adolescents with type I diabetes.
  - Initial manifestation of DKA is between 30% and 40% of children with type I diabetes.
- Pathogenesis (Figure 19.1)
  - DKA results from the lack of, or ineffectiveness of, insulin with a concomitant elevation of counterregulatory hormones.
    - Counterregulatory hormones: glucagon; catecholamines; cortisol; growth hormone
    - Characteristics: hyperglycemia; metabolic acidosis; increased circulating total body ketone concentration
    - Elevated hepatic glucose production represents the primary pathogenic disruption responsible for hyperglycemia in clients with DKA.

BOX 19.1	Interprofessional Management: Diabetic Ketoacidosis and Hyperosmolar Hyperglycemic Syndrome

Diagnostic Assessment
- History and physical examination
- Blood studies, including immediate blood glucose, complete blood count, pH, ketones, electrolytes, blood urea nitrogen, arterial or venous blood gases
- Urinalysis, including specific gravity, glucose, and acetone

Management
- Administration of intravenous fluids
- Intravenous administration of short-acting insulin
- Electrolyte replacement
- Assessment of mental status
- Recording of intake and output
- Central venous pressure monitoring, if indicated
- Assessment of blood glucose levels
- Assessment of blood and urine for ketones
- Electrocardiographic monitoring
- Assessment of cardiovascular and respiratory status

From Lewis, S. L., Bucher, L., Heitkemper, M. M., Harding, M. M., Kwong, J., & Roberts, D. (2017). *Medical-surgical nursing: Assessment and management of clinical problems* (10th ed.). St. Louis: Elsevier.

- Precipitating factors include infections, poor compliance with therapy, intercurrent illnesses, and psychological stress.
- Infection is the most common precipitating factor for DKA.
  - Urinary tract infection (UTI) and pneumonia account for a majority of the 30% to 50% of the clients with these infections.
  - Other acute conditions may cause DKA.
    - Cerebrovascular accident
    - Pancreatitis
    - Pulmonary embolism
    - Alcohol or drug abuse
    - Myocardial infarction (MI)
    - Trauma
    - Medications that affect carbohydrate metabolism
      - Corticosteroids
      - Thiazides
      - Sympathomimetic agents
      - Pentamidine
- Assessment
  - Physical examination shows dehydration.
    - Loss of skin turgor
    - Tachycardia
    - Dry mucous membranes
    - Hypotension
      - Mental status can vary, from full alertness to profound lethargy.
        - 20% of clients are hospitalized with a loss of consciousness.
  - Respiratory assessment
    - Acetone on the breath, which causes the client's breath to smell similar to nail poli[sh] (sweet and fruity odor)
    - Labored Kussmaul respirations (deep, labored breathing pattern)
- Diagnostics
  - Clinical signs usually rapidly develop over a period of less than 24 hours.

PATHOPHYSIOLOGY MAP

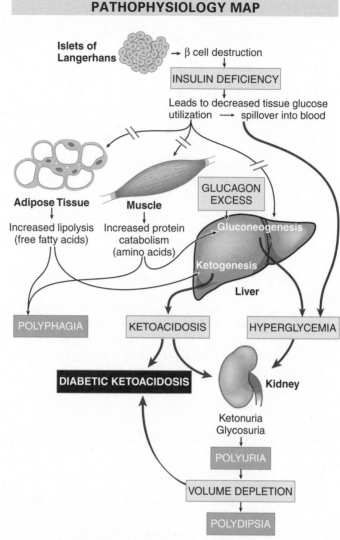

FIGURE 19.1 Metabolic events leading to diabetic ketoacidosis. (From Kumar, V., Abbas, A. K., Fausto, N., & Aster, J. C. [2010]. *Robbins and Cotran pathologic basis of disease* [8th ed.]. Philadelphia: Saunders.)

- Consist of the triad: hyperglycemia; hyperketonemia; metabolic acidosis
- Diagnostic criteria
  - Mild DKA
    - Plasma glucose: greater than 250 mg/dL
    - Arterial pH: between 7.25 and 7.30
    - Serum bicarbonate: between 15 and 18 mEq/L
    - Positive urine ketone
    - Positive serum ketone
    - Variable effective serum osmolality
    - Anion gap: greater than 10 mEq/L
    - Alteration in sensorium or mental obtundation (alertness)

- Moderate DKA
  - Plasma glucose: greater than 250 mg/dL
  - Arterial pH: between 7.00 and less than 7.24
  - Serum bicarbonate: between 10 and 15 mEq/L
  - Positive urine ketone
  - Positive serum ketone
  - Variable effective serum osmolality
  - Anion gap: greater than 12 mEq/L
  - Alteration in sensorium or mental obtundation (alert or drowsy)
- Severe DKA
  - Plasma glucose: greater than 250 mg/dL
  - Arterial pH: less than 7.00
  - Serum bicarbonate: less than 10 mEq/L
  - Positive urine ketone
  - Positive serum ketone
  - Variable effective serum osmolality
  - Anion gap: greater than 12 mEq/L
  - Alteration in sensorium or mental obtundation (stuporous or comatose)
- Signs and symptoms
  - May be exhibited for several days before the development of DKA
    - Polyuria: abnormally large amounts of urine
    - Polydipsia: intense thirst, despite adequate intake of fluids
    - Polyphagia: increased hunger accompanied by weight loss
  - Presenting symptoms
    - Vomiting
    - Abdominal pain; reported in 40% to 75% of cases
- Goals of care
  - Insulin therapy is the cornerstone of DKA management.
- Treatment
  - Administer IV fluids.
    - Determine hydration status.
      - Hypovolemic shock: Administer 0.9% sodium chloride (1 liter per hour).
      - Mild hypotension
        - Evaluate corrected serum sodium level.
          - High serum sodium level: 0.45% sodium chloride (4 to 14 mL/kg/hr), depending on the hydration status
          - Normal serum sodium level: 0.45% sodium chloride (4 to 14 mL/kg/hr), depending on hydration status
          - Low serum sodium level: 0.9% sodium chloride (4 to 14 mL/kg/hr), depending on hydration status
        - When serum glucose reaches 250 mg/dL, change to 5% dextrose with 0.45% sodium chloride at 150 to 250 mL/hr with adequate insulin (0.05 to 0.10 U/kg/hr) intravenous (IV) subcutaneous (SC) infusion or 5 to 10 U every 2 hours to maintain a serum glucose level between 150 and 200 mg/dL until metabolic control is achieved.
      - Cardiogenic shock: monitoring hemodynamics
  - Insulin (IV route)
    - Insulin: regular 0.15 U/kg as IV bonus

- 0.1 U/kg/hr IV insulin infusion
  - If the serum glucose level does not fall between 50 and 70 mg/dL within the first hour, double the insulin infusion hourly until the glucose level falls between 50 and 70 mg/dL within the first hour.
- Insulin (SC and intramuscular [IM] routes)
  - Insulin: regular 0.4 U/kg, ½ IV bonus, ½ SC or IM
  - 0.1 U/kg/hr regular insulin SC or IM
    - If serum glucose does not fall between 50 and 70 mg/dL within the first hour, administer hourly IV insulin bolts (10 U) until the glucose level falls between 50 and 70 mg/dL.
- Potassium
  - If serum potassium is less than 3.3 mEq/L, hold the insulin and administer 40 mEq/L of potassium until the level is equal to or greater than 3.3 mEq/L.
  - If serum potassium is equal to or greater than 5.0 mEq/L, do not administer potassium, but recheck the potassium level every 2 hours.
  - If serum potassium is equal to or greater than 3.3 mEq/L but less than 5.0 mEq/L, administer between 20 and 30 mEq/L of potassium in each liter of IV fluid to keep the serum potassium level between 4 and 5 mEq/L.
- Assess the need for sodium bicarbonate.
  - Dilute 100 mmol of sodium bicarbonate in 400 mL of water, infuse at 200 mL/hr.
    - pH less than 6.9: Repeat sodium bicarbonate administration every 2 hours until pH is greater than 7.0, and monitor serum potassium.
    - pH greater than 7.0: Administer no sodium bicarbonate.
    - pH between 6.9 and 7.0: Dilute 50 mmol of sodium bicarbonate in 200 mL of water, infuse at 200 mL/hr.
      - Repeat the administration of bicarbonate every 2 hours until the pH level is greater than 7.0.
      - Monitor serum potassium.
- Complications
  - Hypoglycemia
    - Is the most common complication during insulin infusion; reported in 10% to 25% of clients
    - Risk factor: failure to reduce insulin infusion rate and/or to use dextrose-containing solutions when glucose levels reach 250 mg/dL
  - Hypokalemia
    - Insulin therapy and the correction of acidosis decrease serum potassium levels by stimulating potassium uptake in the peripheral tissues.
      - Prevention
        - Replace potassium loss with IV potassium as soon as the serum level is less than or equal to 5.0 mEq/L.
    - Clients with normal and decreased serum potassium levels
      - Insulin replacement may precipitate profound hypokalemia (initial serum level less than or equal to 3.3 mEq/L).
      - IV infusion replacement of potassium should begin immediately.
  - Cerebral edema
    - Is a rare, serious complication
    - Occurs in approximately 1% of children with a mortality rate between 40% and 90%
    - Characteristics
      - Decreased level of consciousness (LOC)

- Headache
- Seizures
- Sphincter incontinence
- Pupillary changes
- Papilledema
  - Increased pressure in and around the brain, causing the optic nerve inside the eye to swell
  - Symptoms: visual disturbances; headache; vomiting
- Bradycardia
- Respiratory arrest
- Nursing interventions
  - Check Chem-7 (four electrolytes [sodium, potassium, chloride, and bicarbonate]), and blood urea nitrogen (BUN), creatinine, and glucose levels every 2 to 4 hours until stable.
  - After resolution, if the client is not orally intaking fluids or foods (NPO; nothing by mouth [*nil per os*]), continue IV insulin and supplements with SC regular insulin as needed (PRN [*pro re nata*]).
  - When the client is able to eat, initiate a multidose insulin regimen and adjust PRN.
  - Continue IV insulin infusion for 1 to 2 hours after SC insulin is started to ensure adequate plasma insulin levels.
  - Continue to look for precipitating causes.
- Prevention
  - Client education
    - Importance of early contact with the client's primary care provider
    - Importance of insulin during an illness: Never discontinue insulin without contacting the client's primary care provider.
    - Goals and the use of supplemental short- or rapid-acting insulin
    - Treatment of acute illnesses: fever suppression; treatment of infection
    - During nausea episodes: prompt initiation of liquid diet containing carbohydrates and salt
    - Recordkeeping: temperature; respiratory rate; pulse; blood glucose; insulin doses; oral intake; weight
    - Information on the signs and symptoms of new onset and decompensated diabetes for friends, family, school personal, and health care workers
  - Effective follow-up treatment programs
    - Approximately 50% of admissions could be prevented with improved follow-up treatment and adherence to self-care standards.

APPLICATION AND REVIEW

1. Which catecholamines have the opposite action to that of insulin? *(Select all that apply.)*
   1. Cortisol
   2. Glucagon
   3. Epinephrine
   4. Norepinephrine
   5. Growth hormone
2. Which is the nurse's initial treatment goal when managing a client diagnosed with DKA?
   1. Identification of precipitating cause
   2. Treatment of metabolic complications
   3. Restoration of normal insulin function
   4. Assessment of long-term cardiac-associated complications

3. Which client is at greatest risk for developing DKA?
   1. 23-year-old client diagnosed with type 2 diabetes
   2. 45-year-old female client diagnosed with type 1 diabetes as a 15-year-old child
   3. 7-year-old child diagnosed with type 2 diabetes, secondary to pancreatitis
   4. 10-year-old child whose type 1 diabetes is being managed by an insulin pump
4. Which condition is supportive of a diagnosis of DKA?
   1. Hypoglycemia
   2. Hypoketonemia
   3. Metabolic acidosis
   4. Respiratory alkalosis
5. The nurse is providing information on the development of DKA to a client who has been diagnosed with diabetes. Which instructions should the nurse include in the discussion? *(Select all that apply.)*
   1. Avoid consuming alcohol.
   2. Limit the consumption of sugar.
   3. Practice some form of stress management.
   4. Engage in regular, cardio-focused exercises.
   5. Recognize the early signs of common infections.
6. Which assessment question asked by the nurse during an interview with a client diagnosed with diabetes demonstrates an understanding of the most common cause of DKA?
   1. "Are you experiencing chest pain?"
   2. "Do you take a corticosteroid medication on a regular basis?"
   3. "Do you have any signs of a urinary tract infection?"
   4. "How much alcohol do you consume in a typical week?"
7. Which assessment findings documented in a client's medical record support a diagnosis of DKA? *(Select all that apply.)*
   1. Fruity smelling breath
   2. Heart rate: 106 beats per minute
   3. Serum glucose: 200 mg/dL
   4. Blood pressure: 89/58 mm Hg
   5. 24-hour urine output: 1800 mL
8. When treating DKA, what is the goal of IV fluids and insulin therapies?
   1. Maintaining the serum glucose levels between 150 and 200 mg/dL
   2. Restoring the client's hydration status
   3. Normalizing urinary output
   4. Reversing hypotension
9. The nurse is administering both insulin and potassium to a client experiencing DKA. Which intervention should the nurse implement when the client's serum potassium level is currently 5.2 mEq/L?
   1. Hold the potassium, and recheck the serum potassium level every 2 hours.
   2. Immediately notify the primary health care provider.
   3. Hold the insulin until serum potassium level is less than 3.3 mEq/dL.
   4. Administer between 20 and 30 mEq of potassium in each liter of prescribed IV fluid.
10. The nurse is caring for a client diagnosed with type 1 diabetes who is experiencing nausea. Which information should the nurse provide to this client?
    1. Hold the insulin until the nausea subsides.
    2. Start a liquid diet that contains both carbohydrates and salt.
    3. Avoid consuming food or liquids to minimize the risk of vomiting.
    4. Immediately visit the emergency department of the nearest hospital.

See Answers on pages 357–360.

Hyperglycemic Hyperosmolar Syndrome

- Most clients with hyperglycemic hyperosmolar syndrome (HHS) have type 2 diabetes.
- Initial manifestation of diabetes develops in 7% to 17% of clients.
  - Commonly, clients with HHS have undiagnosed diabetes, are between the ages of 55 and 70 years old, and are frequently nursing home residents.
- Clients diagnosed with HHS have a decreased concentration of free fatty acids (FFAs), cortisol, growth hormone, and glucagon, compared with clients with DKA.
- Precipitating factors
  - Infection
    - Infection is the major factor, occurring in 30% to 60% of clients with DKA.
    - UTIs and pneumonia are the two most common infections.
  - Acute illnesses: cerebrovascular accident; MI
  - Medications: glucocorticoids; thiazides diuretics; phenytoin; beta blockers
- Assessment
  - Physical examination reveals volume depletion.
  - Neurological findings (may cause a misdiagnosis of stroke)
    - Hemiparesis: unilateral muscle weakness or partial paralysis
    - Hemianopsia: visual disturbance, producing decreased vision or anopsia (blindness) in one half of the visual field
- Diagnostics
  - Most clients develop symptoms over several weeks.
  - Diagnostic criteria
    - Plasma glucose: greater than 600 mg/dL
    - Arterial pH: greater than 7.30
    - Serum bicarbonate: greater than 15 mEq/L
    - Small urine ketone
    - Small serum ketone
    - Effective serum osmolality: greater than 320 mOsm/kg
    - Anion gap: 12 mEq/L
    - Alteration in sensorium or mental obtundation (stuporous or comatose)
- Signs and symptoms
  - Altered sensorium: most common presentation
  - Polyuria: abnormally large amounts of urine
  - Polydipsia: intense thirst, despite adequate intake of fluids
  - Progressive decline in LOC
- Goals of care
  - Insulin therapy is the cornerstone of HHS management.
- Treatment
  - Administer IV fluids.
    - Determine hydration status.
      - Hypovolemic shock: Administer 0.9% sodium chloride (1 liter per hour).
      - Mild hypotension
        - Evaluate corrected serum sodium level.
          - High serum sodium level: 0.45% sodium chloride (4 to 14 mL/kg/hr), depending on the hydration status
          - Normal serum sodium level: 0.45% sodium chloride (4 to 14 mL/kg/hr), depending on hydration status

- ○ Low serum sodium level: 0.9% sodium chloride (4 to 14 mL/kg/hr), depending on hydration status
- ○ When serum glucose reaches 300 mg/dL, change to 5% dextrose with 0.45% sodium chloride and decrease insulin to 0.05 to 0.10 U/kg/hr to maintain a serum glucose level between 250 and 300 mg/dL until plasma osmolality is less than 315 mOsm/kg and the client is mentally alert.
  - ▪ Cardiogenic shock: monitoring hemodynamics
- Insulin
  - ▪ Regular 0.15 U/kg as IV bonus
  - ▪ 0.1 U/kg/hr IV insulin infusion
  - ▪ Check the serum glucose level hourly. If the serum glucose level does not fall to at least 50 mg/dL in the first hour, double the insulin dose hourly until the serum glucose level falls at a steady hourly rate to between 50 and 70 mg/dL.
- Potassium
  - ▪ If serum potassium is less than 3.3 mEq/L, hold the insulin and administer 40 mEq/L of potassium until the level is equal to or greater than 3.3 mEq/L.
  - ▪ If serum potassium is equal to or greater than 5.0 mEq/L, do not administer potassium, but recheck the potassium level every 2 hours.
  - ▪ If serum potassium is equal to or greater than 3.3 mEq/L but less than 5.0 mEq/L, administer between 20 and 30 mEq of potassium in each liter of IV fluid to keep the serum potassium level between 4 and 5 mEq/L.
- Complications
  - Hyperglycemic clients with severe potassium deficiency
    - ▪ Insulation administration may precipitate profound hypokalemia, which may induce life-threatening arrhythmias and respiratory muscle weakness.
    - ▪ If the initial serum potassium level is less than 3.3 mEq/L, potassium replacement should begin promptly.
    - ▪ Insulin therapy should be delayed until the potassium level is greater than or equal to 3.3 MEq/L.
  - Hypoglycemia
    - ▪ Is not frequently observed in clients diagnosed with HHS.
  - Hypokalemia
    - ▪ Insulin therapy and the correction of acidosis decrease serum potassium levels by stimulating potassium uptake in the peripheral tissues.
      - ▪ Prevention
        - ○ Replace potassium loss with IV potassium as soon as the serum level is less than or equal to 5.0 mEq/L.
    - ▪ Clients with normal and decreased serum potassium levels
      - ▪ Insulin replacement may precipitate profound hypokalemia (initial serum level less than or equal to 3.3 mEq/L).
      - ▪ IV replacement of potassium should begin immediately.
- Nursing interventions
  - Check Chem-7 (four electrolytes [sodium, potassium, chloride, and bicarbonate]), BUN, creatinine, and glucose levels every 2 to 4 hours until stable.
  - After resolution, if client is NPO, continue IV insulin and supplements with SC insulin PRN.
  - When the client is able to eat, initiate a multidose SC insulin regimen or previous treatment regimen, and assess metabolic control.

- Continue IV insulin for 1 to 2 hours to ensure control after initiating the daily regimen.
- Continue to look for precipitating causes.
- Prevention
  - Client education
    - Importance of early contact with the client's primary care provider
    - Importance of insulin during an illness: Never discontinue insulin without contacting the client's primary care provider.
    - Goals and the use of supplemental short- or rapid-acting insulin
    - Treatment of acute illnesses: fever suppression; treatment of infection
    - During nausea episodes: prompt initiation of liquid diet containing carbohydrates and salt
    - Recordkeeping: temperature; respiratory rate; pulse; blood glucose; insulin doses; oral intake; weight
    - Information on the signs and symptoms of new onset and decompensated diabetes for friends, family, school personal, and health care workers
  - Effective follow-up treatment programs
    - Approximately 50% of admissions could be prevented with improved follow-up treatment and adherence to self-care standards.

Electrolyte Imbalance

- Sodium
  - Sodium levels in clients diagnosed with DKA and HHS
    - Osmotic diuresis (increased urination)
      - Causes sodium loss
      - Hyperglycemia (excess glucose in the bloodstream) causes osmotic shifts of water from the intracellular space to the extracellular space, causing relative dilutional hyponatremia.
  - Sodium lays a primary role in the body's fluid balance and also in the functioning of the body's muscles and central nervous system (CNS).
  - Normal sodium range: between 135 and 145 mEq/L
    - Hypernatremia: sodium level higher than 145 mEq/L
      - Possible causes: diabetes insipidus; dehydration (fever, vomiting, diarrhea, Cushing syndrome, extensive or excessive exercise, prolonged exposure to environmental heat, diaphoresis)
      - Signs and symptoms: agitation; restlessness; thirst; edema; dry mucous membranes; confusion; seizure and coma (in severe cases)
      - Goal of treatment: to correct and manage the underlying causes and dietary sodium restrictions
      - Treatment
        - Provide oral rehydration therapy and IV fluid replacement.
      - Complications: Rapid reduction may lead to a rapid flow of water, which can result in cerebral edema, permanent brain damage (central pontine myolysis), and possible death.
      - Nursing interventions
        - Know the foods that are high in salt (butter, bacon, canned food, cheese, hot dogs, processed foods, lunch meat, and table salt), and restrict sodium intake.
        - Maintain client safety; the individual client may be confused and/or agitated.
        - Slowly administer hypotonic fluids.
          - The risk to brain tissue is increased, attributable to shifting fluids back into the cells.

- ○ Cells are dehydrated with hypernatremia.
  - ▪ Prevention
    - ○ Adhere to a low-sodium diet.
  - ▪ Hyponatremia: sodium level lower than 135 mEq/L
  - ▪ Possible causes: syndrome of inappropriate antidiuretic hormone (SIADH) secretion; medications (diuretics, antidepressants); water intoxication; a result of disease; thyroid gland disorder; cirrhosis; heart failure; pneumonia; renal failure; cerebral disorders; cancer; severe diarrhea and/or vomiting; diabetes insipidus; Addison disease; hypothyroidism; primary polydipsia
    - ▪ Signs and symptoms: confusion; nausea and vomiting; muscle weakness; seizures; headaches; low energy level and/or fatigue; restlessness; irritability
    - ▪ Goal of treatment: to correct and manage the underlying causes
    - ▪ Treatment
      - ○ Administer IV sodium.
        - ○ Hormone replacement may be necessary (Addison disease).
    - ▪ Complications: If sodium levels drop too rapidly, the individual is at risk of cerebral edema.
    - ▪ Nursing interventions
      - ○ Monitor cardiac, respiratory, neuromuscular, renal, and gastrointestinal (GI) status.
    - ▪ Prevention
      - ○ Treat conditions that may contribute to hyponatremia, such as adrenal gland insufficiency.
- Potassium
  - Potassium levels in clients diagnosed with DKA and HHS
    - ▪ Initial serum potassium level is typically elevated in clients with DKA and HHS.
    - ▪ High levels of potassium develop when a shift of potassium occurs from the intracellular space to the extracellular space due to insulin deficiency, acidemia, and hypertonicity.
    - ▪ Insulin therapy and a correction of acidosis decrease potassium levels by activating cellular uptake in the peripheral tissues.
    - ▪ Prevention: Administer IV potassium during the course of DKA therapy.
  - Potassium is an abundant intracellular electrolyte.
  - Potassium promotes and facilitates electrical impulses responsible for normal functioning of the brain and also for muscular contractions.
  - Normal potassium range: between 3.7 and 5.2 mEq/L
    - ▪ Hyperkalemia: potassium levels higher than 5.2 mEq/L
      - ▪ Possible causes: renal disease; some medications
      - ▪ Signs and symptoms: nausea; muscular weakness; fatigue; paralysis; cardiac dysrhythmias (life-threatening)
      - ▪ Goal of treatment: to correct and manage underlying causes
      - ▪ Treatment
        - ○ Restrict potassium-containing foods.
        - ○ Administer potassium-lowering medications (kayexalate) to promote GI sodium absorption, which causes potassium secretion; consideration of renal dialysis
      - ▪ Complications can be life threatening.
      - ▪ Nursing interventions
        - ○ Monitor cardiac, respiratory, neuromuscular, renal, and GI status.
        - ○ Hold or stop any IV or oral potassium supplements.

- Restrict foods high in potassium (potatoes, pork, tomatoes, avocados, strawberries, spinach, fish, mushrooms, cantaloupe, carrots, raisins, bananas).
  - Prevention
    - Adjust the diet to decrease the potassium dietary load.
    - Manage medications that exacerbate hyperkalemia.
  - Hypokalemia: potassium level lower than 3.7 mEq/L
    - Possible causes
      - Commonly the result of bodily fluid loss: diarrhea; vomiting; diaphoresis
      - Medications: diuretics and laxatives
      - Ketoacidosis
    - Signs and symptoms
      - Mild: asymptomatic
      - Moderate or severe: muscular weakness; tingling and numbness; muscle spasms; fatigue; dizziness and light-headedness; palpitations; constipation; bradycardia; cardiac arrest (severe cases)
    - Goal of treatment: to correct and manage the underlying causes
    - Treatment
      - Provide supplemental potassium.
    - Complications: cardiac arrest in severe cases
    - Nursing interventions
      - Monitor cardiac, respiratory, neuromuscular, renal, and GI status.
      - Check serial potassium levels.
    - Prevention
      - Encourage adherence to a diet rich in potassium.
- Calcium
  - Calcium levels in clients diagnosed with DKA and HHS
    - Phosphate replacement increases the risk of hypocalcemia.
    - Calcium levels should be monitored during infusion.
  - Calcium is essential for bone health and other functions.
  - Normal calcium range: between 8.5 and 10.6 mg/dL
    - Hypercalcemia: calcium level higher than 10.6 mg/dL
      - Possible causes; hyperparathyroidism (endocrine disorder); medications (thiazidine, diuretics, lithium); certain forms of cancer of the lungs; Paget disease; multiple myeloma; non–weight-bearing activity; elevated levels of calcitriol (can occur with sarcoidosis and tuberculosis)
      - Signs and symptoms: thirst; anorexia; renal stones; parenthesis; urinary frequency; bone pain; confusion; abdominal pain; muscular weakness; depression; fatigue; constipation; nausea and/or vomiting; lethargy
      - Goal of treatment: to correct and manage the underlying causes
      - Treatment
      - Provide IV fluid hydration.
      - Administer medications (prednisone, diuretics, bisphosphonates). Severe cases may require dialysis.
      - Complications: increased pain level (administering analgesia may be helpful); pathogenic bone fractures, occurring secondary to the bone decalcification
      - Nursing interventions
        - Magnesium levels are highly associated with calcium levels; correcting and treating magnesium levels is necessary before calcium levels can be corrected.

- ○ Keep the client hydrated, which will help decrease the chances of renal stone formation.
  - ○ Assess for flank or abdominal pain and straining in search for stone formation.
- ○ Monitor cardiac, neuromuscular, renal, and GI status.
- ▪ Prevention
  - ○ Encourage a decrease in calcium-rich foods.
  - ○ Assess the intake of calcium-preserving drugs, such as thiazides, supplements, and vitamin D.
- ▪ Hypocalcemia: calcium level lower than 8.5 mg/dL
  - ▪ Possible causes: renal disease; inadequate dietary calcium; vitamin D deficiency (essential for the absorption of calcium); low magnesium level; hypoparathyroidism; eating disorder; pancreatitis; medications (anticonvulsants, alendronate, bisphosphonates [ibandronate], rifampin, phenytoin, phenobarbital, corticosteroids, plicamycin)
  - ▪ Signs and symptoms: muscular aches and pains; tingling sensation in the feet, fingers, tongue, and lips; bronchospasm, leading to respiratory problems; seizures; tetany; cardiac arrhythmias (can be life threatening)
  - ▪ Goal of treatment: to correct and manage the underlying causes
  - ▪ Treatment
    - ○ Administer calcium supplements, coupled with vitamin D.
  - ▪ Complications: life-threatening cardiac arrhythmias
  - ▪ Nursing interventions
    - ○ Monitor cardiac and respiratory status.
    - ○ Provide client safety; individual client may be at increased risk for bone fractures.
    - ○ Initiate seizure precautions.
    - ○ Administer calcium with vitamin D supplements after meals or at bedtime with a full glass of water.
  - ▪ Prevention
    - ○ Encourage the intake of foods high in calcium (yogurt, sardines, cheese, spinach, collard greens, tofu, milk, rhubarb).
- • Magnesium
  - • Magnesium levels in clients diagnosed with DKA and HHS
    - ▪ Hypomagnesemia is prevalent during a DKA episode, decreases after a partial correction of ketoacidosis, and is resolved after the complete correction of ketoacidosis.
  - • Magnesium plays an essential role in the body's enzyme activities, brain neuron activities, contraction of skeletal muscles, and relaxation of respiratory smooth muscles, as well as in the metabolism of calcium, potassium, and sodium.
  - • Normal magnesium range: between 1.7 and 2.2 mg/dL
    - ▪ Hypermagnesemia: magnesium level higher than 2.2 mg/dL
      - ▪ Possible causes: renal failure; diabetic acidosis; dehydration; hyperparathyroidism; Addison disease; excessive and/or prolonged use of magnesium-containing laxatives or antacids
      - ▪ Signs and symptoms: nausea and/or vomiting; weakness; cardiac arrhythmias; respiratory disturbances (possible respiratory paralysis); CNS depression; hypotension
      - ▪ Goal of treatment: to correct and manage the underlying causes
      - ▪ Treatment
        - ○ Stop administering causative agents (magnesium-containing laxatives; renal dialysis).
        - ○ Administer calcium gluconate, calcium chloride, IV dextrose, and insulin.

- Complications: abnormal heart rhythms
- Nursing interventions
  - Monitor cardiac, respiratory, neuromuscular, renal, and GI status.
  - Watch for electrocardiographic (ECG) changes.
  - Provide for client safety; the individual client may be lethargic or drowsy.
- Prevention
  - Avoid magnesium antacids and laxatives with clients in renal failure.
  - Encourage the client to avoid foods high in magnesium.
- Hypomagnesemia: magnesium level lower than 1.7 mg/dL
  - Possible causes: uncontrolled diabetes; prolonged use of diuretics; hypoparathyroidism; diarrhea; GI disorders (Crohn disease); severe burns; malnutrition; alcoholism; medications (cisplatin, cyclosporine, amphotericin, proton pump inhibitors, aminoglycoside antimicrobial drugs)
  - Signs and symptoms: muscular weakness; tingling and/or numbness; conclusions; muscle spasms; cramps; fatigue; nystagmus (involuntary eye movement, which may cause the eye to move rapidly)
  - Goal of treatment: to correct and manage the underlying causes
  - Treatment
    - Provide pain management.
    - Administer IV fluids and magnesium.
  - Complications: pain and discomfort
  - Nursing interventions
    - Monitor cardiac, respiratory, neuromuscular, renal, and GI status.
    - Assess potassium levels.
      - If potassium level is low, magnesium levels will be hard to elevate.
    - Closely monitor magnesium levels. A client may become magnesium toxic, resulting in depression and a loss of deep tendon reflexes.
    - Initiate seizure precautions.
  - Prevention
    - Encourage foods rich in magnesium, such as avocado, green leafy vegetables, peanut butter, pork, potatoes, oatmeal, nuts, oranges, and milk.
- Phosphate
  - Phosphate in clients diagnosed with DKA and HHS
    - Phosphate deficiency is common in clients with DKA and HHS.
      - Benefits of replacement therapy remain uncertain.
      - Replacement may be indicated in clients with cardiac dysfunction, respiratory depression, anemia, and a serum phosphate level lower than between 1.0 and 1.5 mg/dL.
      - Phosphate replacement increases the risk of hypocalcemia.
        - Calcium levels should be monitored during infusion.
  - Phosphate is necessary for the formation of bone and teeth.
  - Phosphate plays an important role in the body to make protein for growth, maintenance, and repair of cells and tissues.
  - Normal phosphate range: between 0.81 and 1.45 molecules per liter (mol/L)
    - Hyperphosphatemia: phosphate level higher than 1.45 mol/L
      - Possible causes: severe or advanced renal disease; hypothyroidism; DKA; rhabdomyolysis (destruction of muscular tissue); systemic infections

- Signs and symptoms: weakness; muscle spasms and/or cramping; tetany; crystal accumulations in the circulatory system and in the body's tissue, which may lead to severe itching and palpable calcifications in the SC tissue
- Goal of treatment: to correct and manage the underlying causes
- Treatment
  - Restrict dietary foods containing phosphates (milk, egg yolks).
  - Administer phosphate binders (lanthanum, sevelamer) to make it hard for the body to absorb phosphates.
- Complications: impaired circulation; cerebrovascular accidents; MI; atherosclerosis
- Nursing interventions
  - Phosphate binders should be taken with or immediately after meals.
- Prevention
  - Avoid using phosphate-containing medications (laxatives, enema).
  - Encourage the restriction of foods high in phosphate.
- Hypophosphatemia: phosphate level lower than 0.81 mol/L
- Possible causes: severe burns; diarrhea; severe malnutrition; hyperparathyroidism; pronounced alcoholism; lymphoma; leukemia; hepatic failure; genetic predisposition; osteomalacia; prolonged use of certain diuretics; prolonged use of aluminum antacids; long-term use of theophylline
- Signs and symptoms: respiratory alterations (respiratory alkalosis); irritability; cardiac dysrhythmias; confusion; coma; death
- Goal of treatment: to correct and manage the underlying causes
- Treatment
  - Administer oral and IV potassium phosphates.
  - Encourage an increased intake of foods high in phosphorous (milk, eggs).
- Complications
  - Assess renal status (BUN, creatinine) before administering phosphorous.
    - If kidneys are not functioning properly, the client will not be able to clear the phosphate.
- Nursing interventions
  - Monitor cardiac, respiratory, neuromuscular, renal, and GI status.
  - Administer oral phosphorus with supplemental vitamin D. Vitamin D aids in the absorption of phosphate.
  - Provide client safety; individual client may be at increased risk of bone fractures.
- Prevention
  - Encourage the intake of foods high in phosphate and low in calcium (fish, organ meats, nuts, chicken, pork, beef, whole grains).

- Chloride
  - Essential part of digestive juices, needed to maintain proper balance of body fluids
  - Normal chloride range: between 97 and 107 mEq/L
    - Hyperchloremia: chloride level higher than 107 mEq/L
      - Possible causes: dehydration; renal disease; diabetes; certain medications (supplemental hormones, some diuretics); vomiting; diarrhea; hyponatremia; hyperparathyroidism
      - Signs and symptoms: pitting edema; extreme thirst; vomiting; diarrhea; dehydration; dyspnea; Kussmaul breathing (deep, labored breathing pattern); tachypnea; hypertension; decreased cognition; coma

- Goal of treatment: to correct and manage the underlying causes
- Treatment
  - Cautiously administer fluids.
  - Eliminate problematic medications.
  - Correct any renal disease and hyperglycemia.
- Complications: can adversely affect the oxygen transportation in the body
- Nursing interventions
  - Fluids must be administered with caution. Too rapid rehydration may lead to cerebral edema and other complications.
- Prevention
  - Eliminate problematic foods and medications.
  - Maintain adequate hydration.
- Hypochloremia: chloride level lower than 97 mEq/L
  - Possible causes: vomiting; hypoventilation; metabolic alkalosis; respiratory acidosis; cystic fibrosis; hyponatremia; respiratory acidosis; high bicarbonate levels
  - Signs and symptoms: dehydration; muscular spasticity; nausea and/or vomiting; hyponatremia; tetany; muscular weakness and/or twitching; respiratory depression; diaphoresis; elevated temperature
  - Goal of treatment: to correct and manage the underlying causes
  - Treatment
    - Administer chloride replacements.
    - Possibly administer hydrochloride acid and a carbonic anhydrase inhibitor (acetazolamide).
  - Complications: respiratory arrest; seizures; coma
  - Nursing interventions
    - Monitor cardiac, respiratory, neuromuscular, renal, and GI status.
    - Provide client safety; individual client may have increased agitation and irritability.
  - Prevention
    - Offer foods high in chloride (table salt or sea salt, seaweed, rye, celery, olives, lettuce tomatoes).
    - Use dietary supplements.

APPLICATION AND REVIEW

11. Which client is at highest risk for developing HHS?
    1. 53-year-old woman with a history of type 2 diabetes recovering from DKA
    2. 76-year-old resident in a long-term care facility who has resident with no history of diabetes
    3. 45-year-old man newly diagnosed with type 2 diabetes
    4. 8-year-old girl with a history of type 1 diabetes
12. Which condition should the nurse expect in a client with HHS?
    1. Lipolysis
    2. Ketogenesis
    3. Hyperglycemia
    4. Increased FFAs
13. The nurse monitors the medications prescribed to a client diagnosed with type 2 diabetes. Which types of medications require further assessment by the nurse? *(Select all that apply.)*
    1. Beta blockers
    2. Glucocorticoids
    3. Thiazide diuretics
    4. Sympathomimetics
    5. Calcium channel blockers

14. The nurse assesses a client diagnosed with HHS. Which finding requires further nursing assessment? *(Select all that apply.)*
    1. Moderate muscle weakness noted on the left side
    2. Frequent requests for "a drink of water"
    3. Disoriented to both time and place
    4. Vomited 30 mL of clear liquid
    5. Hyperalertness

15. Which serum glucose range is the target goal for the client being treated for HHS?
    1. Between 100 and 150 mg/dL
    2. Between 200 and 250 mg/dL
    3. Between 250 and 300 mg/dL
    4. Between 400 and 450 mg/dL

16. Which information should the nurse provide to the client experiencing both DKA and HHS?
    1. Importance of adequate hydration and nutrition
    2. Recognition of early signs and symptoms
    3. Need for regular medical follow-up
    4. Need for treatment adherence

17. Which assessment finding in a client with diabetes indicates a serum sodium level of 149 mEq/L?
    1. Oral temperature of 101° F
    2. Completing a 10K running race
    3. Diarrhea that started 36 hours ago
    4. Having a history of Cushing syndrome
    5. Skiing in snowy, 10° F weather for 5 hours

18. Which complication can occur in a client whose serum sodium level drops rapidly?
    1. Cerebral edema
    2. Cardiac arrest
    3. Vomiting
    4. Seizures

19. The nurse should provide which dietary instruction to a client with a serum potassium level of 5.9 mEq/L?
    1. Avoid consuming tomatoes, avocados, and pork.
    2. Preferred fruits include strawberries and bananas.
    3. Organ meats should replace beef as a protein source.
    4. Vegetables of choice should include carrots and potatoes.

20. A client is prescribed phenobarbital. Which electrolyte imbalance should the nurse monitor in this client?
    1. Hyponatremia
    2. Hypocalcemia
    3. Hypochloremia
    4. Hypomagnesemia

See Answers on pages 357–360.

ANSWER KEY: REVIEW QUESTIONS

1. **Answers: 3, 4**

   3 A catecholamine is an amine derived from catechol that has important physiological effects as neurotransmitters and hormones. Epinephrine is a catecholamine that has a counterregulatory affect on insulin. **4** A catecholamine is an amine derived from catechol that has important physiological effects as neurotransmitters and hormones. Norepinephrine is a catecholamine that has a counterregulatory affect on insulin.

   1 Although cortisol has a counterregulatory affect on insulin, it is not a catecholamine. **2** Although glucagon has a counterregulatory affect on insulin, it is not a catecholamine. **5** Although growth hormone has a counterregulatory affect on insulin, it is not a catecholamine.

   Client Need: Health Promotion and Maintenance; **Cognitive Level:** Understanding; **Integrated Process:** Teaching and Learning

2. **1 The initial treatment goal for DKA is the prompt identification of the precipitating causes of the condition.**

   2 Cause of death in clients with DKA and HHS is rarely the result of a metabolic complication; rather, it is related to the underlying medical illness that precipitated the metabolic decompensation. 3 Under the conditions associated with diabetes, normal insulin function is not necessarily achievable. 4 Such additional assessments are important, but the identification of acute factors have priority over the assessment of long-term complications.

   Client Need: Physiological Integrity; **Cognitive Level:** Analysis; **Nursing Process:** Planning

3. **1 Although most clients diagnosed with DKA have type 1 diabetes, this client's type 2 diabetes increase the risk of developing this complication.**

   2 Although most clients diagnosed with DKA have type 1 diabetes, the female gender does not include the risk of developing this complication. 3 Although most clients diagnosed with DKA have type 1 diabetes, adults are more at risk than children. 4 Most clients diagnosed with DKA have type 1 diabetes with adults more at risk than children. The method of successful management is not a risk factor.

   Client Need: Health Promotion and Maintenance; **Cognitive Level:** Analysis; **Nursing Process:** Assessment

4. **3 Metabolic acidosis is a clinical characteristic of DKA.**

   1 Hyperglycemia is a clinical characteristic of DKA. 2 Hyperketonemia is a clinical characteristic of DKA. 4 Metabolic acidosis is a clinical characteristic of DKA.

   Client Need: Physiological Integrity; **Cognitive Level:** Application; **Nursing Process:** Assessment

5. **Answers: 3, 5**

   3 Psychological stress is a precipitating factor in the development of DKA. 5 Infection is a precipitating factor in the development of DKA.

   1 Although avoiding or minimizing alcohol consumption is suggested, it is a factor in the general management of diabetes, not specifically a precipitating factor in the development of DKA. 2 Although avoiding or minimizing sugar consumption is necessary, it is a factor in the general management of diabetes, not specifically a precipitating factor in the development of DKA. 4 Although engaging in regular exercise is suggested, it is a factor in the general management of diabetes, not specifically a precipitating factor in the development of DKA.

   Client Need: Health Promotion and Maintenance; **Cognitive Level:** Applying; **Integrated Process:** Teaching and Learning

6. **3 Infections, including UTIs and pneumonia, are identified as the triggering factors in up to 50% of clients diagnosed with DKA.**

   1 Although an MI is a recognized acute condition that may trigger DKA, infection is the most common cause. 2 Corticosteroid therapy can affect carbohydrate metabolism and cause DKA, but infection is the most common cause. 4 Alcohol or drug abuse can trigger DKA, but an infection is the most common cause.

   Client Need: Physiological Integrity; **Cognitive Level:** Application; **Nursing Process:** Evaluation

7. **Answers: 1, 2, 4**

   1 Clinical signs of DKA include a sweet, fruity breath resulting from acetone. 2 Tachycardia is a clinical sign associated with DKA. 4 Hypotension is a clinical sign associated with DKA.

   3 Serum glucose levels above 250 mg/dL are associated with DKA. 5 Normal urine output ranges between 800 and 2000 mL per day. Polyuria is associated with DKA.

   Client Need: Physiological Integrity; **Cognitive Level:** Applying; **Nursing Process:** Assessment

8. **1 When serum glucose reaches 250 mg/dL, 5% dextrose with 0.45% sodium chloride and adequate insulin is administered to maintain serum glucose levels between 150 and 200 mg/dL until metabolic control is achieved.**

   2 Although restoring hydration is a goal, the IV fluid and insulin therapies are directed at maintaining serum glucose levels between 150 and 200 mg/dL. 3 Although normalizing urinary output is a goal, the IV fluid and insulin therapies are directed at maintaining serum glucose levels between 150 and

200 mg/dL. **4** Although reversing hypotension is a goal, the IV fluid and insulin therapies are directed at maintaining serum glucose levels between 150 and 200 mg/dL.
Client Need: Physiological Integrity; **Cognitive Level:** Application; **Nursing Process:** Planning

9. **1 If serum potassium is greater than 5.0 mEq/L, potassium is not administered, but the levels are rechecked every 2 hours.**

2 The treatment protocol provides the nurse with directions on how to address this situation. **3** If serum potassium is less than 3.3 mEq/L, insulin is held and 40 mEq/L of potassium is administered until the level is greater than 3.3 mEq/L. **4** If serum potassium is greater than 3.3 mEq/L but less than 5.0 mEq/L, between 20 and 30 mEq of potassium is administered in each liter of IV fluid to keep the serum potassium between 4 and 5 mEq/L.
Client Need: Physiological Integrity; **Cognitive Level:** Applying; **Nursing Process:** Implementation

10. **2 During nausea episodes, the client should be instructed to promptly initiate a liquid diet containing carbohydrates and salt.**

1 Never discontinue insulin without first contacting the primary care provider. **3** Hydration is vital; this client should not eliminate liquids. **4** If fluids are effectively consumed, immediate hospitalization is generally not necessary.
Client Need: Health Promotion and Maintenance; **Cognitive Level:** Applying; **Integrated Process:** Teaching and Learning

11. **2 Commonly, clients with HHS have undiagnosed diabetes, are between the ages of 55 and 70 years old, and are frequently residents of a long-term care facility.**

1 Although HHS occurs most commonly among clients diagnosed with type 2 diabetes, neither the client's age or history of DKA are considered risk factors. **3** Although HHS occurs most commonly among clients diagnosed with type 2 diabetes, neither the client's age nor gender are considered risk factors. **4** HHS is more common among clients with type 2 diabetes.
Client Need: Physiological Integrity; **Cognitive Level:** Analysis; **Integrated Process/Nursing Process:** Assessment

12. **3 HHS results in a deficiency of insulin resulting in hyperglycemia.**

1 HHS results in a deficiency of insulin but at levels that prevent lipolysis from occurring. **2** HHS results in a deficiency of insulin but at levels that prevent ketogenesis from occurring. **4** HHS results in a decrease in the concentration of FFAs.
Client Need: Physiological Integrity; **Cognitive Level:** Understanding; **Nursing Process:** Assessment

13. **Answers: 1, 2, 3**

Beta blocker therapy, glucocorticoid therapy, and thiazide diuretic therapy would increase the client's risk for developing HHS.

4 Sympathomimetic therapy would increase the client's risk for developing DKA, not HHS. **5** Calcium channel blockers are not known to increase the risk for developing HHS.
Client Need: Physiological Integrity; **Cognitive Level:** Understanding; **Nursing Process:** Planning

14. **Answers: 1, 2**

1 HHS exhibits a neurological finding that includes unilateral muscle weakness or partial paralysis. **2** Polydipsia is associated with HHS.

3, 4, 5 Cognitive impairment, vomiting, and hyperalertness are not associated with HHS.
Client Need: Physiological Integrity; **Cognitive Level:** Analysis; **Nursing Process:** Assessment

15. **3 The treatment goal for HHS is to maintain the serum glucose level between 250 and 300 mg/dL.**

1, 2, 4 The treatment goal for HHS is to maintain the serum glucose level between 250 and 300 mg/dL.
Client Need: Physiological Integrity; **Cognitive Level:** Knowing; **Nursing Process:** Evaluation

16. **2 Educating the friends and family regarding the early signs and symptoms of DKA and HHS will help ensure prompt medical treatment that will greatly improve the client's prognosis.**

1 Although hydration and nutrition are important, they are factors that affect the prevention not the treatment of DKA and HHS. **3** Although regular medical follow-up is important, it is a factor in the general management of the client's diabetic state, not specifically to the treatment of DKA and HHS.

4 Although treatment adherence is important, it is a factor in the general management of the client's diabetic state, not specifically to the treatment of DKA and HHS.

Client Need: Physiological Integrity; **Cognitive Level:** Analysis; **Integrated Process:** Teaching and Learning

17. **Answers: 1, 2, 3, 4**

1 A serum sodium level of 149 mEq/L indicates hypernatremia. Dehydration triggered by a fever is a possible cause of hypernatremia. **2** A serum sodium level of 149 mEq/L indicates hypernatremia. Dehydration triggered by extreme exercise is a possible cause of hypernatremia. **3** A serum sodium level of 149 mEq/L indicates hypernatremia. Dehydration triggered by diarrhea is a possible cause of hypernatremia. **4** A serum sodium level of 149 mEq/L indicates hypernatremia. Dehydration triggered by the Cushing syndrome is a possible cause of hypernatremia.

5 A serum sodium level of 149 mEq/L indicates hypernatremia. Dehydration is a trigger for hypernatrium. An extremely cold environment is not a cause of dehydration.

Client Need: Physiological Integrity; **Cognitive Level:** Analysis; **Nursing Process:** Assessment

18. **1 If sodium levels drop too rapidly, the individual is at risk of cerebral edema.**

2 Cardiac arrest is not a likely complication of a rapid drop in serum sodium since it not directly related to fluid or electrolyte imbalances. **3** Vomiting is a possible cause of hyponatremia, not a complication. **4** Seizures are a sign of hyponatremia, not a complication.

Client Need: Physiological Integrity; **Cognitive Level:** Understanding; **Integrated Process:** Teaching and Learning

19. **1 A serum potassium level of 5.9 mEq/L is indicative of hyperkalemia. Tomatoes, avocados, and pork are high in potassium and should be avoided.**

2 A serum potassium level of 5.9 mEq/L is indicative of hyperkalemia. Both strawberries and bananas are high in potassium and should be avoided. **3** A serum potassium level of 5.9 mEq/L is indicative of hyperkalemia. Organ meat is high in potassium and should be avoided. **4** A serum potassium level of 5.9 mEq/L is indicative of hyperkalemia. Carrots and potatoes are high in potassium and should be avoided.

Client Need: Physiological Integrity; **Cognitive Level:** Applying; **Integrated Process:** Teaching and Learning

20. **2 Hypocalcemia can be triggered by phenobarbital therapy.**

1 Hyponatremia is not triggered by phenobarbital therapy. **3** Hypochloremia is not triggered by phenobarbital therapy. **4** Hypomagnesemia is not triggered by phenobarbital therapy.

Client Need: Health Promotion and Maintenance; **Cognitive Level:** Applying; **Nursing Process:** Implementation

FLUIDS AND ELECTROLYTES IN ACUTE INFECTION OVERVIEW

Acute Infection

- Microorganisms are living microscopic organisms found throughout the environment.
- Microorganisms are responsible for causing infections when very specific circumstances fall into place.
- An infection may stay contained within an individual host or spread to other individuals, even infecting entire populations.
  - Endemic refers to a constant rate of infection in a specific population.
  - Epidemic refers to infection rates higher than normal in a certain population in a certain area.
  - Pandemic refers to a larger spread of infection to multiple populations in multiple areas.
    - National
    - Global
- Understanding the chain of infection and infection prevention is key to stopping the spread of disease.
- Electrolyte balance is essential for normal body functions, including the body's ability to prevent and fight infection.
- Imbalances may result in symptoms similar to those caused by infections, making it difficult to distinguish the cause.
- Quickly identifying and treating electrolyte imbalances will assist with preventing further deterioration during an infectious process.

Pathophysiological Factors

- Microorganisms (microbes) are microscopic living organisms not visible to the naked eye.
- Classifications of microorganisms
  - Viruses
    - Small
    - Intracellular
    - Replication
      - A live host cell is required.
      - Viruses mutate with replication.
    - Vaccinations are not effective against viruses.
    - Viruses take over the host cell and may change the deoxyribonucleic acid (DNA) of the host cell.
      - Malignancies may be due to a virus (human papillomavirus [HPV]).
    - Viruses transfer DNA or ribonucleic acid (RNA) into the host cell.
      - Most viruses contain DNA.
      - Viruses are the most common cause of human illness.
      - Viruses can stay dormant in the host and reproduce at later time: influenza A and B; herpes; hepatitis A, B, and C; poliomyelitis; measles; mumps; rabies; hantavirus; human immunodeficiency virus (HIV); HPV

- Bacteria (Table 20.1)
  - Unicellular (single-cell) organisms without a nuclear membrane
  - Are able to reproduce
  - Are able to survive on nonliving objects
  - Some bacteria are nonpathogenic (they do not cause disease).
  - Bacteria have cell walls.
    - Human cells do not have cell walls.
    - Treatment targets the cell walls and is therefore not harmful to human cells.
    - The cell wall regulates the movement of substances in and out of the cell.
  - Two groups of bacteria are identified by a laboratory test that uses a gram-stain technique.
    - Gram-positive bacteria
      - Cell wall takes on the color of the stain.
      - Gram-positive bacteria are more susceptible to antibiotics.
    - Gram-negative bacteria
      - Cell membrane does not take on the color of the stain.
      - Has hairlike projections
        - Pili: are responsible for genetic material transfer
        - Fimbriae: are responsible for cell-to-surface attachment
  - Flagella, a threadlike structure with a whiplike movement, allows the bacteria to swim.
  - Bacteria are identified by the shape of the cells.
    - Rod-shaped *Bacillus* bacteria
    - Spiral-shaped *Spirillum* bacteria (spirochetes)
    - Spherical-shaped *Coccus* bacteria
  - Bacteria are categorized by diplo (paired cells), staphylo (irregular cluster of cells), strepto (chains of cells), tetras (four cells grouped in a square), and palisade (cells lying parallel).
  - Toxic secretions are released by bacteria.
    - Endotoxins
      - Gram-negative bacteria released after bacterial death
      - Symptoms: fever; weakness; circulatory effects
    - Exotoxins
      - Gram-positive bacteria found in body fluids
      - Symptoms: impaired nerve conduction
  - Antibiotic-resistant bacteria are referred to as "super bugs" because they are difficult to fight.
    - Methicillin-resistant *Staphylococcus aureus* (MRSA)
    - Vancomycin-resistant *Enterococcus* (VRE)
- Fungi
  - Are abundant in the environment: humans; animals; plants; foods (bread, cheese, fruit); mold
    - Hyphae: long strands
    - Mycelium: hyphae twisted together; visible to naked eye
    - Spores
      - Resilient; can survive in many environmental conditions
        - Aerobic (mold)
        - Anaerobic (yeast)
      - Able to travel through the air
      - Cause allergic reactions

TABLE 20.1 Disease-Causing Bacteria	
Bacteria	**Diseases Caused**
Chlamydia trachomatis	Chlamydia, lymphogranuloma venereum
Clostridia	
• *Clostridium botulinum*	Food poisoning with progressive muscle paralysis
• *Clostridium tetani*	Tetanus (lockjaw)
Corynebacterium diphtheriae	Diphtheria
Escherichia coli	Urinary tract infections, peritonitis, hemolytic-uremic syndrome
Haemophilus	
• *Haemophilus influenzae*	Nasopharyngitis, meningitis, pneumonia
• *Haemophilus pertussis*	Pertussis (whooping cough)
Helicobacter pylori	Peptic ulcers, gastritis
Klebsiella-Enterobacter organisms	Urinary tract infections, peritonitis, pneumonia
Legionella pneumophila	Pneumonia (Legionnaires' disease)
Mycobacteria	
• *Mycobacterium leprae*	Hansen disease (leprosy)
• *Mycobacterium tuberculosis*	Tuberculosis
Neisseria	
• *Neisseria gonorrhoeae*	Gonorrhea, pelvic inflammatory disease, proctitis
• *Neisseria meningitidis*	Meningococcemia, meningitis
Proteus species	Urinary tract infections, peritonitis
Pseudomonas aeruginosa	Urinary tract infections, meningitis
Salmonella	
• *Salmonella typhi*	Typhoid fever
• Other *Salmonella* organisms	Food poisoning, gastroenteritis
Shigella	Shigellosis; diarrhea, abdominal pain, and fever (dysentery)
Staphylococcus aureus	Skin infections, pneumonia, urinary tract infections, acute osteomyelitis, toxic shock syndrome
Streptococci	
• *Streptococcus faecalis*	Genitourinary infection, infection of surgical wounds
• *Streptococcus pneumoniae*	Pneumococcal pneumonia
• *Streptococcus pyogenes* (group A β-hemolytic streptococci)	Pharyngitis, scarlet fever, rheumatic fever, acute glomerulonephritis, erysipelas, pneumonia
• *S. pyogenes* (group B β-hemolytic streptococci)	Urinary tract infections
• *Streptococcus viridans*	Bacterial endocarditis
Treponema pallidum	Syphilis

From Lewis, S. L., Bucher, L., Heitkemper, M. M., Harding, M. M., Kwong, J., & Roberts, D. (2017). *Medical-surgical nursing: Assessment and management of clinical problems* (10th ed.). St. Louis: Elsevier.

- o Resistant to changes in temperature
- o Resistant to many chemicals used for sanitizing
  - ▪ Few are pathogenic.
  - ▪ Some cause infection on the skin and in the mucous membranes.
  - ▪ Some cause damage to tissue by secreting enzymes and by activating an inflammatory response.
  - ▪ Single cell or chains
  - ▪ Rigid, thick cell wall
- • Protozoa
  - ▪ Parasites
    - ▪ Unicellular
    - ▪ Without a cell wall
    - ▪ May morph into many shapes (single life cycle)
    - ▪ May be visible to naked eye
      - o Helminths (worms)
      - o Eggs and larva are microscopic.
      - o Three life-cycle stages: ovum (egg), larva, and adult
  - ▪ Diseases caused by protozoa include malaria (mosquito bites), amebic dysentery (contaminated food or water source), trichomoniasis (sexually transmitted), and giardia (contaminated food or water source).
- • Other groups of disease-causing microorganisms include mycoplasmas, *Rickettsiae*, and *Chlamydiae*.
- • Resident flora
  - • Normal microbes living on and in the body (indigenous)
  - • Some are beneficial.
  - • Semipermanent or permanent
  - • Not usually pathogenic
  - • Become pathogenic when transmitted to another location
    - ▪ Host is susceptible if immunity is impaired.
  - • Opportunistic infection (immunocompromised host)
    - ▪ Normal flora invades, causing secondary disease.
- • Microorganisms are responsible for causing infections when conditions in the human body are optimal.
  - • Most are not able to live outside of the body.
  - • Three components must be present for a microorganism to cause an infection.
    - ▪ Disease-causing microbes
    - ▪ Host environment
    - ▪ Successful transmission
- • Some microorganisms are more prone to cause infection than others.
  - • Pathogen: disease-causing microorganism
  - • Pathogenicity: strength of the pathogen to cause infection
    - ▪ Some cause diseases all of the time.
    - ▪ Some rarely cause diseases.
  - • Virulence: amount of damage caused by the pathogen
    - ▪ Capacity to invade tissues
    - ▪ Toxic qualities of the pathogen
    - ▪ Strength of the attachment
    - ▪ Ability to evade the host's defense mechanisms through mutation

- Chain of infection
  - Understanding the chain of infection is important to prevent infection and to control its spread.
- A series of six indicators are necessary for the infection to spread.
  - Causative agent
    - Source of infection
    - Pathogen
  - Reservoir
    - Host: human; animal; water; soil; carrier (does not develop the infection)
    - Pathogens must have environment conducive to live and replicate.
    - Colonization
      - Microorganisms replicate on or in a host.
      - No infection or illness occurs.
      - Host susceptibility is dependent on resistance.
    - Infection
      - Microorganisms invade a susceptible host, and the body responds.
        - Immune response
        - Infection may or may not develop.
        - Immune system either eliminates the pathogen or is unable to clear the pathogen.
  - Susceptible host
    - Pathogens enters the host.
    - Factors that increase the risk of susceptibility include injury; medical history; co-morbidities (illnesses, chronic diseases); age (infants, older adults); gender; genetic predisposition; nutritional status; immunization (exposure to a microorganism through injection); antibodies (resistance to exposure); and immune suppression.
    - Health care environments (clients, health care workers)
  - Port of entry
    - Route for a pathogen to enter the host
      - Mucous membranes (mouth, nose)
      - Skin
      - Respiratory tract
      - Gastrointestinal tract
      - Genitourinary tract
  - Transmission
    - Transmission must occur from one source to another.
    - Avenues of transmission
      - Skin-to-skin contact (scabies)
      - Droplet contact
        - Respiratory
        - Large droplets
        - Cough and sneeze droplets
        - Direct contact with the hands
        - Inhalation
      - Bloodborne contact
    - Direct transmission: Susceptible host has direct contact with the causative agent.
      - Causative agents include urine, blood, feces, sputum, emesis, wound drainage, and semen.

- Indirect transmission: Causative agent passes to a source that then encounters a susceptible host.
  - Hand hygiene is the best preventive measure against indirect transmission.
  - Sources may include food, contaminated hands, clothing, toys, and surgical equipment.
- Inhalation
  - Airborne
    - Very small particles float through air for long distances and/or for up to hours.
    - Airborne particles are inhaled by the host through a port of entry (mouth, nose).
- Inoculation (immunization)
- Ingestion
- Placental transfer (mother to fetus)
- Vector-borne
  - Carried by an intermediate live host
    - Animals (rodents)
    - Insects (mosquitoes, mites, ticks)
- Port of exit
  - Avenue through which the pathogen leaves the host to enter another host (specific to the pathogen)
    - Hepatitis A exits through feces.
    - Hepatitis B exits through blood.
- Stages of infection
  - Incubation period
    - Can be present in host for a long period without causing symptoms
    - Pathogen has entered the host.
      - No clinical symptoms are exhibited.
      - Reproduction begins.
  - Prodromal period
    - Clinical symptoms are present.
  - Acute period
    - Infectious disease is fully developed.
      - Symptoms are at their peak.
    - May be a slow onset with a long prodromal period
    - May be a quick onset with a severe prodromal period
    - Length of the acute period is dependent on the specific pathogen and the host resistance.
  - Convalescent period
    - Recovery begins.
    - Signs and symptoms improve.
- Nosocomial infections
  - Infections spread in health care facilities.
    - Common nosocomial infections
      - Upper respiratory tract infection
      - Pneumonia
        - Primary cause: ventilators
      - Urinary tract infection
        - Primary cause: indwelling catheters
      - *Clostridium difficile* (*C-diff*)
      - Surgical wound infections

- Bloodstream infections (bacteremia)
- Antibiotic-resistant infections
  - Contributing factors
    - Abundance of microorganisms
    - Contagions
    - Antibiotic resistance
    - Multiple hosts
    - Contamination from one individual to another
- Chronic infection
  - Immune system is unable to eradicate the infection completely.
  - Microbes continue to reproduce.
  - Mild clinical symptoms are continually exhibited.
  - Periods of acute exacerbation of symptoms occur.
  - Chronic infection may result in damage to tissues after prolonged disease.
- Subclinical infection
  - Microbes reproduce in the body.
  - Symptoms are not present (chickenpox).
- Septicemia
  - Systemic infection
    - Infection overwhelms the immune defense system.
  - Septic shock
    - Bacterial infection in the bloodstream
      - Release of bacterial toxins
      - Gram-negative bacteria most common cause
      - Most frequent source of infections
        - Respiratory system (pneumonia)
        - Genitourinary system (urinary tract infections)
    - Older adults are particularly susceptible to septic shock.
    - Blood pressure drops
    - Life threatening
- Immune system
  - The immune response is a natural defense mechanism that attempts to prevent pathogen entry and attempts to clear the pathogen that has gained entry.
  - Natural defense system
    - Innate
    - First line of defense
    - Reaction to all pathogens
    - Same reaction every time
    - Barriers (skin)
      - Epidermis (thick, tough outer layer)
      - Dermis (sebaceous glands, sweat glands)
        - Secretes substances that prevent some microorganisms from reproducing
        - Some bacteria, that are normal on the skin's surface, are not damaged by these secretions.
    - Mucous membranes (antimicrobial)
    - Fever (inflammatory response)
      - Normal body temperature: 37° C (98.6° F)
      - Is regulated by the hypothalamus

- Higher-than-normal temperature
  - Fever is a systemic response to microorganisms.
  - Pyrogens (chemicals that produce heat) are released into the blood.
  - Mild increase in temperature
    - Is beneficial in fighting infection
    - Slows the rate of bacterial cell division
- Fever 40° C (104° F)
  - Causes nerve cell damage
- Antimicrobial proteins
  - Complement proteins: interferon and acute-phase proteins
  - Innate (nonspecific) responses
    - Antimicrobial proteins assist in lysis, the disintegration of foreign cells by breaking down the cell wall.
    - Also aid in the inflammation response
    - Phagocytosis (ingestion of bacteria)
- Phagocytes
  - Phagocytes destroy foreign matter by ingesting bacteria.
  - Two types of phagocytes
    - Macrophages: found throughout the body in tissues and organs
    - Neutrophils: largest concentration found in bloodstream; travel to the site of infection
- Lymphocytes
  - Innate (nonspecific) response
    - Lymphocytes destroy viruses and cancer cells.
- Inflammation
  - Is the natural response to injuries and infections
  - Function: to prepare the site for repair, clearing the site of foreign material and pathogens
  - Injury initiates a cascade of events.
    - Various chemicals are released.
    - Localized arteriole dilation occurs, increasing permeability and the number of phagocytes.
    - Signs of inflammation include heat, swelling, redness, and pain.
  - The body's inability to clear foreign matter results in chronic inflammation.
- Acquired defense system
  - Second line of defense
    - Is initiated when the first-line defenses become overwhelmed
    - Both responses work at the same time.
  - Requires a previous exposure to a specific pathogen
    - Produces specific antibodies that react to a specifically recognized antigen
  - Response stops when the threat is no longer present.
  - The body's acquired defense system recognizes the pathogen.
    - The response is faster and stronger with each exposure.
  - Macrophages
    - Type of white blood cell that ingests pathogens
    - Play a key role in the immune response to infectious microorganisms
  - B lymphocytes (B cells)
    - Provide antibody-mediated immunity

- Produce and secrete antibodies
- Found in the blood and body fluids
- Attach to foreign microorganisms before entering the host cells
- Initial exposure
  - Primary response
  - Natural defense mechanism
  - B cells are specific to the antigen
- Second and/or subsequent exposure
  - Secondary response
  - Acquired defense mechanism
  - Immunizations
  - T lymphocytes (T cells)
  - Directly attack the foreign cells, assisting in lysis of the cells
  - Aid in the inflammatory response
  - Risk of illness is high with a low T cell count.

APPLICATION AND REVIEW

1. Which statement concerning viruses is true?
   1. Viruses are incapable of changing the host cell DNA.
   2. Viruses are seldom associated with cancer development.
   3. Viruses are the most common cause of human illnesses.
   4. Viruses can live and duplicate in both live and dead host cells.
2. Which conditions are caused by viral infections? *(Select all that apply.)*
   1. Poliomyelitis
   2. Rabies
   3. Herpes
   4. Malaria
   5. Measles
3. Which statement concerning bacteria is true?
   1. Bacteria are multicellular organisms.
   2. Bacteria are, by their nature, pathogenic.
   3. Bacteria can survive on inorganic objects.
   4. Bacteria need ideal situations to reproduce.
4. Antibiotic therapy is most effective for a client with which classification of bacterial infection?
   1. Bacilli
   2. Tetras
   3. Endotoxins
   4. Gram positive
5. Which assessment data is characteristic of an exotoxin bacterial infection?
   1. Tingling in the fingers
   2. Fever higher than 101° F
   3. Impaired hand grip
   4. Poor pedal pulse
6. Which client behavior results in a pathogenic situation involving resident flora bacteria?
   1. Aspirating vomitus
   2. Scratching an itchy rash
   3. Drinking contaminated water
   4. Sharing infected body fluids
7. Which characteristic of a microorganism causes infection?
   1. Virulence
   2. Resilience
   3. Pathogenicity
   4. Attachment strength

8. Which elements are necessary for an infection to spread? *(Select all that apply.)*
   1. Pathogen
   2. Reservoir
   3. Entry point
   4. Point of exit
   5. Ineffective treatment

9. Which finding suggests that a child is in the prodromal period of a measles infection?
   1. Attending a day care facility where a measles outbreak has occurred
   2. Demonstrating a low-grade fever and malaise
   3. An observable measles rash that is clearing visible
   4. A noticeable lessening of both fever and rash

10. Which hospital-based interventions are often associated with nosocomial infections? *(Select all that apply.)*
    1. Mechanical ventilation
    2. Intravenous therapy
    3. Cardiac monitoring
    4. Indwelling catheter
    5. Antibiotic therapy

11. Which structures located in the dermis layer of the skin serve to support the body's first line of defense against infections? *(Select all that apply.)*
    1. Sebaceous gland
    2. Sweat glands
    3. Blood vessels
    4. Hair follicle
    5. Nail bed

12. Which clinical observations tend to confirm the presence of inflammation? *(Select all that apply.)*
    1. Redness at the site of a laceration
    2. Heat radiating from a great toe
    3. Pus at an incision site
    4. Swelling in an ankle
    5. Chills and fever

See Answers on pages 378–381.

Signs and Symptoms of Infection

- Most symptoms are due to the inflammatory response of the individual.
  - Severity of the symptoms are dependent on the specific pathogen, the affected organ system, and the intensity of inflammatory response.
  - Local signs of infection are exhibited in the area immediately surrounding the site of infection.
    - Inflammation: heat; swelling; redness; pain
    - Serous (clear, yellow) drainage and tissue necrosis (caused by viruses)
    - Purulent (thick, white or yellow) drainage containing white blood cells (WBCs) and pus (caused by bacteria)
    - Lymphadenopathy (tender, swollen lymph nodes)
  - Systemic signs of infection include fever, fatigue, weakness, body aches, nausea, and headache.
    - Altered mental status: disorientation; confusion; seizures; loss of consciousness
    - Symptoms are directly related to organ system affected.
      - Sepsis
      - Can progress to septic shock
        - Initial signs and symptoms of sepsis shock: fever; shaking; chills; flushed skin; bounding pulse; tachypnea (rapid respirations, greater than 20 respirations per minute)

○ Progressive symptoms of sepsis shock
  ○ Body temperature is below normal (98.6° F [37° C]) body temperature.
  ○ Body loses more heat through rapid respirations than it can absorb or maintain.
  ○ Weak and thready pulse
  ○ Pale and cool skin

APPLICATION AND REVIEW

13. Which statement made by a client supports the presence of a systemic infection? *(Select all that apply.)*
1. "I'm feeling hot."
2. "My entire body aches."
3. "I hear ringing in my ears."
4. "I'm too nauseated to eat."
5. "I'm too tired to even take a shower."

14. Which assessment data indicate that the client is demonstrating progressive signs of septic shock? *(Select all that apply.)*
1. Flushed skin
2. Thready pulse
3. Pale, cool skin
4. Temperature of 97.2° F
5. Respirations at 22 breaths per minute

See Answers on pages 378–381.

Types of Infection

- Mild-to-severe infections can occur throughout the body in any body system in any organ.
  - Integumentary infections
    - Dermatitis: superficial bacterial infection
    - Scabies: parasitic infection
    - Ringworm: fungal infection
    - Cellulitis: bacterial infection of the skin and underlying soft tissue
    - Impetigo: infection from disease-causing bacteria such as *Streptococcus pyogenes* and *Staphylococcus aureus*
    - Necrotizing fasciitis: bacterial ("flesh eating") infection that kills tissues
      - Rapid progression
      - Septic shock
      - Death
  - Orthopedic infections
    - Postsurgical infection
      - Open surgical reduction of a fracture
      - Joint replacement: hip; knee; shoulder
      - Spinal surgery
    - Open fracture infection: contamination from environmental exposure
    - Osteomyelitis: infection within the bone
  - Cardiovascular infections
    - Bacteremia: bloodstream infection
    - Intravascular catheter–associated infection
    - Phlebitis: inflammation of vessels (chemical-induced infection)
    - Endocarditis: infection of the endocardium
      - Invasive cardiac procedure
      - Intravenous drug use

- Prosthetic heart valve
- Underlying heart disease
  - Pericarditis: infection of the pericardium (lining surrounding the heart)
- Central nervous system infections
  - Meningitis: infection of the lining surrounding the brain and spinal cord
    - Skull fracture
  - Encephalitis: infection of the brain tissue
    - Cerebrospinal fluid (CSF) shunts to treat hydrocephalus
    - Traumatic brain injury
- Respiratory tract infections
  - Pneumonia: bacterial or viral infection of the lungs
    - Health care–associated (hospital) acquired infection
    - Community-acquired infection
  - Sinusitis: infection of the paranasal sinuses
  - Bronchitis: infection of the mucous membranes in the bronchial tubes
  - Tuberculosis: infection from disease-causing bacteria, *Mycobacterium tuberculosis*
- Gastrointestinal infections
  - C-diff: infection from disease-causing bacteria, *Clostridium difficile*
  - Gastritis: infection of the lining of the stomach
  - Colitis: infection of the colon (large intestine)
  - Cholecystitis: infection of the gallbladder
  - Pancreatitis: infection of the pancreas
  - Appendicitis: infection of the appendix
  - Peritonitis: infection of the peritoneum (serous membrane lining covering the abdominal organs)
- Urinary tract infections
  - Commonly caused by indwelling catheters
  - Cystitis: infection of the urinary bladder
  - Pyelonephritis: infection of the urinary kidney

Assessment

- Complete history
  - Age of the individual
    - Older adults may not mount as intense of an inflammatory response attributable to the decline in the defense capabilities of the immune system.
      - Older adults are more susceptible to infection.
  - Information regarding the current illness
    - Onset of symptoms
      - Recent injuries, including recent surgeries and hospitalizations
      - Changes in bodily functions
      - Exposure to other infected individuals (travel)
  - Information regarding previous infections and illnesses
  - Current medications
  - Immunization history
  - Living environment such as retirement communities and long-term nursing facilities (high risk of exposure)
  - Lifestyle: work; family; tobacco use; alcohol use; activity level
  - Fever: high grade; low grade

- Heart rate: tachycardia (abnormally rapid pulse)
- Respiratory rate: tachypnea (abnormally rapid breathing)
- Nausea
- Vomiting
- Inflammation (trend changes)
- Pain level
- Malaise
- Altered mental status: confusion; disorientation
- Body fluids: amount; color; odor; clarity
- Complete blood cell (CBC) count with differential
  - Differentiates WBC concentrations
- Diagnostic tests
  - Laboratory tests
    - Culture and sensitivities
      - Aerobic bacteria
      - Anaerobic bacteria
      - Microbes, such as sputum, urine, stool, wound exudate, and blood, obtained from a specimen are grown in a petri dish.
      - Staining identifies gram-positive or gram-negative bacteria.
      - Once identified, the pathogen is tested against different antibiotic agents to narrow the antibiotic options and to relate, specifically, to the sensitivity of the microbe.
    - Viruses need a living host to grow.
    - Blood testing
      - Bacterial: leukocytosis (elevated WBC count)
      - Viral: leukopenia (low WBC count)
      - Antibodies detection
      - Acute infection: elevated neutrophilic WBC count
      - Chronic infection: elevated lymphocytes (small WBCs) and monocytes (large phagocytic WBCs)
  - Radiological imaging
    - Identify the site and size of the infection.
    - Assist with identifying the pathogen related to the location.
    - Modalities: chest x-ray image, computed tomography (CT) scan; magnetic resonance imaging (MRI)

Treatment

- Goal of treatment is to eliminate the microorganism-causing infection.
- The body's own immune system is the first line of defense and may eradicate the pathogen without other interventions.
- Antimicrobial therapy or antibiotic medications
  - The goal is to be as specific as possible to the identified pathogen.
    - Initial treatment is the administration of broad-spectrum antibiotics specific to the suspected microbe.
    - Narrow the antibiotic options.
      - Perform the gram-stain procedure to differentiate the microbe into either gram-positive or gram-negative bacteria.
      - Determine the sensitivity to the antibiotic.

- Factors affecting the appropriate antibiotic
  - Definitive identification of the pathogen causing the infection and its virulence and susceptibility or resistance to the antibiotic
  - Host
    - Age
      - Decreased kidney function
      - Decreased absorption
      - Drug interactions
    - Allergies and/or adverse reactions
    - Genetics
    - Metabolic abnormalities (co-morbidities)
    - Pregnancy
      - All antimicrobials cross the placental barrier, exposing the fetus.
      - Antimicrobials are secreted in breast milk.
    - Renal function
    - Liver function
    - Site of infection
      - Antibiotic must have adequate concentration to be able to penetrate the site (bone, prostate, heart, CSF).
    - Serum concentration of the antibiotic
    - Antibiotic-resistant organisms
      - Prolonged hospitalization
      - Recent antibiotic use
      - Health care–associated infection
    - Antimicrobial properties: ability to penetrate the site; susceptibility of the pathogen; toxicity risk; bioavailability (intravenous versus oral route); frequency of dosing; interaction with other medications; aggressive nature to eradicate the pathogen; renal or hepatic metabolism; side effects; route of administration; fat solubility; protein-binding degree; cost
- Viral infections
  - Most viral illnesses will subside without medication.
  - Treat the symptoms.
  - Some antiviral medications exist.
    - Do not destroy virus
    - Specific antiviral for specific virus
    - Prevent the virus from replicating
    - Shorten the duration of the illness
    - May decrease severity of symptoms
      - Human immunodeficiency virus (HIV)
      - Influenza
      - Herpes
- Fungal infections
  - Antifungal medications
    - Increase permeability of the membrane
    - Interfere with mitosis
    - Fungal cells are similar to human cells; the risk for toxicity is high.
- Protozoa infections
  - Antiprotozoal medications

- Risk of toxicity is high.
- Most antiprotozoal medications are synthetically manufactured.
- Medications differ, based on the stage of the protozoa.
- Antibiotic prophylaxis
  - Is administered before a surgical procedure to reduce postoperative infections and to ensure that the antibiotics are present in the tissue before intervention
- Passive immunotherapy
  - Administration of antibodies to assist the host in fighting an infection

Infection Prevention

- Infections are not always identified in individuals prior to contact with others.
- Preventing transmission is key to stopping the spread of disease.
- Infection control (Table 20.2)
  - Universal Precautions
    - Protocol for health care workers
    - Applies to every client, regardless of diagnosis or symptoms when handling body fluids
    - Hand hygiene
      - Strict and frequent handwashing procedures
      - Alcohol-based hand sanitizer before and after each client contact
    - Personal protective equipment
      - Wearing proper garments for clients with isolation precautions
    - Waste disposal and safe injection practices
      - Do not recap needles.
      - Protect broken skin.
      - Use available equipment with safety features, such as needleless systems and splash guards.

TABLE 20.2 Types of Isolation Precautions Used in Health Care Settings	
Type	**Examples**
Standard Precautions • Used for care of all clients, regardless of their diagnosis or presumed infection status	Includes the use of handwashing and appropriate personal protective equipment
Transmission-Based Precautions • Recommended to provide additional precautions beyond Standard Precautions to prevent the transmission of pathogens • Can be used for clients with known infections or suspected to be infected or colonized with pathogens that can be transmitted by airborne or droplet transmission or by contact with dry skin or contaminated surfaces. • These precautions should be used in addition to Standard Precautions.	**Airborne Precautions:** Used for infections spread in small particles in the air such as chickenpox (varicella), measles, and tuberculosis **Droplet Precautions:** Used for infections spread in large droplets by coughing, talking, or sneezing, such as influenza and bacterial meningitis **Contact Precautions:** Used for infections spread by skin-to-skin contact or contact with other surfaces such as *Clostridium difficile*, MRSA, and VRE.

From Lewis, S. L., Bucher, L., Heitkemper, M. M., Harding, M. M., Kwong, J., & Roberts, D. (2017). *Medical-surgical nursing: Assessment and management of clinical problems* (10th ed.). St. Louis: Elsevier.
MRSA, Methicillin-resistant *Staphylococcus aureus*; *VRE*, vancomycin-resistant *Enterococcus*.

- Vaccinations
  - Protect against the spread of disease
- Aseptic technique
  - Antiseptics
    - Chemical solutions
    - Destroy microbes on living tissue.
  - Proper cleaning
    - Wounds
    - Tools used from one client to the next, such as scissors and stethoscopes
- Sterilization procedures
  - Chemical disinfectant
    - Kills microorganisms on inanimate surfaces
    - Requires adequate exposure time
    - Requires appropriate concentrations
  - Autoclave
    - Destroys microorganisms using high temperatures
  - Proper packaging
- Environmental prevention
  - Vector (insect) population control
  - Community sanitation facilities
  - Clean water source
  - Clean food supply
- Childhood immunizations
  - Recommended boosters

APPLICATION AND REVIEW

15. What is the primary goal of a culture and sensitivity diagnostic test?
    1. Speedy identification of the pathogen
    2. Determining effective antibiotic therapy
    3. Minimizing the need for additional blood testing
    4. Determining the effectiveness of the client's immune system
16. Which is a risk associated with antibiotic therapy during pregnancy?
    1. Fetal exposure to the antibiotic
    2. Creation of fetal antibiotic resistance
    3. Dose must be increased to account for dual circulations
    4. Mother is more likely to experience an allergic reaction
17. What is the fundamental basis for the implementation of Universal Precautions when considering client and staff safety?
    1. Should be implemented when encountering bodily fluids
    2. Applies to every client, regardless of his or her diagnosis
    3. Requires effective handwashing procedures
    4. Prohibits the recapping of used needles

See Answers on pages 378–381.

Electrolytes and Infection

- Electrolyte balance is essential for normal body functions, including the body's ability to prevent and fight infection.

- Imbalances may result in symptoms similar to those caused by infections, making it difficult to distinguish the cause.
- Quick identification and treatment of electrolyte imbalances prevent further deterioration during the infectious process.
  - Efficacy of medications is best when the body's pH levels are maintained within the normal range.
- Electrolyte imbalance in relation to an infection most commonly occur with excess fluid loss.
  - Vomiting
  - Diarrhea
  - Perspiration (high fever)
  - Antibiotics
  - Systemic involvement associated with severe infection
    - Acute kidney injury
    - Liver injury (medication toxicity, hepatitis)
- Symptoms of imbalances correspond with electrolyte functions within the body.
  - Calcium functions: bone health; teeth health; nerve impulses; muscle movement; blood clotting; intestinal function
  - Sodium functions: fluid balance; blood pressure regulation; muscle contraction; nerve conduction
  - Potassium functions: cardiac conduction; blood pressure; electrolyte balance; nerve transmission; bone health; muscle contraction
  - Magnesium functions: production of DNA and RNA; nerve function; muscle function; heart rhythm; regulation of blood glucose levels; supports immune system
  - Chloride functions: electrolyte balance; pH balance
  - Phosphorous functions: bone strength; teeth strength; adenosine triphosphate (ATP) production (energy, growth, repair)
- Common symptoms to all electrolyte imbalances
  - Cardiac disturbances: irregular heart rhythm (tachycardia); fatigue; lethargy; seizures; nausea; vomiting
  - Gastrointestinal disturbances: diarrhea; constipation; abdominal cramping
  - Musculoskeletal disturbances: muscle weakness; muscle cramping
  - Central nervous system disturbances: altered mental status (irritability, confusion); headaches; numbness; tingling
- Imbalances in septicemia
  - Metabolic acidosis
    - Inadequate perfusion
    - Anaerobic metabolism
    - Increased lactic acid
  - Hyperkalemia (increased potassium level greater than 5.3 mmol/L)
    - Decreased renal function: muscle cramping (early sign); weakness (late sign); low blood pressure; bradycardia
  - Respiratory alkalosis
    - Early compensatory mechanism to reverse metabolic acidosis
      - pH level: greater than 7.45
      - Partial pressure of carbon dioxide ($PaCO_2$) level: less than 35 mm Hg
    - Tachypnea (hyperventilation)
      - Loss of carbon dioxide

- Respiratory acidosis
  - Respiratory failure (decompensated)
    - Decreased respiratory rate
    - Decreased volume
    - Decreased oxygenation
    - pH level: less than 7.35
    - $PaCO_2$ level: greater than 45 mm Hg
- Increased anion gap
  - Due to metabolic acidosis
  - Accumulation of acid
- Decreased pH less than 7.35 (acidosis)

APPLICATION AND REVIEW

18. Which client electrolyte imbalance should prompt the nurse to conduct a functional assessment? *(Select all that apply.)*
    1. Phosphorous
    2. Magnesium
    3. Potassium
    4. Calcium
    5. Chloride
19. Which question should the nurse ask when attempting to assess a client for a possible electrolyte imbalance? *(Select all that apply.)*
    1. "Do you have problems with diarrhea or constipation?"
    2. "How often do you experience muscle cramping?"
    3. "Would you say that you have a normal appetite?"
    4. "Do you have problems emptying your bladder?"
    5. "Would you consider yourself depressed?"
20. Which conditions should be regularly assessed in a client diagnosed with septicemia? *(Select all that apply.)*
    1. Hyperkalemia
    2. Hypokalemia
    3. Metabolic acidosis
    4. Respiratory alkalosis
    5. Respiratory acidosis

See Answers on pages 378–381.

ANSWER KEY: REVIEW QUESTIONS

1. **3 Viruses are the cause of the most human illnesses.**

   1 Viruses are capable of changing DNA in their host cells. **2** Malignancies are commonly associated with viruses. **4** Replication requires a live host cell.

   Client Need: Health Promotion and Maintenance; **Cognitive Level:** Understanding; **Integrated Process:** Teaching and Learning

2. **Answers: 1, 2, 3, 5**

   1 Poliomyelitis is caused by a virus. **2** Rabies is caused by a virus. **3** Herpes is caused by a virus. **5** Measles is a viral infection.

   4 Malaria is a bacterial infection.

   Client Need: Health Promotion and Maintenance; **Cognitive Level:** Knowing; **Integrated Process:** Teaching and Learning

3. **3 Bacteria can survive on inorganic (nonliving) objects.**

   1 Bacteria are unicellular organisms. **2** Not all bacteria are pathogenic. **4** Reproduction of bacteria is common.

Client Need: Health Promotion and Maintenance; **Cognitive Level:** Understanding; **Integrated Process:** Teaching and Learning

4. **4 The cell wall of gram-positive bacteria make them more susceptible to treatment with antibiotics.**

   1 Bacilli are a type of bacteria shape; shape does not affect susceptibility to antibiotics. **2** Tetras make up a group of four bacteria that form a square; grouping does not affect susceptibility to antibiotics. **3** Endotoxic bacteria are gram-negative bacteria; gram-negative bacteria with cell walls are more resistant to antibiotics.

   Client Need: Health Promotion and Maintenance; **Cognitive Level:** Understanding; **Integrated Process:** Teaching and Learning

5. **1 Impaired nerve conduction is a symptom of exotoxin bacterial infection.**

   2 Fever is associated with endotoxin, not exotoxin, bacterial infections. **3** Muscle weakness is associated with endotoxin, not exotoxin, bacterial infections. **4** Impaired circulation is associated with endotoxin, not exotoxin, bacterial infections.

   Client Need: Physiological Integrity; **Cognitive Level:** Applying; **Nursing Process:** Assessment

6. **1 For the most part, normal (or friendly) flora will not become pathogenic unless they end up in a place where they should not be. For example, choking on vomit might introduce the gut flora into the lungs, which is bad. Even if an individual survived the choking, he or she might die from a virulent pneumonia caused by his or her own flora.**

   2 Residential flora normally reside in specific locations inside the body and are not pathogenic unless they end up in a place where they should not be. **3** Contaminated water does not contain resident flora unique to a specific body and/or location in the body. **4** Sharing body fluids that are contaminated introduces nonresidential flora into the body.

   Client Need: Health Promotion and Maintenance; **Cognitive Level:** Analysis; **Integrated Process:** Teaching and Learning

7. **3 Pathogenicity refers to the microorganism's strength to cause an infection.**

   1 Virulence refers to the amount of damage the pathogen causes. **2** Resilience is the ability to adapt and resist destruction. **4** Attachment strength is associated with virulence.

   Client Need: Physiological Integrity; **Cognitive Level:** Understanding; **Integrated Process:** Teaching and Learning

8. **Answers: 1, 2, 3, 4**

   1 The chain of infection requires the presence of a causative agent or pathogen. **2** The chain of infection requires the existence of a host that provides the pathogen with an environment in which to live and reproduce. **3** The chain of infection requires a location or way for the pathogen to enter the host. **4** The chain of infection requires a way for the pathogen to leave the host to enter another host.

   5 Treatment is not a factor in the chance of infection.

   Client Need: Health Promotion and Maintenance; **Cognitive Level:** Understanding; **Integrated Process:** Teaching and Learning

9. **2 The prodromal period is characterized by the onset of clinical symptoms.**

   1 The incubation period occurs when the pathogen enters the body and before the onset of clinical symptoms. **3** The acute period occurs when fully developed symptoms occur. **4** The recovery period exhibits improved signs and symptoms.

   Client Need: Physiological Integrity; **Cognitive Level:** Applying; **Nursing Process:** Evaluation

10. **Answers: 1, 2, 4, 5**

    Mechanical ventilation, intravenous therapy, an indwelling catheter, and antibiotic therapy are common sources of nosocomial pneumonia.

    3 Cardiac monitoring is noninvasive and not a common source of nosocomial-associated infections.

    Client Need: Health Promotion and Maintenance; **Cognitive Level:** Applying; **Integrated Process:** Teaching and Learning

11. **Answers: 1, 2**

    1 The sebaceous glands secrete substances that prevent some microorganisms from reproducing, thus helping prevent infections. **2** The sweat glands secrete substances that prevent some microorganisms from reproducing, thus helping prevent infections.

    3 Although blood vessels are located in the dermis, they are not a factor in the prevention of infections. **4** Although hair follicles are in the dermis, they are not a factor in the prevention of infections. **5** Although the nail bed is in the dermis, it is not a factor in the prevention of infections.
    Client Need: Health Promotion and Maintenance; **Cognitive Level:** Understanding; **Integrated Process:** Teaching and Learning

12. **Answers: 1, 2, 4**
    Localized redness, heat, and swelling are signs of inflammation.
    3 Pus and drainage are signs of an infection. **5** Chills and fever are signs of an infection.
    Client Need: Physiological Integrity; **Cognitive Level:** Applying; **Nursing Process:** Assessment

13. **Answers: 1, 2, 4, 5**
    1 A fever and the accompanying feeling of heat is associated with a systemic infection. **2** Body aches are associated with a systemic infection. **4** Nausea is associated with a systemic infection. **5** Fatigue is associated with a systemic infection.
    3 Tinnitus is not associated with a systemic infection.
    Client Need: Physiological Integrity; **Cognitive Level:** Applying; **Nursing Process:** Assessment

14. **Answers: 2, 3, 4**
    2 Thready pulse is a progressive sign of septic shock. **3** Pale, cool skin is a progressive sign of septic shock. **4** A below normal temperature is a progressive sign of septic shock.
    1 Flushed skin is an initial sign of septic shock. **5** Rapid respirations are an initial sign of septic shock.
    Client Need: Physiological Integrity; **Cognitive Level:** Applying; **Nursing Process:** Assessment

15. **2 A culture and sensitivity test allows for the identification of the most effective antibiotic to treat an infection.**
    1 The primary goal of this diagnostic test is to identify the most effective antibiotic to eradicate the pathogen causing the infection. **3** This diagnostic test does not necessarily rule out the need for further diagnostic blood testing. **4** This diagnostic test does not assess the client's immune system.
    Client Need: Physiological Integrity; **Cognitive Level:** Applying; **Integrated Process:** Teaching and Learning

16. **1 The placenta is an ineffective antibiotic barrier, exposing the fetus to the direct effects of the medication.**
    2 Antibiotic resistance is not a risk in this situation. **3** An increased dose is not required in this situation. **4** The mother is not at an additional risk for an allergic reaction.
    Client Need: Physiological Integrity; **Cognitive Level:** Understanding; **Nursing Process:** Planning

17. **2 The safety of both the client and staff requires the implementation of Universal Precautions when providing care to any client.**
    1 Universal Precautions must be implemented when performing any intervention on any client. **3** Effective handwashing is only one of several Universal Precaution practices. **4** Proper handling of needles is only one of several Universal Precaution practices.
    Client Need: Health Promotion and Maintenance; **Cognitive Level:** Applying; **Integrated Process/Nursing Process:** Planning

18. **Answers: 1, 3, 4**
    Phosphorous, potassium, and calcium influence bone strength.
    2, 5 Magnesium and chloride do not influence bone health.
    Client Need: Physiological Integrity; **Cognitive Level:** Applying; **Nursing Process:** Planning

19. **Answers: 1, 2**
    1 Gastrointestinal disturbances, such as constipation and diarrhea, may be signs of an electrolyte imbalance. **2** Muscle cramping may be a sign of an electrolyte imbalance.
    3 Changes in appetite are not usually a sign of an electrolyte imbalance. **4** Ineffective bladder emptying is not usually a sign of an electrolyte imbalance. **5** Depression is not associated with an electrolyte imbalance.
    Client Need: Physiological Integrity; **Cognitive Level:** Analysis; **Nursing Process:** Assessment

20. Answers: 1, 3, 4, 5

   1 Hyperkalemia is an imbalance associated with septicemia. **3** Metabolic acidosis is an imbalance associated with septicemia. **4** Respiratory alkalosis is an imbalance associated with septicemia. **5** Respiratory acidosis is an imbalance associated with septicemia.

   2 Hypokalemia is an imbalance not associated with septicemia.

   Client Need: Physiological Integrity; **Cognitive Level:** Knowing; **Nursing Process:** Assessment

References

Abdo, W. F., & Heunks, L. M. (2012). Oxygen-induced hypercapnia in COPD: myths and facts. *Critical Care, 16*(5), 323.

Alexander, K., & Lewis, S. L. (2015). Nursing management: Fluid, electrolyte, and acid-base imbalances. In *Lewis's Medical surgical nursing: Assessment and management of clinical problems* (4th ed., pp. 262–293). New York: Elsevier.

Anderson, C. A., Appel, L. J., Okuda, N., Brown, I. J., Chan, Q., Zhao, L., et. al. (2010). Dietary sources of sodium in China, Japan, the United Kingdom, and the United States, women and men aged 40 to 59 years: The INTERMAP study. *Journal of the American Dietetic Association, 110*(5), 736–745.

Arneson, W. (2014). Electrolytes: The salts of the earth. *Laboratory Medicine, 45*(1), e11–e15.

Baird, M. S. (2015). *Manual of critical care nursing: Nursing interventions and collaborative management* (7th ed.). St. Louis: Elsevier.

Ball, J. W., Dains, J. E., Flynn, J. A., Solomon, B. S., & Stewart, R. W. (2015). *Seidel's guide to physical examination* (8th ed.). St. Louis: Elsevier.

Berend, K., van Hulsteijn, L. H., & Gans, R. O. (2012). Chloride: The queen of electrolytes? *European Journal of Internal Medicine, 23*(3), 203–211.

Boron, W. F., & Boulpaep, E. L. (2012). *Medical physiology: A cellular and molecular approach* (updated 2nd ed.). Philadelphia: Elsevier.

Brown, D., Edwards, H., Seaton, L., & Buckley, T. (2017). *Lewis's medical-surgical nursing: Assessment and management of clinical problems* (4th ed.). New York: Elsevier.

Brunelli, S. M., & Goldfarb, S. (2007). Hypophosphatemia: Clinical consequences and management. *Journal of American Society of Nephrology, 18*(7), 1999–2003.

Cairo, J. M. (2014). *Mosby's respiratory care equipment.* (9th ed.). St. Louis: Elsevier.

Chernecky, C. C, & Berger, B. J. (2013). *Laboratory tests and diagnostic procedures* (6th ed.). St. Louis: Elsevier.

Chernecky, C. C, Macklin, D., & Murphy-Ende, K. (2006). *Laboratory tests and diagnostic procedures.* St. Louis: Elsevier.

Copsteam, L., & Banasik, J. (2013). *Pathophysiology* (5th ed.). St. Louis: Elsevier.

Curtis, K., & Ramsden, C. (2016). *Emergency and trauma care for nurses and paramedics* (2nd ed.). Australia: Elsevier.

Daly, K., & Farrington, E. (2013). Hypokalemia and hyperkalemia in infants and children: Pathophysiology and treatment. *Journal of Pediatric Health Care, 27*(6), 486–496.

Davis, A. (2016). Traumatic brain injury. In M. S. Baird (Ed.), *Manual of critical care nursing: Nursing interventions and collaborative management* (7th ed., pp. 368–389). St. Louis: Elsevier.

De Vasconcelos, K. (2015). Hyperchloraemia: Ready for the big time? *Southern African Journal of Anaesthesia and Analgesia, 21*(4), 91–95.

Edwards, S. L. (2008). Pathophysiology of acid base balance: The theory practice relationship. *Intensive & Critical Care Nursing, 24*(1), 28–40.

El-Sharkawy, A. M., Sahota, O., Maughan, R. J., & Lobo, D. N. (2014). The pathophysiology of fluid and electrolyte balance in the older adult surgical patient. *Clinical Nutrition, 33*(1), 6–13.

Ferri, F. F. (2018). Nutritional trace elements and their clinical implications. In F. F. Ferri (Ed.), *Ferri's clinical advisor* (pp. 1934–1936). Philadelphia: Elsevier.

Forbes, H., & Watt, E. (2016). *Jarvis's physical examination and health assessment* (2nd ed.). Philadelphia: Saunders.

Gahart, B. L., & Nazareno, A. R., Ortega, M. Q. (2016). *2017 Intravenous medications: A handbook for nurses and health professionals.* St. Louis: Elsevier.

Hanberg, J. S., Rao, V., Ter Maaten, J. M., Laur, O., Brisco, M. A., Perry Wilson, F., et. al. (2016). Hypochloremia and diuretic resistance in heart failure: mechanistic insights. *Circulation Heart Failure, 9*(8), e003180.

Haynes, A. (2018). Cardiovascular disorders. In L. D. Urden, K. M. Stacy, M. E. Lough (Eds.). *Critical care nursing: Diagnosis and management* (8th ed., pp. 290–358). St. Louis: Elsevier.

Hazinski, M. F. (2013). *Nursing care of the critically ill child* (3rd ed.). St. Louis: Elsevier.

Heitz, U., & Horne, M. M. (2005). *Mosby's pocket guide series: Fluid, electrolyte, and acid-base balance.* (5th ed.). St. Louis: Elsevier.

Heuer, A. J., & Scanlan, C. L. (2013). *Wilkins' clinical assessment in respiratory care* (7th ed.). St. Louis: Elsevier.

Hockenberry, M. J., & Wilson, D. (2015). *Wong's nursing care of infants and children* (10th ed.). St. Louis: Elsevier.

Huether, S. E., & McCance, K. L., Brashers, V. L., & Rote N. S. (2017). *Understanding pathophysiology* (6th ed.). St. Louis: Elsevier.

Ignatavicius, D. D., & Workman, M. L. (2016). *Medical-surgical nursing: Patient-centered collaborative care* (8th ed.). St. Louis: Elsevier.

Kamel, K. S., & Halperin, M. L. (2016). *Fluid, electrolyte, and acid-base physiology: A problem-based approach* (5th ed.). Philadelphia: Elsevier.

Kataoka, H. (2017). Treatment of hypochloremia with acetazolamide in an advanced heart failure patient and importance of monitoring urinary electrolytes. *Journal of Cardiology Cases, 17*(3), 80–84.

Lewis, S. L., Bucher, L., Heitkemper, M. M., Harding, M. M., Kwong, J., & Roberts, D. (2017). *Medical-surgical nursing: Assessment and management of clinical problems* (10th ed.). St. Louis: Elsevier.

Lima-Oliveira, G., Lippi, G., Salvagno, G. L., Montagnana, M., Picheth, G., & Guidi, G. C. (2012). Different manufacturers of syringes: A new source of variability in blood gas, acid-base balance and related laboratory test? *Clinical biochemistry, 45*(9), 683–687.

Pizzorno J. E., Murray, M. T. (2013). Mineral status evaluation. In C. Masur (Ed.). *Textbook of natural medicine* (4th ed., pp. 200–205). St. Louis: Elsevier Churchill Livingstone.

McCance, K. L., Huether, S. E., Brashers, V. L., & Rote, N. S. (2015). *Pathophysiology: The biologic basis for disease in adults and children* (7th ed.). St. Louis: Elsevier.

McDowell, J. R. S., Matthews, D. M., Brown, F. J., & Matthews, D. (2007). *Diabetes: A handbook for the primary healthcare team*. London: Elsevier Churchill Livingstone.

McLafferty, E., Johnstone, C., Hendry, C., & Farley, A. (2014). Fluid and electrolyte balance. *Nursing Standard, 28*(29), 42–49.

McQuillan, K. A., & Thurman, P. A. (2009). Traumatic brain injuries. In K. A. McQuillan, M. B. F. Makic, & E. Whalen (Eds.), *Trauma nursing* (4th ed., pp. 448–518). Philadelphia: Saunders.

Monahan, F. D., Neighbors, M., & Green, C. (2017). Neurologic disorders. In F. D., Monahan, M. Neighbors, & C. Green (Eds.), *Swearingen's manual of medical-surgical nursing: A care planning resource* (7th ed., pp. 229–376). St. Louis: Elsevier.

Murat, I., Humblot, A., Girault, L., & Piana, F. (2010). Neonatal fluid management. *Best Practice & Research. Clinical Anaesthesiology, 24*(3), 365–374.

MyFoodData. Top 10 foods highest in phosphorus. Retrieved from https://www.myfooddata.com/articles/high-phosphorus-foods.php

National Institutes of Health. Magnesium: Fact sheet for health professionals. Retrieved from https://ods.od.nih.gov/factsheets/Magnesium-HealthProfessional/

Oh, W. (2012). Fluid and electrolyte management of very low birth weight infants. *Pediatrics and Neonatology, 53*(6), 329–333.

Potter, P. A., Perry, A. G., Stockert, P., & Hall, A. (2016). *Fundamentals of nursing* (9th ed.). St. Louis: Elsevier.

Speakman, E., & Weldy, N. J. (2002). *Body fluids and electrolytes: A programmed presentation* (8th ed.). St. Louis: Mosby.

Touhy, T. A., Jett, K. F. (2014). *Ebersole and Hess' gerontological nursing & healthy aging* (4th ed.). St. Louis: Elsevier.

Verklan, M. T., & Walden, M. (2014). *Core curriculum for neonatal intensive care nursing* (5th ed.). St. Louis: Elsevier.

Walker, M. D. (2016). Fluid and electrolyte imbalances: Interpretation and assessment. *Journal of Infusion Nursing, 39*(6), 382–386.

Yunos, N. M., Bellomo, R., Story, D., & Kellum, J. (2010). Bench-to-bedside review: Chloride in critical illness. *Critical Care, 14*(4), 226.

Zerwekh, J., Claborn, J. C., Gaglione, T. Miller, C. J. (2010). *Mosby's fluids and electrolytes, memory NoteCards: Visual, mnemonic, and memory aids for nurses* (2nd ed.). St. Louis: Elsevier.

Index